Respiratory Medicine

Respiratory Medicine

Recent advances

Edited by

Peter J. Barnes
Professor and Director of Thoracic Medicine, National Heart and Lung Institute, London, and Honorary Consultant Physician, Royal Brompton National Heart and Lung Hospital, London, UK

BUTTERWORTH
HEINEMANN

Butterworth-Heinemann Ltd
Linacre House, Jordan Hill, Oxford OX2 8DP

A member of the Reed Elsevier group

OXFORD LONDON BOSTON
MUNICH NEW DELHI SINGAPORE SYDNEY
TOKYO TORONTO WELLINGTON

First published 1993

British Library Cataloguing in Publication Data

A catalogue record for this book is available from the British Library

Library of Congress Cataloguing in Publication Data

A catalogue record for this book is available from the Library of Congress

ISBN 0 7506 0712 2

Typeset by Jane Bryant, Hindhead, Surrey
Printed and bound in Great Britain by
Biddles Ltd, Guildford and King's Lynn

Contents

Preface to the Series

Shortly after the end of the Second World War, separate Institutes for Postgraduate Education were established as part of the University of London to encourage research into diseases of the chest and of the heart. Each Institute was associated with well-established hospitals – the Institute for Diseases of the Chest with the Brompton and London Chest Hospitals, and the Institute of Cardiology with the National Heart Hospital.

Although these various Institutes and hospitals were scattered throughout London, certain farsighted physicians noted the advantages to be gained by unifying their efforts. In the 1960s, therefore, the Institutes joined together as the Cardiothoracic Institutes, while the hospitals also adopted a central administration. The sites themselves, however, remained separate, although plans were established to bring them together. Within the last 2 years, these plans have finally come to fruition.

In 1988, the Lord Flowers, Vice-Chancellor of the University of London, opened the new premises of the Institute, which was renamed the National Heart and Lung Institute. In February 1991, Her Majesty the Queen opened the Sydney Street wing of the new Royal Brompton National Heart and Lung Hospital, while the London Chest Hospital, still separate, was renamed the Victoria Park branch of the hospitals.

We believe that these amalgamations now give us the opportunity to realize the potential envisaged by our predecessors when they proposed our union. They bring together cardiologists, chest physicians, surgeons, paediatricians, research workers, and all their associated specialities, on one site: a site with considerable potential for still further expansion. Already, since the Institute has been united on one site, it has become associated with the Thrombosis Research Institute and the Wynn Institute for Metabolic Research. Taken together, this combination makes us the largest postgraduate organization dedicated exclusively to diseases of the heart and lungs within Europe. As such, we believe we have need of a forum in which to discuss and disseminate the major researches and advances being made by our staff and their collaborators throughout the world. Thanks to the enthusiastic support of Butterworth-Heinemann, this will now be possible through the *Royal Brompton Reviews*.

It is our intention to produce two series of these reviews, one concerned with diseases of the heart and the other with diseases of the lung. The first review was devoted to the patterns of disease occurring in the continuum which extends from coronary arterial atherosclerosis, through ischaemic heart disease, to heart failure. This second review deals with recent advances in diseases of the lungs. In the future we will alternate between heart and lung diseases and may select topics common to both areas.

Robert H. Anderson
Peter J. Barnes
Series Editors

Preface

This is the second in the Royal Brompton Review Series and the first to deal with respiratory medicine. There have been striking advances in all areas of respiratory medicine which have led to greater understanding of diseases such as asthma, cystic fibrosis and fibrosing lung diseases. there have also been marked changes in therapy as a result of these advances and the development of new approaches to management of lung diseases. Respiratory diseases impose a considerable health burden on society and deserve increased research funding to reflect their importance in the community. this volume is based on contributions by research and clinical staff who are currently working, or who have recently worked, at the National heart and Lung Institute and the Royal Brompton National Heart and Lung Hospital. There has always been a close association between Institute and Hospital and many of the chapters reflect the close links between basic science and clinical respiratory medicine. Topics covered include asthma, cystic fibrosis, respiratory infections (including HIV), fibrosing lung disease, home ventilation and respiratory muscles. While this is not a comprehensive coverage of respiratory medicine, it provides an overview of developments in the most active areas of research and reflects the research currently taking place in Europe's largest institute devoted to lung diseases.

We hope this will be the first of several volumes on lung diseases and, in the future, plan to focus on specific areas of active clinical interest and to highlight areas of research common to cardiovascular and pulmonary medicine.

Peter J. Barnes
Department of Thoracic Medicine,
National Heart and Lung Institute

Contributors

Peter J. Barnes, MA, DM, DSc, FRCP
Professor and Director of Thoracic Medicine, Royal Brompton National Heart and Lung Institute, London and Honorary Consultant Physician, Royal Brompton National Heart and Lung Hospital, London

K.F. Chung, MD, FRCP
Senior Lecturer in Thoracic Medicine and Honorary Consultant Physician, Department of Thoracic Medicine, National Heart and Lung Institute, London

Peter Cole, BSc, FRCP, FRCPath
Professor of Respiratory Medicine, National Heart and Lung Institute, London and Honorary Consultant Physician, Royal Brompton National Heart and Lung Hospital, London

John Collins, MD, FRCP
Consultant Physician, Royal Brompton National Heart and Lung Hospital, London

C.J. Corrigan, MA, PhD, MRCP
Clinical Lecturer, Department of Allergy and Clinical Immunology, National Heart and Lung Institute, London and Honorary Senior Registrar, Royal Brompton National Heart and Lung Hospital, London

R.M. du Bois, MA, MD, FRCP
Consultant Physician, Royal Brompton National Heart and Lung Hospital, London and Honorary Senior Lecturer, National Heart and Lung Institute, London

S.R. Durham, MD, MRCP
Senior Lecturer, Department of Allergy and Clinical Immunology,National Heart and Lung Institute, London and Honorary Consultant Physician, Royal Brompton National Heart and Lung Hospital, London

T.W. Evans, MD, MRCP, PhD
Senior Lecturer in Thoracic Medicine, National Heart and Lung Institute; Consultant in Intensive Care, Royal Brompton National Heart and Lung Hospital, London

R.W. Fuller, MD, MRCP
Department of Respiratory Medicine, Glaxo Group Research Ltd, Greenford

Duncan M. Geddes, MD, FRCP
Consultant Physician, Royal Brompton national Heart and Lung Hospital, London

Malcolm Green, DM, FRCP
Consultant Physician, Royal Brompton National Heart and Lung Hospital, London

N.K. Harrison, MD, MRCP
Honorary Lecturer, Biochemistry Unit, Department of Thoracic Medicine, National Heart and Lung Institute, London and Senior Registrar, Royal Brompton National Heart and Lung Hospital, London

Margaret E. Hodson, MD, MSc, FRCP, DA
Reader, Department of Cystic Fibrosis, National Heart and Lung Institute, London and Honorary Consultant Physician, Royal Brompton National Heart and Lung Hospital, London

A.B. Kay, PhD, FRCP
Professor and Director, Department of Allergy and Clinical Immunology, and Honorary Consultant Physician, Royal Brompton National Heart and Lung Hospital, London

G.J. Laurent, PhD
Reader, Biochemistry Unit, Department of Thoracic Medicine, National Heart and Lung Institute, London

Mark Messent, FCAnaes
BUPA Research Fellow in Intensive Care and Honorary Registrar in Anaesthetics and Intensive Care, Royal Brompton National Heart and Lung Hospital, London

John Moxham, MD, FRCP
Professor of Thoracic Medicine, King's College School of Medicine and Dentistry; Senior Lecturer, National Heart and Lung Institute, London

A.J. Newman Taylor, OBE, FRCP, FFOM
Professor of Occupational and Environmental Medicine, National Heart and Lung Institute, London and Consultant Physician, Royal Brompton National Heart and Lung Hospital, London

Anita K. Simonds, MD, MRCP
Consultant in Respiratory Medicine, Royal Brompton National Heart and Lung Hospital, London

John Wiggins, MD, MRCP
Consultant Physician, Wexham Park Hospital, Slough

Robert Wilson, MD, MRCP
Senior Lecturer, Department of Thoracic Medicine, National Heart and Lung Institute, London and Consultant Physician, Royal Brompton National Heart and Lung Hospital, London

1

Immunology of airways allergic disease

C. J. Corrigan, S. R. Durham and A. B. Kay

Introduction

It is widely accepted that chronic mucosal inflammation plays an important role in the pathogenesis of allergic diseases and asthma, although the precise relationship of inflammation to symptoms, or to objective measures of disease severity, remains unclear. In the early 20th century, following the discovery of histamine and its link with allergy and anaphylaxis, asthma was regarded essentially as intermittent spasm of bronchial smooth muscle, although 'vascular turgescence' of the bronchial mucosa and increased secretion of mucous glands were also acknowledged. With the discovery of glucocorticoid therapy, it became clear that the bronchi were not normal between attacks, in the sense that glucocorticoids could often 'open up' the airways even in ostensibly well controlled patients. It was realized that, for many patients, asthma is a chronic disease with intermittent acute exacerbations. Similarly, while it was recognized relatively early that the immediate release of mediators from IgE-sensitized mast cells is characteristic of allergic reactions, it has only recently become clear that allergic diseases are also characterized by chronic inflammation of the mucosa at sites exposed to sensitizing allergens. This new concept of allergy and asthma as chronic inflammatory diseases with intermittent acute exacerbations has had very important implications for therapeutic management. In this chapter the immunobiology of the leucocytes involved in the inflammatory response in asthma and allergic disease, and how the various leucocytes and their products may contribute to the observed pathological features, will be discussed. These cells do not act in isolation but interact both with each other and with resident tissue cells and local neural networks. It is very unlikely, therefore, that one particular cell or mediator is fully responsible for the pathogenetic mechanisms underlying asthma and allergic inflammation, but rather that the combined effects of a number of cells and their products must be taken into consideration.

Evidence for mucosal inflammation in asthma and allergic disease

Asthma

The classic studies of bronchial histopathology in patients who died of asthma [1–3] showed intense invasion of the bronchial mucosa with inflammatory cells, particularly eosinophils, macrophages and lymphocytes. Neutrophils were present but in fewer numbers. Deposition of eosinophil products in and around the bronchial epithelium was a particularly prominent feature [4]. Other features noted in these studies which appear to be typical of asthma include loss of surface lining epithelium, collagen deposition in the reticular layer beneath the basement membrane of the epithelium, dilatation of blood vessels, mucosal oedema and hypertrophy of both submucosal glands and bronchial smooth muscle.

More recent studies have been performed on mild asthmatic volunteers, utilizing the techniques of bronchoalveolar lavage (BAL) and bronchial biopsy through the flexible fibreoptic bronchoscope. These studies have shown that many of the inflammatory changes observed in asthma deaths are also a feature of milder, apparently well controlled disease. Elevated numbers of eosinophils, in both the bronchial mucosa and in BAL fluid, were constant features of mild asthma [5–7]. Similarly, increased numbers of activated lymphocytes, identified by transmission electron microscopy as irregular, atypical lymphocytes [8] or shown by immunocytochemistry to be CD25 (IL-2 receptor) bearing cells [5] were also invariably seen. Evidence exists that activation of T lymphocytes and subsequent eosinophil recruitment and secretion may contribute to epithelial damage and possibly also to bronchial hyperresponsiveness in asthma [9–12]. In contrast, recent studies of the bronchial mucosa of patients with mild asthma associated with atopy demonstrated no significant changes in the numbers of mast cells or their subtypes in the bronchial mucosa [13, 14], nor any increase in number of bronchial mucosal neutrophils in these patients [8, 12, 14].

Immunohistochemical and electron microscopic studies [8, 14, 15] have shown that the apparent thickening of the epithelial basement membrane in the asthmatic bronchial mucosa is in fact a consequence of subepithelial deposition of reticular collagen. This suggests that fibroblast activation, rather than epithelial cell dysfunction, might account for this phenomenon.

Asthma has been traditionally subdivided clinically according to its apparent aetiology (intrinsic, extrinsic and occupational), implying possible variability in its pathogenesis. One important question therefore relates to whether these clinical distinctions are apparent in histopathological terms. Preliminary studies addressing this question would suggest that they are not: a post-mortem study of the bronchial mucosa of a patient who had died with severe occupational asthma showed histological changes similar to those seen in fatal non-occupational asthma [16], while a recent immunocytochemical study [17] showed that bronchial biopsies from extrinsic and occupational asthmatics were indistinguishable in terms of their inflammatory cell infiltrate – in both cases the biopsies showed increased numbers of activated eosinophils and T lymphocytes, but not of neutrophils and monocyte/macrophages, compared with normal control subjects. Similarly, BAL fluid obtained from a group of 'intrinsic' asthmatics [18] showed increased numbers of activated T lymphocytes, eosinophils and neutrophils compared with normal controls. These observations suggest that the bronchial response in patients with asthma is uniform, regardless of the nature of the provoking agent, and support the hypothesis that the pathogenesis of asthma is independent of coexisting atopy.

Allergic rhinitis

The most common manifestations of allergic disease are allergic rhinitis and conjunctivitis, both of which are responsible for considerable and increasing morbidity. These diseases are more clearly associated with inappropriate IgE responses than asthma (although perennial non-allergic rhinitis is also well described).

Surprisingly few studies have investigated the histopathology of chronic allergic rhinitis and conjunctivitis. Some [19, 20] have shown increased numbers of mast cells and basophils in nasal secretions of patients with allergic rhinitis. Quantitative studies on the numbers of mast cells in the nasal mucosa after exposure to allergen have given widely divergent conclusions, ranging from an overall decrease through redistribution to an overall increase [21–24]. Allergen provocation has also been shown to result in an influx of inflammatory cells into nasal washings [25]. These cells were predominantly eosinophils, although mononuclear cells and neutrophils were also increased. No systematic studies of the numbers and activation status of T lymphocytes and monocyte/macrophages in the nasal mucosa in allergic rhinitis have to date been performed. Allergen challenge of the ocular conjunctiva of patients with allergic conjunctivitis [26] resulted in an inflammatory cell influx similar to that described in allergic rhinitis, with eosinophils predominating.

Human experimental models of asthma and allergy

Most of the studies that have been performed on allergic and asthmatic inflammation have concentrated on the possible inflammatory roles of granulocytic leucocytes, particularly eosinophils and mast cells. Furthermore, many of these investigations have been based on comparisons of the numbers and activation status of these cells and the concentrations of their mediators before and after experimental allergen challenge, although a few have compared diseased patients with normal controls. The clinical response to acute allergen challenge in some allergic subjects is biphasic, consisting of an early and late phase response. The early phase response develops within 10 min, usually resolves within 1–3 h, and is generally attributed to degranulation of cells sensitized by binding of allergen-specific IgE (principally mast cells). The late phase response begins as the early phase response resolves, reaches a maximum within 6-10 h and can last for 24 h or more if untreated. It is associated with an influx of various inflammatory cells into the challenged mucosa. The clinical characteristics of the early and late phase responses depend on the organ challenged: bronchospasm in the lungs; erythema and induration (the 'flare' reaction) in the skin; rhinorrhoea, sneezing and congestion in the nose; erythema, swelling, lacrimation and itching in the conjunctiva [27–30]. The traditional view has been that late phase responses occur as an all-or-nothing event in a given individual: recent studies, however, indicate that the development of late asthmatic responses could occur as a continuous spectrum of severity depending on the dose of allergen administered [31, 32]. It seems likely therefore that all sensitive subjects would develop late responses if it were possible to administer a sufficiently high dose of allergen.

It has been argued by many that the late phase response represents a valid clinical model of the expression and severity of 'real' atopic asthma and allergic inflammation, and various experimental observations have been cited to justify this conclusion:

1. The development of late phase responses in children was associated with a higher frequency of asthmatic attacks in the preceding year [33].
2. In patients with occupational asthma, the development of exposure-related symptoms was unusual unless the patient also developed late phase responses after laboratory challenge [34].
3. Successful abrogation of asthmatic symptoms after immunotherapy in children sensitive to house dust mites was associated with suppression of the late asthmatic response following repeated allergen challenge [35].
4. An increase in non-specific bronchial hyperresponsiveness was observed to occur 3 h after allergen challenge, just before the development of the late phase response [32] and was shown to persist for several days [36]. This correlated with the magnitude of the subsequent late phase fall in FEV_1.
5. Glucocorticoids, which reduce bronchial hyperresponsiveness in 'real' asthma, were shown to inhibit development of the late phase response whereas bronchodilators, including β_2-agonists and theophylline, with no effect on hyperresponsiveness, did not [37-39].

There is therefore clear evidence that the late phase bronchoconstrictor response following laboratory allergen challenge is accompanied by increased bronchial responsiveness, thereby ostensibly fulfilling the criteria for the definition of 'real' asthma. Nevertheless, some doubts must remain concerning the validity of this model. One major problem is the uncertainty as to how far events associated with the late phase reaction are dependent on the IgE-mediated events of the preceding immediate reaction. On the one hand, the modest correlation between the magnitudes of the two reactions, at least in the skin [40], and their differential susceptibility to inhibition by drugs such as glucocorticoids suggest that different mechanisms may be operating in their pathogenesis, but on the other hand, late asthmatic responses have been observed to follow challenge with non-specific stimuli such as exercise [41]. Furthermore, at least in the skin, passive cutaneous sensitization with allergen-specific IgE-containing serum conferred the ability to mount late phase reactions to subsequent challenge with the same allergen or with anti-IgE [42, 43]. These observations raise the possibility that events such as cell activation and recruitment observed in association with the late phase reaction in various tissues are no more than a non-specific consequence of the local release of mast cells and other mediators. In other words, the late phase response may be a model for the *exacerbation* of, rather than the *pathogenesis* of asthma and allergic disease.

Immunobiology of specific leucocytes and evidence for their involvement in asthma and allergic disease

General

The basic strategies used to implicate particular leucocytes in the pathogenesis of allergic diseases are based on demonstrating an increase in the number and/or the activation status of these cells, or increased concentrations of their mediators in patients with disease compared with controls. These studies may be static and observational, but more commonly address changes in cell numbers and activation after experimental allergen challenge. The possible relevance of experimental allergen challenge studies, particularly to the pathogenesis of asthma, has already been discussed.

In the case of asthma, cell numbers and function are often related to bronchial hyperresponsiveness. Bronchial hyperresponsiveness is widely regarded as a useful measurement of the severity of asthma because it is invariably observed in asthmatics and its degree can be correlated with both the severity of symptoms and the amount of anti-asthma therapy required for disease control [44, 45]. Nevertheless, because the precise cause of bronchial hyperresponsiveness is unknown, observations linking cell numbers and their activation status with the degree of bronchial hyperresponsiveness in asthmatics can only provide circumstantial evidence for the involvement of these cells or their products.

Eosinophils

Immunobiology of eosinophils

Eosinophils are non-dividing, granular cells arising principally in the bone marrow. It is generally assumed that eosinophils have been phylogenetically retained because of their particular ability to combat helminthic parasitic infections [46, 47], but this is by no means certain: a recent study showed that parasite-induced eosinophilia in mice could be abolished by the administration of antibody against interleukin-5 (IL-5) with no obvious effect on the immune response to the parasite infection [48].

Eosinophil differentiation, like that of all leucocytes, is under the influence of cytokine growth factors: interleukin-3 (IL-3), granulocyte/macrophage colony-stimulating factor (GM-CSF) and IL-5 have all been shown to promote eosinophil differentiation [49, 50], but whereas IL-3 and GM-CSF act on the precursors of a number of leucocytes, IL-5 appears to be specific for eosinophils. IL-5 may be the most important cytokine for eosinophil differentiation because it is released principally, if not exclusively, by T lymphocytes [51] and it has been shown that the eosinophilia associated with parasitic infections is T-lymphocyte dependent [50]. This hypothesis is further supported by the observation that transgenic mice constitutively expressing the gene for IL-5 developed a marked peripheral blood eosinophilia [52]. If IL-5 alone were sufficient to mediate the eosinophilia associated with helminthic infections, asthma and allergic diseases, this might explain why expansion of eosinophils in these diseases is typically seen without expansion of other leucocyte lineages.

One of the fundamental problems when investigating the pathogenesis of asthma and allergic disease has been to explain why eosinophils, rather than other granulocytes such as neutrophils, preferentially accumulate in the inflamed mucosa. Established eosinophil chemoattractants such as platelet-activating factor (PAF) and C5a, although highly potent [53], are non-specific in that they also attract neutrophils. It now seems likely that this phenomenon will be at least partly explained by a better understanding of how eosinophils migrate from the vascular space into the tissues. Migration is initiated by an interaction between receptors on the cell surface with their ligands on the surface of vascular endothelial cells. At least three such ligands have now been characterized: intercellular adhesion molecule 1 (ICAM-1, CD54), endothelial leucocyte adhesion molecule 1 (ELAM-1) and vascular cell adhesion molecule 1 (VCAM-1). The best characterized adhesion receptors on leucocytes belong to the integrin superfamily of receptors, heterodimers which are subdivided into three families according to the structure of their β-chains: β_1 (CD29), β_2 (CD18) and β_3 (CD61). Each β-chain associates at the cell surface with a variable number of α-chains. The β_1 family has six members, α_1–α_6 (CD49a–f), also known as VLA-1–6, the β_2 family three members, LFA-1, Mac-1 and p150,95 (CD11a–c) and the β_3 family two members (CD41 and CD51). *In vitro* assays of leucocyte adhesion to monolayer cultures of human umbilical vein endothelial cells (HUVEC) have clarified the role of the individual receptors and their ligands. Both resting and activated leucocytes adhere to HUVEC. Adhesion is augmented by prior stimulation of the HUVEC with inflammatory mediators such as IL-1, which increases the expression of endothelial adhesion receptors. Adhesion was shown to be inhibited by monoclonal antibodies against ICAM-1 and ELAM-1 on the endothelium and also by monoclonal antibodies against LFA-1 and Mac-1 on leucocytes [51]. These mechanisms apply to both eosinophils and neutrophils, since both express LFA-1 and Mac-1. Two further mechanisms were recently described, however, which appear to be unique to eosinophils:

1. IL-3 and IL-5 up-regulated eosinophil, but not neutrophil, adhesion to unstimulated HUVEC [54].
2. Eosinophils, but not neutrophils, were shown to express $\alpha_4\beta_1$ (VLA-4), which is a ligand for VCAM-1 on the surface of stimulated endothelial cells [55]. Eosinophil, but not neutrophil, adhesion both to IL-1-stimulated HUVEC and to COS cells transfected with cDNA encoding VCAM-1 was inhibited by monoclonal antibody against $\alpha_4\beta_1$.

These mechanisms offer the first explanations as to how eosinophils accumulate preferentially in tissues in allergic diseases and asthma. The important role of lymphokines, particularly IL-5, is self-evident. It remains possible that highly potent but non-specific chemoattractants such as PAF act in concert with selective agents such as IL-5 to effect specific eosinophil accumulation.

In addition to receptors for adhesion molecules, eosinophils express a number of other immunologically important receptors, including receptors for the Fc portions of IgG, IgA, IgD and IgE. Eosinophils were shown to bind IgE in a specific manner [56] and to exhibit a number of IgE-dependent functions including killing of schistosomula opsonized with specific IgE [57]. This raises the possibility that eosinophils might be activated directly by IgE-dependent mechanisms in asthma and allergic disease. Of the three receptors for the Fc portion of IgG (the high-affinity receptor Fc-γ RI, CD64, and the two low-affinity receptors Fc-γ RII and RIII, CD32 and CD16), eosinophils were shown to express only CD32 to a significant degree [58], in contrast to neutrophils which constitutively express CD16. The physiological significance of this is unknown. The CD32 receptor was shown to mediate a number of eosinophil effector functions including schistosomula killing, phagocytosis, secretion of granule proteins and synthesis of lipid mediators such as PAF and LTC_4. Eosinophil IgA receptors, when engaged with IgA-coated Sepharose beads, trigger release of eosinophil granule proteins [59], which may be of physiological significance at mucosal surfaces. It is likely that further eosinophil surface molecules will be described with important physiological functions. Of interest are the recent demonstrations that eosinophils, after prolonged culture with cytokines expressed HLA-DR [60], raising the possibility that these cells have the potential to present antigenic fragments to T lymphocytes. Eosinophils were also shown to express CD4 after cytokine stimulation [61].

Eosinophils can secrete a number of lipid mediators and proteins which may have a role to play in the pathophysiology of asthma and allergic diseases (Figure 1.1), and have been shown to elaborate eicosanoids derived from the 5- and 15-lipoxygenase pathways, especially LTC_4, as well as PAF [62–64]. Both LTC_4 and PAF were shown to cause bronchoconstriction [65, 66] whilst LTC_4 was shown to be a mucus secretagogue [67]. PAF also increases vascular permeability. Inhaled PAF was shown to increase bronchial hyperresponsiveness in humans [65], although whether this was accompanied by bronchial inflammation has not been studied. Eosinophils store four basic proteins in their granules: major basic protein (MBP), eosinophil-derived neurotoxin (EDN), eosinophil cationic protein (ECP) and eosinophil peroxidase (EPO) [68]. MBP was shown to be toxic for human respiratory epithelial cells and pneumocytes [69, 70]. Inhalation of MBP, albeit at high concentrations, caused bronchial hyperresponsiveness in a primate model of asthma [71]. EPO has also been shown to be toxic for respiratory epithelium and pneumocytes, particularly in combination with peroxide and halide ions [72]. Degranulation of eosinophils with release of these proteins follows engagement of their IgG, IgA and IgE receptors [59, 73], or direct stimulation with soluble mediators such as PAF and LTB_4 [74]: however, the precise cause of eosinophil degranulation *in vivo* is not clear. It has recently been demonstrated that eosinophils also have the capacity to elaborate certain cytokines including TGF-α, GM-CSF and IL-3 [75–77]. GM-CSF secreted by eosinophils was shown to exert an autocrine effect on cell survival [77]. Finally, eosinophils were shown to undergo a respiratory

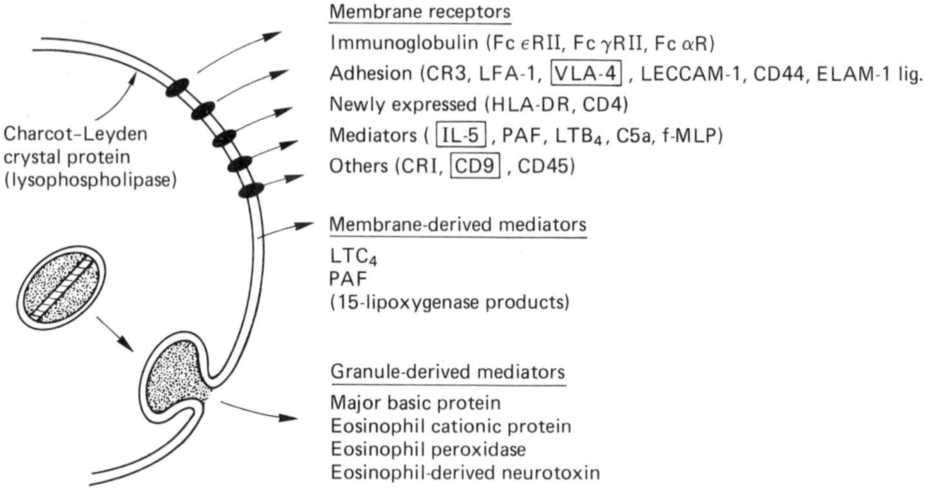

Figure 1.1 Diagrammatic representation of eosinophil mediators and membrane receptors. The precise nature of Fc-ε receptors on eosinophils remains uncertain. Certain receptors expressed on eosinophils but not neutrophils, e.g. VLA-4, IL-5 and CD9, are represented in boxes on the diagram

burst reaction, releasing superoxide ions and peroxide in response to physiological stimuli, a process that was augmented in patients with allergic rhinitis [78].

These extensive inflammatory properties of eosinophils, along with their abundance at sites of asthmatic and allergic inflammation, have given rise to the current consensus of opinion that they are prime inflammatory effector cells in these diseases.

Eosinophils in asthma and allergic diseases

In addition to the evidence from histopathological studies strong circumstantial evidence suggests that eosinophils are important pro-inflammatory cells in asthma. A blood and sputum eosinophilia is often, though not invariably, associated with asthma of diverse aetiology. Longitudinal [79] and cross-sectional [80] studies of asthmatic patients suggest that blood eosinophil counts correlate with the degree of bronchial hyperresponsiveness. Immunostaining of the bronchial mucosa of patients who died from severe asthma revealed large amounts of MBP deposited in the airways [4]. In atopic asthmatics developing a late phase bronchoconstrictor response following allergen challenge, the degree of associated bronchial hyperresponsiveness correlated with the peripheral blood eosinophil count [81]. These observations were extended [82] to show that the proportion of hypodense eosinophils in the peripheral blood of asthmatics was elevated and that the numbers of these cells better reflected the severity of asthma than the total eosinophil count. The numbers of eosinophils in peripheral blood, BAL fluid and bronchial biopsies in a group of asthmatics were elevated compared with normal controls, and it was possible to demonstrate an increasing degree of eosinophilia with clinical severity [83]. Concentrations of MBP in BAL fluid from atopic asthmatics were found to be higher than in normal controls [6, 84], and in one of these studies [6], correlations were observed between the concentration of MBP, the numbers of denuded epithelial cells in BAL fluid and the degree of bronchial hyperresponsiveness. Two studies employing allergen bronchial challenge of atopic asthmatics showed that late phase bronchoconstriction was accompanied by an influx of eosinophils and neutrophils into BAL fluid, whereas subjects developing an isolated early phase response showed no such influx [85, 86]. Similar observations were found in a study using local allergen challenge through the bronchoscope [87]. Inhalation of plicatic acid by subjects with red cedar asthma elicited a BAL eosinophilia together with sloughing of bronchial epithelial cells [88]. A placebo-controlled double-blind study of asthmatics showed that sodium cromoglycate suppressed the accumulation of eosinophils in bronchial mucus and BAL fluid, coinciding with clinical improvement [89].

The eosinophil membrane-derived lipid mediators PAF and LTC_4 have a number of properties which give them a possible role in asthma and allergic disease, but it has been difficult to demonstrate the presence of these mediators in asthma, possibly because of their low concentrations and rapid metabolism. Small elevations in LTC_4 concentrations were noted in BAL fluid from patients with mild asthma [90] and during late phase reactions when fluid from diluent challenge was compared with that obtained from allergen challenge [89], but no studies to date have shown convincing PAF elaboration in association with clinical asthma.

Eosinophils were frequently observed in nasal smears from patients with allergic and non-allergic rhinitis and nasal polyps but not from unaffected controls [91]. Regional variations in the number of eosinophils in the nasal mucosa in rhinitis may be significant [92]. Eosinophil influx was also observed in association with late phase reactions to allergen challenge of the nose [93]. In one study, eosinophils were also described in the normal nasal mucosa [94]. These studies take no account of possible functional heterogeneity of the eosinophils.

In summary, many studies associate increased numbers of eosinophils and concentrations of their granule products with bronchial hyperresponsiveness and allergic rhinitis but, as discussed above, such observations can only provide circumstantial evidence for a role for eosinophils in these diseases. However, inhibition of the migration of eosinophils into the airways of allergen-challenged non-human primates using a monoclonal antibody against the adhesion molecule ICAM-1 was observed to inhibit the development of airways hyperresponsiveness [95], which provides more direct evidence for a role for eosinophils in this phenomenon.

CD4 T lymphocytes

Pro-inflammatory role of CD4 T lymphocytes

CD4 T lymphocytes have a central role to play in any antigen-driven inflammatory process (cell or antibody mediated), because they are the only cells capable of recognizing 'foreign' antigenic material after processing by antigen-presenting cells. Once CD4 T lymphocytes have been activated by antigen, they elaborate a wide variety of protein mediators (lymphokines) which have the capacity to orchestrate the differentiation, recruitment, accumulation and activation of specific granulocyte effector cells at mucosal surfaces. A full description of the properties of individual lymphokines is beyond the scope of this chapter, but the general properties responsible for their pro-inflammatory actions are summarized below:

1. Lymphokines increase the production of specific granulocytes from precursor cells both in the bone marrow and at sites of inflammation.
2. They can prolong the survival of specific granulocytes, bringing about granulocyte accumulation in tissues.
3. Some lymphokines are directly chemotactic for specific granulocytes and can cause preferential adherence of specific granulocytes to vascular endothelium.
4. They can prime specific granulocytes for an enhanced response to physiological activating stimuli.
5. Lymphokines influence the activation of B lymphocytes and the classes of antibodies that they produce in immune responses.

To take eosinophils as an example, CD4 T lymphocytes are a major source of IL-5, which has been demonstrated to promote the differentiation of mature eosinophils from precursor cells [49, 96]; prolong the *in vitro* survival of eosinophils from days to weeks, especially in the presence of fibroblasts or endothelial cells [97, 98]; exhibit chemotactic activity *in vivo* for eosinophils, but not neutrophils, although this effect was weak and requires further confirmation [99]; enhance the adhesion of eosinophils, but not neutrophils, to vascular endothelial cells, a vital initial step in tissue emigration; prime eosinophils for increased activity in a number of subsequent effector responses, including antibody-mediated killing of parasitic larvae, elaboration of lipid mediators and activation by PAF [98, 100].

Similar effects are exhibited by IL-3 [101] and GM-CSF [102, 103], although these lymphokines are not eosinophil specific. Interferon-γ has been shown to enhance eosinophil cytotoxicity [104]. The observations that T-lymphocyte clones from patients with the hyper-eosinophilic syndrome demonstrated IL-5-like activity [105] and that T lymphocytes cultured from patients with asthma spontaneously secreted lymphokines which could prolong eosinophil survival [106] directly support the hypothesis that eosinophil numbers and function may be regulated *in vivo* by T lymphocytes.

Expansion and differentiation of mast cells in tissues was shown to be dependent on IL-3 and IL-4 [107]. A deficiency of mucosal mast cells (see below) was demonstrated in the gastrointestinal tract of humans with defective T-lymphocyte function [108]. In nude mice, IL-3 restored the intestinal mucosal mast cell response to *Strongyloides* infection and facilitated worm expulsion [109].

These studies emphasize the facts that activated CD4 T lymphocytes can bring about *selective* accumulation and activation of specific granulocytes in tissues and that T-lymphocyte-mediated granulocyte accumulation and activation need not be dependent on the presence of antibodies, including IgE. CD4 T lymphocytes are therefore pro-inflammatory cells *in their own right* and can no longer be regarded simply as 'helper' cells for antibody production.

It is worth bearing in mind that T lymphocytes are the principal, but not the only, source of lymphokines: for example, GM-CSF has been shown to be elaborated by macrophages and endothelial cells [110]. The potential of granulocytes, including eosinophils and mast cells, to produce lymphokines is discussed elsewhere in this chapter.

T lymphocytes and the regulation of IgE synthesis

Individuals are said to be 'atopic' if they synthesize inappropriately elevated quantities of IgE. Some of this IgE may be specific for certain environmental antigens or 'allergens'. IgE-mediated mechanisms may not be indispensable for the development of asthma and *chronic* allergic inflammation, although there is little doubt that they are responsible for the acute exacerbation of symptoms sometimes observed in asthmatics and rhinitics after allergen exposure. To this extent at least the regulation of IgE synthesis is relevant to the pathogenesis of these diseases.

Early observations showed that certain T-lymphocyte clones derived from both atopic and non-atopic individuals by non-specific activation with phytohaemagglutinin, when added to autologous or allogeneic B lymphocytes could enhance the synthesis of IgE (rather than IgG) by the B lymphocytes [111]. It was later discovered that the amount of preferential IgE synthesis induced by T-lymphocyte clones is directly related to the amount of IL-4 secreted by the clones, and inversely related to the amount of interferon-γ secreted [112, 113]. Physical contact between T and B lymphocytes is also essential, because exogenous IL-4 alone was not found to increase IgE synthesis by pure B-lymphocyte populations. The fact that contact with T lymphocytes and presence of IL-4 can induce preferential IgE synthesis in B lymphocytes, regardless of their antigen specificity [114] may partly explain why polyclonal as well as allergen-specific IgE synthesis occurs in atopics. Other lymphokines, including $BCGF_{low}$ and IL-2 further enhance IL-4 induced IgE synthesis in these *in vitro* systems [114], probably through their non-specific enhancement of B-lymphocyte proliferation.

However, it is still unclear why certain individuals synthesize allergen-specific IgE and others do not. At the population level, atopy shows a strong tendency to be inherited, and recent data suggest that it may be inherited as an autosomal dominant trait with a high degree of penetrance [116, 117]. For this reason, researchers have looked for global differences in the regulation of IgE synthesis between atopic and non-atopic individuals, in particular an increased synthesis of IL-4 by T lymphocytes derived from atopic individuals. Such differences are hard to find: only one of three patients with atopic dermatitis demonstrated T-lymphocyte clones which were deficient in interferon-γ production [118], while a study of T-lymphocyte clones derived from a patient with the hyper-IgE syndrome failed to show distinct patterns of lymphokine secretion [119].

It may be possible that only allergen-specific T lymphocytes in atopic individuals show abnormal lymphokine synthesis. This has been regarded as unlikely, as allergens apparently show no particular structural features which allow them to be distinguished from other antigens, but it was recently shown that *Dermatophagoides pteronyssinus*-specific T-lymphocyte clones from two atopic patients secreted large amounts of IL-4 and small amounts of interferon-γ on exposure to specific allergen, whereas stimulation of *D. pteronyssinus*-specific clones from an HLA-matched non-atopic donor resulted in the secretion of large amounts of interferon-γ and little IL-4 [120]. Furthermore, T-lymphocyte clones specific for non-allergen antigens (*Candida albicans* or tetanus toxoid) from the same atopic patients produced small amounts of IL-4 and large amounts of interferon-γ. These observations, if found to be generally applicable in larger numbers of patients and with a wide variety of allergens, would support the above hypothesis.

In summary, CD4 T lymphocytes have an important role to play in the regulation of IgE synthesis. Although some preliminary evidence shows that T-lymphocyte dysfunction contributes to inappropriate IgE synthesis, there is no reason as yet to suppose that this accounts for the strong heritable element of atopy. In fact, it seems more likely that the heritability of atopy operates at the level of the mucosal environment where allergen exposure occurs, rather than at the level of allergen-specific T lymphocytes.

Th1 and Th2 CD4 T lymphocytes

Not all lymphokines are implicated in the pathogenesis of asthmatic and allergic inflammation. IL-3, IL-5 and GM-CSF are strongly implicated in that they can selectively recruit and activate mast cells and eosinophils, and IL-4 is implicated in that it is responsible for the promotion of inappropriate IgE synthesis. The genes encoding these lymphokines are located relatively close together in the human genome, on the long arm of chromosome 5, raising the possibility that their expression may be, at least in part, coordinately regulated. There is already good evidence that this is the case in mouse T lymphocytes. Antigen-activated murine CD4 T-lymphocyte clones can be divided into two broad types, Th1 and Th2, according to the pattern of lymphokines they secrete [121]: Th1 cells secrete IL-2, interferon-γ and TNF-β, but not IL-4, IL-5 or IL-6; Th2 cells secrete IL-4, IL-5 and IL-6 but not IL-2, interferon-γ or TNF-β. Other lymphokines, including IL-3 and GM-CSF are secreted by both cell types (Figure 1.2).

The mechanisms which determine expression of Th1 or Th2 phenotypes are not completely understood. Interferon-γ, when added to antigen-stimulated cultures of mouse CD4 T lymphocytes favoured the expression of the Th1 phenotype [122], whilst another lymphokine secreted by Th2 cells, 'cytokine synthesis inhibitory factor' (or IL-10) inhibited Th1 clone proliferation through an effect on antigen-presenting cells [123, 124]. Thus, products of Th1 clones have the capacity to inhibit the growth of Th2 clones, and vice versa.

The functional capacities of Th1 and Th2 CD4 T-lymphocyte clones differ in a manner which reflects their respective patterns of lymphokine synthesis. Th2 clones, through their secretion of IL-4 and IL-5, serve as excellent helper cells for the synthesis of immunoglobulins including IgE by B lymphocytes *in vitro* [125], because both these lymphokines non-specifically enhance B-lymphocyte activation. In addition, by their secretion of IL-3, IL-4 and IL-5, Th2 clones could activate mast cells and eosinophils, and are therefore strongly implicated in the pathogenesis of allergic and asthmatic inflammation.

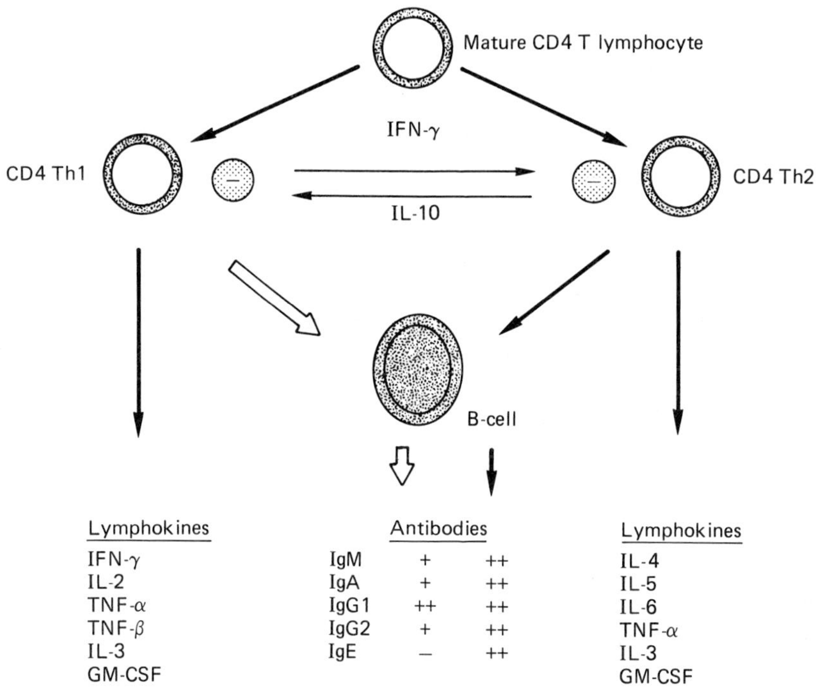

Figure 1.2 Th1 and Th2-type CD4 T lymphocytes in the mouse. Th1 cells mediate DTH reactions, whereas Th2-type cells are better at helping B lymphocytes to make immunoglobulin of all classes (including IgE), and are strongly implicated in asthmatic and allergic inflammation. Th1 and Th2 cells are mutually inhibitory through the release of interferon-α and IL-10 respectively

Th1 clones have been shown to provide help for B lymphocyte IgG synthesis in some, but not all, *in vitro* systems [126]. They strongly suppress IgE production through their release of interferon-γ and also suppresse B-lymphocyte proliferation non-specifically [127]. Th1 cells were also shown to have the capacity to elicit delayed-type hypersensitivity (DTH) reactions *in vivo*. In an experimental system where T lymphocytes and antigen were injected directly into mouse footpads, only Th1 clones were able to elicit antigen-specific swelling [128]. It is not clear why Th2 cells cannot elicit DTH reactions, but one possibility is that the lymphokines produced by these cells are irrelevant to the pathogenesis of DTH.

Human CD4 T-lymphocyte clones stimulated at random using lectins do not fall cleanly into Th1 and Th2 patterns, and there are many examples of clones that secrete a mixture of lymphokines characteristic of both categories [119, 129]. Nevertheless, T lymphocytes with Th1 and Th2 type patterns of lymphokine secretion do appear to exist *in vivo*. These data can be reconciled with those from mice if is assumed that precursor cells (Th0 cells) exist that secrete a mixture of Th1 and Th2 type lymphokines, and that these Th0 cells develop into Th1 or Th2 cells under the influence of extraneous factors such as their antigen specificity, the site of antigen presentation and the nature of the antigen-presenting cells.

This functional dichotomy of activated CD4 T lymphocytes, which either mediate DTH reactions and suppress IgE synthesis (Th1) or mediate allergic and asthmatic inflammation and promote IgE synthesis (Th2) is likely to have a profound impact on our future understanding of allergic inflammation and inappropriate IgE synthesis.

Experimental observations implicating activated CD4 T lymphocytes in the pathogenesis of asthma and allergic inflammation

Two recent studies of bronchial biopsies obtained from mild atopic asthmatics [5, 13] assessed the numbers and activation status of mucosal T lymphocytes by immunostaining with monoclonal antibodies directed against T-lymphocyte phenotypic and activation markers. Interestingly, the total numbers of both CD4 and CD8 T lymphocytes in the bronchial mucosa of these mild asthmatics were not significantly elevated above normal; CD4 cells predominated over CD8 in both cases. In contrast, only cells from the asthmatics showed evidence of IL-2 receptor expression, suggesting activation. Furthermore, the number of activated T lymphocytes in the asthmatics could be correlated with both the total number of eosinophils and the number of activated eosinophils. Finally, the degree of activation could be correlated with disease severity, as assessed by measurement of bronchial hyperresponsiveness.

These observations provide circumstantial evidence to support the hypothesis that activated CD4 T lymphocytes control the numbers and activation status of eosinophils in asthmatic bronchial inflammation, and that the degree of activation is one factor which determines disease severity. Using immunostaining and flow cytometry it was shown that a proportion of CD4 T lymphocytes (but not CD8 cells) in the peripheral blood of patients with acute severe asthma are activated, as assessed by expression of IL-2 receptor, HLA-DR and VLA-1 [130]. The degree of activation of these cells decreased after therapy to an extent that could be correlated with the degree of clinical improvement [131].

An increase has been demonstrated in the relative numbers of lymphocytes found in BAL fluid obtained from patients with mild, stable asthma [132], whereas other studies showed the numbers in asthmatics and normal controls to be similar [6]. Studies on the activation status and the production of lymphokines by these cells are eagerly awaited. In a further study employing allergen bronchial challenge of sensitized atopic asthmatics [87], a selective increase in CD4 cells in BAL fluid was observed 48 h after allergen challenge in subjects who had previously been shown to develop a late phase reaction. These findings complement those of a decrease in levels of CD4 T lymphocytes in the peripheral blood following allergen inhalation by atopic asthmatics [133], and together they suggest that selective recruitment of CD4 T lymphocytes to the lung may occur in association with the late phase asthmatic reaction to allergen bronchial challenge. The possible relevance of this model to the pathogenesis of 'real' asthma has already been discussed. Similarly, in a study employing cutaneous allergen challenge of atopic subjects [134], activated CD4 T lymphocytes were selectively recruited during the course of the late phase reaction.

Despite the fact that sensitive enzyme-linked immunosorbent assay (ELISA) and radioimmunoassay for many lymphokines are now available, measurement of lymphokine secretion *in vivo* is very difficult because of their low concentrations and rapid metabolism. Furthermore, the concentrations of lymphokines in the peripheral blood and BAL fluid of asthmatics may only dimly reflect the local concentrations in the inflamed mucosa. Serum concentrations of interferon-γ have been shown to be elevated in a group of acute severe asthmatics compared with mild asthmatics and normal controls [131]. Interferon-γ secretion is characteristic of a 'TH1-type' response, but because 'Th2-type' lymphokines were not measured in this study it is impossible to assesss the relative contributions of each type of response. Furthermore, TH1-type CD4 T lymphocyte activation could be a superimposed phenomenon in *acute severe* asthma owing, for example, to intercurrent infection.

A useful alternative to the direct measurement of lymphokine concentrations is the detection of the synthesis of their mRNA using the technique of *in situ* hybridization with lymphokine-specific cDNA probes or riboprobes. Although this is not strictly a quantitative technique, it can localize the secretion of lymphokines within cells and tissues. This technique was recently used to demonstrate that IL-5 mRNA was elaborated by cells in the bronchial mucosa of most mild asthmatics but not in normal controls [135] (Figure 1.3). The amount of mRNA detected correlated broadly with the numbers of activated CD4 T lymphocytes and eosinophils in biopsies from the same subjects, providing direct evidence to support the hypothesis that activated CD4 T lymphocytes secrete IL-5 within the asthmatic bronchial mucosa, which regulates the numbers and activation status of

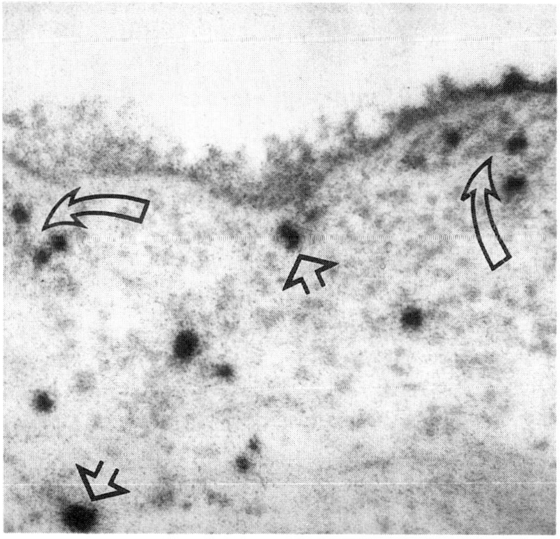

Figure 1.3 Bronchial biopsy hybridized with antisense ^{32}P-labelled riboprobe for IL-5. Specific hybridization signals (some marked by arrows) are seen as dense accumulations of silver grains over cells in the submucosa

eosinophils. In a further study using this technique the cutaneous inflammatory responses to challenge with allergen in atopic subjects and tuberculin in non-atopic subjects were compared [136]. Both late phase allergic and DTH responses were associated with an influx of activated CD4 T lymphocytes, but whereas mRNA molecules encoding IL-2 and interferon-γ were abundant within the tuberculin reactions, very little mRNA encoding these lymphokines was observed in the late phase allergic reactions. Conversely, mRNA encoding IL-4 and IL-5 was abundant in the late phase allergic but not in the tuberculin reactions. In effect, the profiles of lymphokine secretion in the allergic and tuberculin reactions closely paralleled those of Th2 and Th1 CD4 T lymphocytes, respectively. Furthermore, the relative numbers and types of granulocytes infiltrating these reactions reflected the different patterns of lymphokine release [137].

The detection of mRNA does not necessarily equate with protein synthesis and it will need to be shown that translation and secretion of these lymphokines also occurs. Furthermore, T lymphocytes are not the only potential sources of these lymphokines. Finally, it must be borne in mind that the antigen specificity of the recruited T lymphocytes is unknown, and because the tuberculin response was elicited in non-atopic subjects, it is not certain whether the TH2-type response observed in the allergic reaction was *antigen-specific* or *atopy-specific*. Nevertheless, these observations provide direct evidence in support of the hypothesis that activated T lymphocytes, through their patterns of lymphokine secretion, regulate the types of granulocyte which participate in inflammatory reactions; furthermore, they demonstrate that Th1 and Th2 CD4 T-lymphocyte responses can be detected in humans under physiological conditions and that the antigen specificity of the T lymphocytes may be one factor which determines which type of response is initiated.

Neutrophils

The accumulation of neutrophils at sites of inflammation has the potential to result in significant tissue damage. Neutrophils are associated with tissue injury in many inflammatory conditions [138], by the release of oxygen metabolites, proteases and cationic materials. The neutrophil is also a potential source of a wide variety of mediators, including prostaglandins, thromboxanes, LTB_4 and PAF which may contribute to the genesis and exacerbation of the inflammatory response. Neutrophils may be activated by exposure to inflammatory mediators (including PAF and leukotrienes) and certain lymphokines (including GM-CSF, TNF-α and IL-8).

There have been no systematic studies on the possible role of neutrophils in allergic inflammation. In asthma, those studies which have been performed neither confirm nor exclude the contribution of neutrophils. In terms of numbers, neutrophils appear to be a 'normal' resident of larger airways in both normoresponsive and hyperresponsive individuals. In one study [6], approximately 50% of the cells in the bronchial wash of atopic and non-atopic controls and mild asthmatics were neutrophils, the numbers being approximately equal in all groups. Similar findings were obtained in immunohistochemical studies of the bronchial mucosa in mild atopic asthmatics [13]: approximately equal numbers of neutrophils were observed in biopsies from both asthmatics and normal controls. Neutrophils in asthmatics may, nevertheless, demonstrate a different degree of activation than in normals: numerous studies have shown that peripheral blood neutrophils become 'activated' in association with allergen- and exercise-induced early and late phase asthmatic responses [139–142]. Activation was detected by increased membrane expression of complement receptors and enhanced cytotoxicity for complement-coated targets. The significance of these findings in isolation is hard to assess, as neutrophils (like other granulocytes) may become non-specifically activated by exposure to a variety of stimuli. In contrast to eosinophils, no studies on asthmatics showing that neutrophil numbers and/or activation status can be correlated with disease severity have been reported.

Significant increases in the levels of neutrophils in BAL fluid and bronchial mucosa were observed in association with the late phase response of atopic asthmatics to allergen bronchial challenge [86]. Comparable observations were made in BAL during late phase reactions in sensitized subjects challenged with toluene diisocyanate, in which it was found that increases in the numbers of neutrophils, eosinophils and lymphocytes were diminished by prior administration of oral prednisolone [143]. In contrast, BAL neutrophilia was not a feature of late phase reactions elicited by challenge with plicatic acid in patients with red cedar asthma [88].

Characterization of substances with the ability to attract leucocytes to sites of inflammation is of considerable interest. A high molecular weight (600 kDa) neutrophil chemotactic activity (NCA) factor, which appears in the serum of sensitized asthmatics in association with both early and late phase responses to experimental challenge of allergen or non-specific stimuli such as exercise, has been well documented [144–147]. NCA of similar size, along with a second, smaller (<25 kDa) factor was also observed in the serum of patients with acute severe asthma [148], and a third intermediate (40–60 kDa) sized NCA was observed in both acute severe asthmatics and normal controls. Recent evidence suggests that the intermediate and low molecular weight NCA originate from T lymphocytes and monocytes: when peripheral blood mononuclear cells from patients with acute severe asthma were cultured without stimulation in serum-free medium, NCA of 40–60 kDa and 12–25 kDa was elaborated into the culture supernatants [149]. The 40–60 kDa activity was also observed in cultures from normal controls. The 12–25 kDa molecular weight NCA is distinct from IL-8 [150–153], a well characterized neutrophil chemotactic cytokine, although other chemotactic protein molecules with similar physicochemical characteristics continue to be described [154]. Secretion of chemotactic proteins by activated T lymphocytes and monocytes may be a mechanism whereby granulocytes are attracted to sites of inflammation. The origin and nature of the high molecular weight serum NCA remain unresolved.

Convincing evidence suggesting that neutrophils are capable of altering airways function comes from animal experiments. They have been firmly implicated in the pathogenesis of ozone- and antigen-induced hyperreactivity in dogs [155–159], in antigen-induced late phase responses and hyperresponsiveness in rabbits [160] and in responses to endotoxin [161, 162] and antigen [163] in sheep. Rabbits demonstrate increased responsiveness when airways inflammation is induced with phlogistic fragments of C5, and this too is dependent on neutrophils [164]. The requirement for granulocytes (especially neutrophils) in these experiments has been established by association (lavage and histology), depletion studies (such as with nitrogen mustard) and, most convincingly, by depletion followed by selective repletion with enriched populations of purified neutrophils [157]. In a guinea-pig model of late and 'late-late' phase antigen-induced bronchoconstriction, there was a sevenfold increase in the numbers of neutrophils in BAL fluid at 6 h, and a 17-fold increase at 17 h [165]. However, the relevance of these animal models to the pathogenesis of bronchial hyperresponsiveness in human asthma is impossible to assess.

The question of whether the neutrophil participates in the functional alterations associated with allergic disease and asthma therefore remains unanswered. The frequent recovery of neutrophils from BAL fluid of asthmatic patients [166, 167], the presence of neutrophils in pathological sections of asthmatic airways [10,11] and the ability of neutrophils to alter airways function together suggest that they may indeed have a role.

Mast cells and basophils

Mast cells have long been recognized as major effector cells of the allergic or Type I hypersensitivity reaction by virtue of their high-affinity surface receptors for IgE. The widespread distribution of mast cells throughout the body in general, and at mucosal surfaces in particular, in both atopic and non-atopic individuals, and the recognition that they may be activated by non-immunological means, suggests that mast cells may be involved in inflammatory processes regardless of the presence or absence of atopy. At the same time, the recognition of lower-affinity IgE receptors on other inflammatory cells, such as eosinophils, B lymphocytes and monocytes, has raised the possibility that mast cells and basophils are not necessarily involved in IgE-dependent inflammatory mechanisms. Basophils have not yet been identified in bronchial pathology, although they probably exist as they do in most other organs.

Two types of human mast cells termed T (tryptase-positive, chymase-negative) and TC (tryptase-positive, chymase-positive) have been described based on differences in neutral protease content. T-type cells predominate in nasal scrapings and nasal epithelium of subjects with allergic rhinitis [168, 169], and in the epithelium and lamina propria of bronchi and in BAL fluid [170, 171]. TC-type cells predominate in the gastrointestinal submucosa and the skin [172]. It should be emphasized that these divisions in terms of anatomical sites are relative. They have a similar histamine content [173]. T-type cells probably secrete both LTC_4 and PGD_2 after IgE-dependent activation [174], whereas TC-type cells secrete PGD_2 but little or no LTC_4 [174]. *In vitro* allergen challenge of TC-type cells from the skin of sensitized atopic subjects resulted in histamine release that was insensitive to inhibition by sodium cromoglycate [176]. T-type cells recovered from BAL fluid were more sensitive [171], but even then the concentration of drug required to produce significant inhibition was very high [100 μM]. T-type cells appear to be more dependent on T lymphocyte products for their continued presence in tissues: a study of patients with congenital or acquired immune deficiency showed a severe depletion of T-type mast cells in the gastrointestinal mucosa with normal numbers of TC cells [108].

Mast cell products, particularly lipid-derived mediators, have the propensity to participate in many of the acute clinical features of asthma and allergic disease. In several studies on atopic asthmatics, the numbers of mast cells in BAL fluid were higher than those in normal controls in the absence of allergen challenge [6, 7, 84, 177], but this finding is not specific for asthma because it was also observed in association with a number of other pulmonary diseases [178]. The numbers of mast cells and the concentrations of histamine in BAL fluid could in some studies be correlated with the degree of bronchial hyperresponsiveness [6, 7, 179]. Both spontaneous and stimulated mediator release from mast cells were higher in asthmatics than in normal controls [6, 177]. Quantitative studies on mast cells in the nasal mucosa after allergen challenge have given widely disparate results, ranging from an overall decrease via redistribution to an overall increase [21–24]; on balance however mast cell numbers probably increase in response to challenge.

The early phase response to allergen challenge in both the nose and the bronchi may be accounted for by mast cell products: histamine and PGD_2 release were demonstrated to occur in association with this response [86, 180, 181], whilst the response was almost totally abrogated by a combination of histamine and prostaglandin antagonists [182, 183]. The fact that sodium cromoglycate inhibits the early response has been taken as evidence of mast cell involvement, although the high concentration of drug required for inhibition of BAL fluid mast cells *in vitro* rather weakens this argument. There is little evidence for or against the suggestion that mast cell products contribute to late phase reactions to allergen challenge at any site. Most experiments implicating mast cells in the pathogenesis of asthma have been performed on atopic asthmatics where mechanisms for IgE-mediated release of mediators are assumed to operate. It is less clear what could induce mast cell degranulation in non-atopic asthmatics, although cytokine products of activated T lymphocytes and monocytes related to IL-8 that act directly on mast cells to induce histamine release are beginning to be described [184]. Furthermore, there is some evidence that mast cell degranulation may be provoked by non-specific stimuli such as cold air and hyperventilation [185]. The release of histamine observed in association with late phase responses may reflect basophil rather than mast cell degranulation, since it was not accompanied by the release of other mast cell products such as PGD_2 in the skin [186] or tryptase in the nose [187].

It has recently been shown that IgE-mediated activation of murine mast cells results in the secretion of IL-3 and GM-CSF [188]. Messenger RNAs for several other cytokines including IL-5 and IFN-γ have also been identified in similarly activated mast cell clones [189]. These cytokines have the ability to recruit, prime and activate neutrophils, monocytes and eosinophils. Their elaboration by mast cells in response to allergen may provide a mechanism by which the mast cells participate in late phase responses and ongoing asthma and allergic disease.

Monocytes and macrophages (mononuclear phagocytes)

The role of mononuclear phagocytes as antigen processing and presenting cells is well established. It seems reasonable to assume that in health and disease such cells are present in and around the bronchi where they process inhaled antigen and present it to local T lymphocytes. It is therefore difficult to understand why inflammatory processes are not initiated in the bronchi of *all* individuals. Experiments in rodents suggest that, under normal circumstances, alveolar macrophages play an important *inhibitory* role by attenuating local immune responses [190], and that it is the HLA class II bearing dendritic cells in the bronchial epithelium that are responsible for T-lymphocyte activation [190, 191]. It is possible that asthmatic inflammation involves an escape from this local immune attenuation. Similar HLA class II-bearing cells (Langerhans cells) are also found in the nasal mucosa [192], although there is no obvious counterpart of the alveolar macrophage at this site.

Macrophages form the majority of cells recovered in BAL fluid from normal and asthmatic subjects. In addition to IgG Fc receptors, monocytes and macrophages express low-affinity Fc receptors for IgE [193, 194], raising the possibility that they may be activated directly by IgE-dependent mechanisms. The numbers of these receptors on alveolar macrophages were shown to be higher in both atopic and non-atopic asthmatics than in normal controls [195, 196]. Macrophages isolated from BAL fluid of atopic asthmatics showed enhanced exocytosis in response to anti-IgE and relevant allergen challenge *in vitro* compared with normal controls [194, 197, 198]. Exocytosis of macrophages may be accompanied by elaboration of inflammatory mediators including thromboxane A_2, LTB_4, PGI_2, PGE_2 and PAF [197, 199, 200]. Allergen challenge of atopic asthmatics was shown to increase the concentration of β-glucuronidase in BAL fluid *in vivo* [201]. The macrophage is one but not the only source of this enzyme. The percentages of monocytes in BAL fluid forming complement-mediated erythrocyte rosettes were also shown to increase during the late phase reaction to allergen bronchial challenge [86]. In one study, IgE-dependent activation of macrophages was demonstrated to result in the release of IL-1 [202]. IL-1 has a multitude of pro-inflammatory actions, including the enhancement of leucocyte adherence to vascular endothelium. Macrophages also have the potential to secrete other lymphokines such as TNF-α, GM-CSF, IL-8 and histamine releasing factors.

Thus, although alveolar macrophages appear to be locally inhibitory to T lymphocyte activation they have the capacity to propagate inflammation through alternative mechanisms such as IgE-dependent activation, and it would be surprising if they did not participate in airways responses to inhaled allergens. It is, however, worth bearing in mind that these cells may play an important role in the resolution of inflammation [203]. Because macrophages can manifest many different functional phenotypes it is possible that the airways of asthmatics may contain macrophages which are both contributing to and serving to limit the inflammatory response.

Summary and conclusions

The nature of allergic and asthmatic inflammation

Evidence is accumulating that chronic asthmatic and allergic inflammation represent a specialized form of cell-mediated immunity, in which secretion of specific lymphokines, principally by activated T lymphocytes, brings about local mucosal accumulation and activation of specific granulocytes, particularly eosinophils (Figure 1.4). The release of inflammatory mediators from these cells results in tissue damage and may contribute to further recruitment of inflammatory cells. This scheme does not envisage an indispensable role for antibody-dependent inflammatory mechanisms, including those mediated by IgE. There is little doubt, however, that IgE-mediated mechanisms may *exacerbate* asthma and allergic diseases. Inhaled allergens in sensitized atopic individuals have been shown to increase bronchial hyperresponsiveness both in an experimental setting and on natural exposure [36, 204]. Furthermore, there is increasing evidence that allergen load is important for the development of symptoms of atopy and asthma and that removal of patients from allergens decreases the severity of clinical asthma and bronchial hyperresponsiveness [205, 206]. Nevertheless, the observations that the synthesis of allergen-specific IgE in some individuals does not necessarily result in allergic disease and that not all patients with asthma and rhinitis are demonstrably

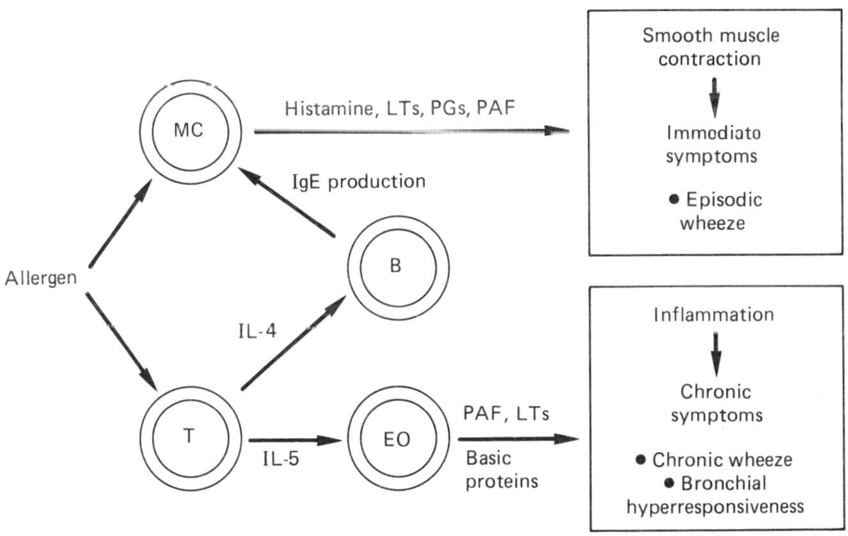

Figure 1.4 Postulated mechanisms in asthmatic and allergic inflammation. Antigen-activated T lymphocytes (T) produce lymphokines which cause the specific accumulation and activation of eosinophils (EO), whose products cause mucosal damage which results in chronic symptoms. Additionally, in atopic individuals, acute release of mediators from IgE-sensitized cells (MC) may cause periodic acute exacerbations of symptoms. The role of T lymphocytes in the control of IgE synthesis by B lymphocytes (B) is also highlighted

atopic would support the argument that allergen-specific IgE synthesis is neither necessary nor sufficient for the development of these diseases. It is possible to hypothesize that asthma and rhinitis result from an inherited defect in the local mucosal environment (such as a defect in epithelial integrity or a dysregulation of local immune tolerance to environmental allergens) which facilitates the development of chronic cell-mediated inflammation, accompanied in some individuals by inappropriate IgE synthesis. It will be important in the future to delineate the relative importance of cell-mediated and IgE-mediated mechanisms in these diseases in order to plan effective therapeutic strategies. Glucocorticoids are very effective as prophylactic therapy for rhinitis and are the only drugs which have been shown unequivocally to reduce bronchial hyperresponsiveness in asthma. They strongly inhibit T lymphocyte and monocyte function, but exert little or no direct inhibitory effect on granulocytes such as mast cells and eosinophils [207]. This might be taken as evidence that suppression of cell-mediated inflammation is more effective for the therapy of these diseases than inhibition of granulocyte function. On the other hand, it is also true to state that drugs which potently inhibit mast cell and eosinophil degranulation *in vivo* do not yet exist.

The precise aetiologies of asthma and allergic disease remain unknown. It is clearly too simplistic to suppose that the question is one of the presence or absence of allergen-specific IgE (although it is of interest that the prevalence of asthma was closely related to the serum IgE level standardized for age and sex [208]). Nevertheless, it is reasonable to suppose that all asthmatic and allergic inflammation is antigen driven. The resident inflammatory cells of the mucosae, after inappropriate antigen recognition might become misdirected, forsaking their probable defensive role for one of tissue damage. The nature of the putative activating antigen(s) is unclear: although inhaled aeroallergens are obvious candidates in allergic rhinitis and 'atopic' asthma, it seems unlikely that they can be implicated in every case; indeed, even in atopic asthmatics exacerbating factors other than allergens (such as viral infections) may be more prominent clinically. A further possibility is that asthma is an 'autoimmune' disease, the driving antigens being normal antigens within the bronchial mucosa which are inappropriately recognized by local T lymphocytes.

Some notes of caution

One very weak link in the chain of asthma research is the exact relationship between inflammation and bronchial hyperresponsiveness. Until the precise cause of bronchial hyperresponsiveness is defined at the cellular level, studies which demonstrate cellular changes in patients with hyperresponsiveness can never provide better than circumstantial evidence for a role for that particular change in asthma. For example, it is currently assumed that bronchial hyperresponsiveness is a consequence of bronchial epithelial damage effected by eosinophil products. These suppositions may be true but they need to be demonstrated clearly. It would perhaps be better to abandon the concept of bronchial hyperresponsiveness and to attempt to define asthma in terms of pathophysiological changes at the cellular level.

Research in allergic disease is confounded by the difficulty of performing experiments, particularly dynamic experiments, in humans. For this reason many experimenters have fallen back on animal 'models' of asthma. The making of a model, however, implies prior knowledge of the structure of that which is being modelled, and so it could be argued that no animal model of disease can be validated until the precise pathophysiology of the disease is known. Animal experiments may nevertheless be invaluable in answering questions about well-defined stages of the inflammatory process (such as whether blockage of an adhesion molecule on endothelial cells inhibits influx of granulocytes into tissues) and in testing the efficacy of drugs.

Caution must also be exercised in the interpretation of experiments on humans. The majority of dynamic human experiments have focused on acute challenge of sensitized atopic individuals, which may not always represent the true pathogenesis of the disease. Whilst the presence of a given cell or mediator is certainly a prerequisite for its involvement in an inflammatory process, the converse does not necessarily follow. Furthermore, static 'snapshots' of what is probably a highly dynamic process give no information as to timing of the influx and egress of inflammatory cells, which are important in determining the inflammatory cell 'load'. Little information is available regarding the temporal course of the inflammatory process in allergic disease and asthma. Although the potential for inflammatory cells to exhibit variable states of priming and activation seems considerable, there are as yet few studies which have addressed this problem. Finally, the precise situation of inflammatory cells within the mucosa might be relevant to an interpretation of their role, with regard to both their possible interactions with resident mucosal cells and the local effects of their mediators. It is by no means clear, for example, that bronchoalveolar lavage samples appropriate airway sites.

The way ahead

Further studies on the temporal course and natural history of allergic and asthmatic inflammation are needed. In view of the emerging importance of T-lymphocyte mediated chronic inflammatory reactions in these diseases, it would undoubtedly be of value to ascertain the antigen specificity and profiles of lymphokine secretion of T lymphocytes within the inflamed mucosa. This might lead to the discovery of pathogenetic subdivisions of the diseases which are as yet unrecognized, and point the way to new therapeutic strategies involving the inhibition of accumulation or activation of particular granulocytes at mucosal surfaces directly or indirectly through inhibition of lymphokine secretion.

References

1. Houston JC, De Navasquez S, Trounce JR. A clinical and pathological study of fatal cases of status asthmaticus. *Thorax* 1953; **8:** 207–213.
2. Dunnill MS. The pathology of asthma with special reference to changes in the bronchial mucosa. *J Clin Pathol* 1960; **13:** 27–33.
3. Dunnill MS, Massarella GR, Anderson JA. A comparison of the quantitative anatomy of the bronchi in normal subjects, in status asthmaticus, in chronic bronchitis and in emphysema. *Thorax* 1969; **24:** 176–179.
4. Filley WV, Holley KE, Kephart GM, Gleich GJ. Identification by immunofluorescence of eosinophil

granule major basic protein in lung tissues of patients with bronchial asthma. *Lancet* 1982; **ii:** 11–16.
5. Azzawi M, Bradley B, Jeffery PK *et al.* Identification of activated T lymphocytes and eosinophils in bronchial biopsies in stable atopic asthma. *Am Rev Respir Dis* 1990; **142:** 1410–1413.
6. Wardlaw AJ, Dunnette S, Gleich GJ, Collins JV, Kay AB. Eosinophils and mast cells in bronchoalveolar lavage in mild asthma: relationship to bronchial hyperreactivity. *Am Rev Respir Dis* 1988; **137:** 62–69.
7. Kirby JG, Hargreave FE, Gleich GJ, O'Byrne PM. Bronchoalveolar cell profiles of asthmatic and non-asthmatic subjects. *Am Rev Respir Dis* 1987; **136:** 379–383.
8. Jeffery PK, Wardlaw AJ, Nelson FC, Collins JV, Kay AB. Bronchial biopsies in asthma: an ultrastructural, quantitative study and correlation with hyperreactivity. *Am Rev Respir Dis* 1989; **140:** 1745–1753.
9. Glynn AA, Michaels L. Bronchial biopsy in chronic bronchitis and asthma. *Thorax* 1960; **15:** 142–153.
10. Salvato G. Some histological changes in chronic bronchitis and asthma. *Thorax* 1968; **23:** 168–172.
11. Laitinen LA, Heino M, Laitinen A, Kava T, Haahtela T. Damage of airway epithelium and bronchial reactivity in patients with asthma. *Am Rev Respir Dis* 1985; **131:** 599–606.
12. Beasley R, Roche W, Roberts JA, Holgate ST. Cellular events in the bronchi in mild asthma and after bronchial provocation. *Am Rev Respir Dis* 1989; **139:** 806–817.
13. Bradley BL, Azzawi M, Assoufi B *et al.* Eosinophils, T-lymphocytes, mast cells, neutrophils and macrophages in bronchial biopsies from atopic asthmatics: comparison with atopic non-asthma and normal controls and relationship to bronchial hyperresponsiveness. *J Allergy Clin Immunol* 1991; **88:** 661–674.
14. Jeffery PK, Godfrey RW, Adelroth E, Nelson F, Rogers A, Johansson S-A. Effects of treatment on airway inflammation and thickening of basement membrane reticular collagen in asthma: a quantitative light and electron microscopic study. *Am Rev Respir Dis* 1992; **45:** 890–899.
15. Roche WR, Beasley R, Williams JH, Holgate ST. Subepithelial fibrosis in the bronchi of asthmatics. *Lancet* 1989; **i:** 520–523.
16. Fabbri LM, Danielli D, Crescioli S *et al.* Fatal asthma in a subject sensitised to toluene diisocyanate. *Am Rev Respir Dis* 1988; **137:** 1494–1498.
17. Bentley AM, Maestrelli P, Fabbri LM *et al.* Activated T-lymphocytes and eosinophils in the bronchial mucosa in isocyanate induced asthma. *J Allergy Clin Immunol* 1992; **89:** 821–829.
18. Mattoli S, Mattoso VL, Soloperto M, Allegra L, Fasoli A. Cellular and biochemical characteristics of bronchoalveolar lavage fluid in symptomatic nonallergic asthma. *J Allergy Clin Immunol* 1991; **87:** 794–802.
19. Okuda M, Otsuka H. Basophilic cells in allergic nasal secretions. *Arch Otorhinolaryngol* 1977; **314:** 283–289.
20. Hastie R, Chir B, Heroy JH, Levy DA. Basophil leukocytes and mast cells in human nasal secretions and scrapings studied by light microscopy. *Lab Invest* 1979; **40:** 554–561.
21. Wihl JA, Mygind N. Studies on the allergen-challenged human nasal mucosa. *Acta Otolaryngol* 1977; **84:** 218–286.
22. Borres MP, Irander K, Bjorksten B. Meatchromatic cells in nasal mucosa after allergen challenge. *Allergy* 1990; **45:** 98–103.
23. Enerback L, Pipkorn U, Granerus G. Intraepithelial migration of nasal mucosal mast cells in hay fever. *Int Arch Allergy Appl Immunol* 1986; **80:** 44–51.
24. Lozewicz S, Gomez E, Claque J, Gatland D, Davies RJ. Allergen-induced changes in the nasal mucous membrane in seasonal allergic rhinitis: effect of nedocromil sodium. *J Allergy Clin Immunol* 1990; **85:** 125–131.
25. Bascom R, Pipkorn U, Lichtenstein LM, Naclerio RM. The influx of inflammatory cells into nasal washings during the late response to antigen challenge: effect of systemic steroid pretreatment. *Am Rev Respir Dis* 1988; **138:** 406–412.
26. Bonini SE, Bonini ST, Vecchione A, Naim DM, Allansmith MR, Balsano F. Inflammatory changes in conjunctival scrapings after allergen provocation in humans. *J Allergy Clin Immunol* 1988; **82:** 462–469.
27. Robertson DG, Kerigan AT, Hargreave FE, Chalmers R, Dolovich J. Late asthmatic responses induced by ragweed pollen antigen. *J Allergy Clin Immunol* 1974; **54:** 244–254.
28. Dvoracek JE, Yunginger JW, Kern EB, Hyatt RE, Gleich GJ. Induction of nasal late-phase reactions by insufflation of ragweed-pollen extract. *J Allergy Clin Immunol* 1984; **73:** 363–368.
29. Richerson HB, Rajtora DW, Penick GD *et al.* Cutaneous and nasal allergic responses in ragweed hay fever: lack of clinical and histopathologic correlations with late phase reactions. *J Allergy Clin Immunol* 1979; **64:** 67–77.
30. Bonini ST, Bonini SE, Todini V, Adriani E, Allansmith MR. Late-phase ocular reaction induced by conjunctival allergen challenge. A dose response study in humans. *J Allergy Clin Immunol* 1988; **82:**

462–468.
31. Crimi E, Brusaco V, Losurdo E, Crimi P. Predictive accuracy of late asthmatic reaction to *Dermatophagoides pteronyssinus*. *J Allergy Clin Immunol* 1986; **78:** 908–913.
32. Durham SR, Craddock CF, Cookson WO, Benson MK. Increases in airway responsiveness to histamine precede allergen-induced late asthmatic responses. *J Allergy Clin Immunol* 1988; **82:** 764–770.
33. Warner JO. Significance of late reactions after bronchial challenge with house dust mite. *Arch Dis Child* 1976; **51:** 905–910.
34. Chan-Yeung M, Lam S. State of the art: occupational asthma. *Am Rev Respir Dis* 1986; **133:** 686–703.
35. Warner JO, Price JF, Soothill JF, Hey EN. Controlled trial of hyposensitisation to *Dermatophagoides pteronyssinus* in children with asthma. *Lancet* 1978; **ii:** 912–915.
36. Cartier A, Thomson NC, Frith PA, Roberts R, Hargreave FE. Allergen-induced increase in bronchial responsiveness to histamine: relationship to the late asthmatic response and change in airway calibre. *J Allergy Clin Immunol* 1982; **70:** 170–177.
37. Burge PS, Efthimiou J, Turner-Warwick M, Nelman PT. Double blind trials of inhaled beclomethasone dipropionate and fluocortin dibutyl ester in allergen-induced immediate and late asthmatic reactions. *Clin Allergy* 1982; **12:** 523–531.
38. Cockcroft DW, Murdock KY. Protective effect of inhaled albuterol, cromolyn, beclomethasone and placebo on allergen-induced early asthmatic responses, late asthmatic responses and allergen-induced increases in bronchial responsiveness to inhaled histamine. *J Allergy Clin Immunol* 1987; **79:** 734–740.
39. Cockcroft DW, Murdock KY, Gore PB, O'Byrne PM, Manning P. Theophylline does not inhibit allergen-induced increase in airway responsiveness to methacholine. *J Allergy Clin Immunol 1989*; **83:** 913–920.
40. Frew AJ, Kay AB. The pattern of human late-phase skin reactions to extracts of aeroallergens. *J Allergy Clin Immunol* 1988; **81:** 1117–1121.
41. Lee TH, Nagakura T, Papageorgiou N, Iikura Y, Kay AB. Exercise-induced late asthmatic reactions with neutrophil chemotactic activity. *N Engl J Med* 1983; **308:** 1502–1505.
42. Solley GO, Gleich GJ, Jordan RE, Schroeter AL. The late phase of the immediate wheal and flare skin reaction. Its dependence upon IgE antibodies. *J Clin Invest* 1976; **58:** 408–420.
43. Dolovich J, Hargreave FE, Chalmers R, Shierk J, Gauldie J, Bienenstock J. Late cutaneous allergic responses in isolated IgE-dependent reactions. *J Allergy Clin Immunol* 1973; **52:** 38–46.
44. Hargreave FE, Ryan G, Thomson NC *et al*. Bronchial responsiveness to histamine or methacholine in asthma: measurement and clinical significance. *J Allergy Clin Immunol* 1981; **68:** 347–355.
45. Juniper EF, Frith PA, Hargreave FE. Airway responsiveness to histamine and methacholine: relationship to minimum treatment to control symptoms of asthma. *Thorax* 1981; **36:** 575–579.
46. Butterworth AE. Cell-mediated damage to helminths. *Adv Parasitol* 1984; **23:** 143–235.
47. Butterworth AE, Sturrock RF, Houba V, Mahmoud AA, Sher A, Rees PH. Eosinophils as mediators of antibody-dependent damage to schistosomula. *Nature* 1975; **256:** 727–729.
48. Sher A, Coffman RL, Hieny S, Scott P, Cheever AW. Interleukin-5 is required for the blood and tissue eosinophilia but not the granuloma formation induced by infection with *Schistosoma mansoni*. *Proc Natl Acad Sci USA* 1990; **87:** 61–65.
49. Sanderson CJ, Warren DJ, Strath M. Identification of a lymphokine that stimulates eosinophil differentiation in vitro: its relationship to interleukin-3 and functional properties of eosinophils produced in cultures. *J Exp Med* 1985; **162:** 60–74.
50. Basten A, Beeson PB. Mechanism of eosinophilia. II: Role of the lymphocyte. *J Exp Med* 1970; **131:** 1288–1305.
51. Kyan-Aung U, Haskard DO, Poston RN, Thornhill MH, Lee TH. Endothelial leukocyte adhesion molecule 1 and intercellular adhesion molecule 1 mediate adhesion of eosinophils to endothelial cells *in vitro* and are expressed by endothelium in allergic cutaneous inflammation *in vivo*. *J Immunol* 1991; **146:** 521–528.
52. Dent LA, Strath M, Mellor AL, Sanderson CJ. Eosinophilia in transgenic mice expressing interleukin-5. *J Exp Med* 1990; **172:** 1425–1431.
53. Wardlaw AJ, Moqbel R, Cromwell O, Kay AB. Platelet activating factor: a potent chemotactic and chemokinetic factor for human eosinophils. *J Clin Invest* 1986; **78:** 1701–1706.
54. Walsh GM, Hartnell A, Wardlaw AJ, Kurihara K, Sanderson CJ, Kay AB. IL-5 enhances the *in vitro* adhesion of human eosinophils, but not neutrophils, in a leukocyte integrin (CD11/18) dependent manner. *Immunology* 1990; **71:** 258–265.
55. Walsh GM, Hartnell A, Mermod J-J, Kay AB, Wardlaw AJ. Human eosinophil, but not neutrophil adherence to IL-1 stimulated HUVEC is $\alpha 4\beta 1$ (VLA-4) dependent. *J Immunol* 1991; **146:** 3419–3423.
56. Capron M, Capron A, Dessaint J-P, Torpier G, Johanson SGO, Prin L. Fc receptors for IgE on human and rat eosinophils. *J Immunol* 1981; **126:** 2087–2092.
57. Capron M, Spiegelberg HL, Prin L, Bennich H, Butterworth AE, Pierce RJ, Ouaissi MA, Capron A.

Role of IgE receptors in effector function of human eosinophils. *J Immunol* 1984; **132:** 462–468.
58. Hartnell A, Moqbel R, Walsh GM, Bradley B, Kay AB. Fc gamma and CD11/CD18 receptor expression on normal density and low density eosinophils. *Immunology* 1990; **69:** 264–270.
59. Abu-Ghazaleh RI, Fujisawa T, Mestecky J, Kyle RA, Gleich GJ. IgA-induced eosinophil degranulation. *J Immunol* 1989; **142:** 2393–2400.
60. Lucey DR, Nicholson-Weller A, Weller PF. Mature human eosinophils have the capacity to express HLA-DR. *Proc Natl Acad Sci USA* 1989; **86:** 1348–1351.
61. Lucey DR, Dorsky DI, Nicholson-Weller A, Weller PF. Human eosinophils express CD4 protein and bind human immunodeficiency virus 1 gp120. *J Exp Med* 1989; **169:** 327-332.
62. Shaw RJ, Walsh GM, Cromwell O, Moqbel R, Spry CJF, Kay AB. Activated human eosinophils generate SRS-A leukotrienes following physiological (IgG-dependent) stimulation. *Nature* 1985; **316:** 150–152.
63. Shaw RJ, Cromwell O, Kay AB. Preferential generation of leukotriene C4 by human eosinophils. *Clin Exp Immunol* 1984; **56:** 716–722.
64. Lee TC, Hanahan DJ, Malone B, Roddy LL, Wasserman SI. Increased biosynthesis of platelet activating factor in activated human eosinophils. *J Biol Chem* 1984; **259:** 5526–5530.
65. Cuss FM, Dixon CMS, Barnes PJ. Effects of inhaled platelet activating factor on pulmonary function and bronchial responsiveness in man. *Lancet* 1986; **ii:** 189–192.
66. Hanna CJ, Back MK, Pane PD, Schellenberg RR. Slow reacting substances leukotrienes contract human airway and vascular smooth muscle *in vitro*. *Nature* 1981; **290:** 343–344.
67. Kaliner M, Shelhamer, Barson B, Nadel J, Patour C, Maram Z. Human respiratory mucus. *Am Rev Respir Dis* 1986; **134:** 612-621.
68. Gleich GJ, Adolphson CR. The eosinophil leukocyte. *Annu Rev Immunol* 1986; **39:** 177–253.
69. Gleich GJ, Frigas E, Loegering DA, Wassom DL, Steinmuller D. Cytotoxic properties of eosinophil major basic protein. *J Immunol* 1979; **123:** 2925–2927.
70. Ayars GH, Altman LC, Gleich GJ, Loegering DA, Baker EB. Eosinophil and eosinophil granule mediated pneumocyte injury. *J Allergy Clin Immunol* 1985; **76:** 595–604.
71. Gundel RH, Letts LG, Gleich GJ. Human eosinophil major basic protein induces airway constriction and airway hyperresponsiveness in primates. *J Clin Invest* 1991; **87:** 1470–1473.
72. Gleich GJ. The eosinophil and bronchial asthma: current understanding. *J Allergy Clin Immunol* 1990; **85:** 422-436.
73. Khaliffe J, Capron M, Cesbron JY *et al.* Role of specific IgE antibodies in peroxidase EPO release from human eosinophils. *J Immunol* 1986; **137:** 1659–1664.
74. Kroegel C, Yukawa T, Dent G, Venge P, Chung FK, Barnes PJ. Stimulation of degranulation from human eosinophils by platelet-activating factor. *J Immunol* 1989; **142:** 3518–3526.
75. Wong DT, Weller PF, Galli SJ *et al.* Human eosinophils express transforming growth factor alpha. *J Exp Med* 1990; **172:** 673–681.
76. Moqbel R, Hamid Q, Ying S *et al.* Expression of mRNA and immunoreactivity for the granulocyte/macrophage colony stimulating factor (GM-CSF) in activated human eosinophils. *J Exp Med* 1991; **174:** 749–752.
77. Kita H, Ohnishi T, Okubo Y, Weiler D, Abrams JS, Gleich GJ. GM-CSF and interleukin-3 release from human peripheral blood eosinophils and neutrophils. *J Exp Med* 1991; **174:** 745–748.
78. Shult PA, Graziano FM, Busse WW. Enhanced eosinophil luminol-dependent chemiluminescence in allergic rhinitis. *J Allergy Clin Immunol* 1985; **77:** 702–708.
79. Horn BR, Robin ED, Theodore J, Van Kessel A. Total eosinophil counts in the management of bronchial asthma. *N Engl J Med* 1975; **292:** 1152–1155.
80. Taylor KJ, Luksza AR. Peripheral blood eosinophil counts and bronchial hyperresponsiveness. *Thorax* 1987; **42:** 452–456.
81. Durham SR, Kay AB. Eosinophils, bronchial hyperreactivity and late-phase asthmatic reactions. *Clin Allergy* 1985; **15:** 411–418.
82. Frick WE, Sedgwick JB, Busse WW. The appearance of hypodense eosinophils in antigen-dependent late phase asthma. *Am Rev Respir Dis* 1989; **139:** 1401–1406.
83. Bousquet J, Chanez P, Lacoste JY *et al.* Eosinophilic inflammation in asthma. *N Engl J Med* 1990; **323:** 1033–1039.
84. Tomioka M, Ida S, Yuriko S, Takishima T. Mast cells in bronchoalveolar lumen of patients with bronchial asthma. *Am Rev Respir Dis* 1984; **129:** 1000–1005.
85. De Monchy JGR, Kauffman HF, Venge P *et al.* Bronchoalveolar eosinophilia during allergen-induced late asthmatic reactions. *Am Rev Respir Dis* 1985; **131:** 373–376.
86. Diaz P, Gonzalez MC, Galleguillos FR *et al.* Leukocytes and lipid mediators in bronchoalveolar lavage during allergen-induced late-phase asthmatic reactions. *Am Rev Respir Dis* 1989; **139:** 1383–1389.

87. Metzger WJ, Zavala D, Richerson HB *et al.* Local allergen challenge and bronchoalveolar lavage of allergic asthmatic lungs: description of the model and local airway inflammation. *Am Rev Respir Dis* 1987; **135:** 433–440.
88. Lam S, LeRiche J, Phillips D, Chan-Yeung M. Cellular and protein changes in bronchial lavage fluid after late asthmatic reaction in patients with red cedar asthma. *J Allergy Clin Immunol* 1987; **80:** 44–50.
89. Diaz P, Galleguillos FR, Gonzalez MC, Pantin C, Kay AB. Bronchoalveolar lavage in asthma: the effect of DSCG on leukocyte counts, immunoglobulins and complement. *J Allergy Clin Immunol* 1984; **74:** 41–48.
90. Wardlaw AJ, Hay H, Cromwell O, Collins JV, Kay AB. Leukotrienes LTC_4 and LTB_4 in bronchoalveolar lavage fluid in bronchial asthma and other respiratory diseases. *J Allergy Clin Immunol* 1989; **84:** 19–26.
91. Mullarkey MF, Hill JS, Webb DR. Allergic and non-allergic rhinitis: their characterization with reference to the meaning of nasal eosinophilia. *J Allergy Clin Immunol* 1980; **65:** 122–126.
92. Valeri E. Nasal allergy with special reference to eosinophils and histopathology. *Acta Allergol* 1956; **203:** 203–210.
93. Naclerio RM, Kagey-Sobotka A, Lichtenstein LM. Observations on nasal late phase reactions. *Immunol Invest* 1987-1988; **16:** 649–685.
94. Thaete LG, Spicer SS, Spock A. Ultrastructure and carbohydrate cytochemistry of surface and glandular epithelium of human nasal mucosa. *Am J Anat* 1981; **162:** 243–263.
95. Wegner CD, Gundel RH, Reilly P, Haynes N, Letts GL, Rothlein R. Intercellular adhesion molecule 1 (ICAM-1) in the pathogenesis of asthma. *Science* 1990; **247:** 456–459.
96. Campbell HD, Tucker WQJ, Hort Y *et al.* Molecular cloning, nucleotide sequence and expression of the gene encoding human eosinophil differentiation factor interleukin-5. *Proc Natl Acad Sci USA* 1987; **84:** 6629–6633.
97. Rothenberg ME, Owen WF, Silberstein DS, Soberman RJ, Austen KF, Stevens RL. Eosinophils cocultured with endothelial cells have increased survival and functional properties. *Science* 1987; **237:** 645–647.
98. Rothenberg ME, Petersen J, Stevens RL *et al.* IL-5 dependent conversion of normodense human eosinophils to the hypodende phenotype uses 3T3 fibroblasts for enhanced viability, accelerated hypodensity and sustained antibody-dependent cytotoxicity. *J Immunol* 1989; **143:** 2311–2316.
99. Wang JM, Rambaldi A, Biondi A, Chen ZG, Sanderson CJ, Mantovani A. Recombinant human interleukin-5 is a selective eosinophil chemoattractant. *Eur J Immunol* 1989; **19:** 701–705.
100. Lopez AF, Sanderson CJ, Gamble JR, Campbell HD, Young IG, Vadas MA. Recombinant human interleukin-5 is a selective activator of eosinophil function. *J Exp Med* 1988; **167:** 219–224.
101. Rothenberg ME, Owen WF, Silberstein DS *et al.* Human eosinophils have prolonged survival, enhanced functional properties and become hypodense when exposed to human interleukin-3. *J Clin Invest* 1988; **81:** 1986–1992.
102. Silberstein DS, Owen WF, Gasson JC *et al.* Enhancement of human eosinophil cytotoxicity and leukotriene synthesis by biosynthetic (recombinant) granulocyte-macrophage colony stimulating factor. *J Immunol* 1986; **137:** 3290–3294.
103. Lopez AF, Williamson DJ, Gamble JR *et al.* Recombinant human granulocyte-macrophage colony stimulating factor stimulates *in vitro* mature human eosinophil and neutrophil function, surface receptor expression and survival. *J Clin Invest* 1986; **78:** 1220–1228.
104. Valerius T, Repp R, Kalden JR, Platzer E. Effects of IFN on human eosinophils in comparison with other cytokines. *J Immunol* 1990; **145:** 2950–2958.
105. Raghavachar A, Fleischer S, Frickhofen N, Heimpel H, Fleischer B. T-lymphocyte control of human eosinophilic granulopoiesis. *J Immunol* 1987; **139:** 3753–3758.
106. Walker C, Virchow J-C, Bruijnzeel PLB, Blaser K. T cell subsets and their soluble products regulate eosinophilia in allergic and nonallergic asthma. *J Immunol* 1991; **146:** 1829–1835.
107. Stevens RL, Austen KF. Recent advances in the cellular and molecular biology of mast cells. *Immunol Today* 1989; **10:** 381–386.
108. Irani AA, Craig SS, De Blois G, Elson CO, Schechter NM, Schwartz LB. Deficiency of tryptase-positive, chymase-negative mast cell type in gastrointestinal mucosa of patients with defective T-lymphocyte function. *J Immunol* 1987; **138:** 4381–4386.
109. Abe T, Nawa Y. Worm expulsion and mucosal mast cell response induced by repetitive IL-3 administration in *Strongyloides ratti* infected nude mice. *Immunology* 1988; **63:** 181–185.
110. Sieff CA. Haematopoietic growth factors. *J Clin Invest* 1987; **79:** 1549–1557.
111. Romagnani S, Maggi E, Del Prete GF, Ricci M. Activation through CD3 molecule leads a number of human T-cell clones from allergic and non-allergic individulas to promote IgE synthesis. *J Immunol* 1987; **138:** 1744–1749.

112. Del Prete GF, Maggi E, Parronchi P *et al.* IL-4 is an essential factor for the IgE synthesis induced *in vitro* by human T-cell clones and their supernatants. *J Immunol* 1988; **140:** 4193–4198.
113. Maggi E, Del Prete GF, Macchia D *et al.* Profile of lymphokine activities and helper function for IgE in human T-cell clones. *Eur J Immunol* 1988; 18: 1045–1050.
114. Parronchi P, Tiri A, Macchia D *et al.* Noncognate contact-dependent B-cell activation can promote IL-4 dependent *in vitro* human IgE synthesis. *J Immunol* 1990; **144:** 2102–2108.
115. De Kruyff RH, Turner T, Abrams JS, Palladino MA, Umetsu DT. Induction of human IgE synthesis by CD4+ T-cell clones. Requirement for interleukin-4 and low molecular weight B-cell growth factor. *J Exp Med* 1989; **170:** 1477–1493.
116. Cookson WOCM, Hopkin JM. Dominant inheritance of atopic IgE responsiveness. *Lancet* 1988; **i:** 86–88.
117. Cookson WOCM, Sharp PA, Faux JA, Hopkin JM. Linkage between IgE responses underlying asthma and rhinitis and chromosome 11q. *Lancet* 1989; **i:** 1292–1295.
118. Romagnani S, Del Prete G, Maggi E *et al.* Role of interleukins in induction and regulation of human IgE synthesis. *Clin Immunol Immunopathol* 1989; **50:** 513–518.
119. Quint DJ, Bolton EJ, MacNamee LA *et al.* Functional and phenotypical analysis of human T-cell clones which stimulate IgE production *in vitro*. *Immunology* 1989; **67:** 68–74.
120. Wierenga EA, Snoek M, de Groot C *et al.* Evidence for compartmentalisation of functional subsets of CD4+ T-lymphocytes in atopic patients. *J Immunol* 1990; **144:** 4651–4656.
121. Mosmann TR, Coffman RL. Th1 and Th2 cells: different patterns of lymphokine secretion lead to different functional properties. *Annu Rev Immunol* 1989; **7:** 145–173.
122. Gajewski TF, Joyce J, Fitch FW. Antiproliferative effect of interferon-γ in immune regulation. III. Differential selection of Th1 and Th2 murine helper T-lymphocyte clones using recombinant IL-2 and recombinant interferon-γ. *J Immunol* 1989; **143:** 15–20.
123. Fiorentino D, Bond HW, Mosmann TR. Two types of mouse T helper cells. IV. Th2 clones secrete a factor that inhibits cytokine production by Th1 clones. *J Exp Med* 1989; **170:** 65–80.
124. Fiorentino DF, Zlotnik A, Vieira P *et al.* IL-10 acts on the antigen-presenting cell to inhibit cytokine production by Th1 cells. *J Immunol* 1991; **146:** 3444–3451.
125. Stevens TL, Bossie A, Sanders VM *et al.* Subsets of antigen-specific helper T-cells regulate isotype secretion by antigen-specific B-cells. *Nature* 1988; **334:** 255–258.
126. Coffman RL, Seymour BW, Lebman DA *et al.* The role of helper T-cell products in mouse B-cell differentiation and isotype regulation. *Immunol Rev* 1988; **102:** 5–28.
127. Reynolds DS, Boom WH, Abbas AK. Inhibition of B-lymphocyte activation by interferon-γ. *J Immunol* 1987; **139:** 767–773.
128. Cher DJ, Mosmann TR. Two types of murine helper T-cell clone. II. Delayed-type hypersensitivity is mediated by Th1 clones. *J Immunol* 1987; **138:** 3688–3694.
129. Paliard X, de Waal Malefijt R, Yssel H *et al.* Simultaneous production of IL-2, IL-4 and IFN-γ by activated human CD4+ and CD8+ T-cell clones. *J Immunol* 1988; **141:** 849–855.
130. Corrigan CJ, Hartnell A, Kay AB. T-lymphocyte activation in acute severe asthma. *Lancet* 1988; **i:** 1129–1131.
131. Corrigan CJ, Kay AB. CD4 T-lymphocyte activation in acute severe asthma. Relationship to disease severity and atopic status. *Am Rev Respir Dis* 1990; **141:** 970–977.
132. Graham DR, Luksza AR, Evans CC. Bronchoalveolar lavage in asthma. *Thorax* 1985; **40:** 717.
133. Gerblich AA, Campbell AE, Schuyler MR. Changes in T-lymphocyte subpopulations after antigenic bronchial provocation in asthmatics. *N Engl J Med* 1984; **310:** 1349–1352.
134. Frew AJ, Kay AB. The relationship between infiltrating CD4+ T-lymphocytes, activated eosinophils and the magnitude of the allergen-induced late phase cutaneous reaction. *J Immunol* 1988; **141:** 4158–4164.
135. Hamid Q, Azzawi M, Ying S *et al.* Expression of mRNA for interleukin-5 in mucosal bronchial biopsies from asthma. *J Clin Invest* 1991; **87:** 1541–1546.
136. Kay AB, Ying S, Varney V *et al.* Messenger RNA expression of the cytokine gene cluster IL-3, IL-4, IL-5 and GM-CSF in allergen-induced late phase cutaneous reactions in atopic subjects. *J Exp Med* 1991; **173:** 775–778.
137. Gaga M, Frew AJ, Varney VA, Kay AB. Eosinophil activation and T-lymphocyte infiltration in allergen-induced late phase skin reactions and classical delayed-type hypersensitivity. *J Immunol* 1991; **147:** 816–822.
138. Henson PM, Johnston RB. Tissue injury in inflammation: oxidants, proteinases and cationic proteins. *J Clin Invest* 1987; **79:** 669–674.
139. Papageorgiou N, Carroll M, Durham SR, Lee TH, Walsh GM, Kay AB. Complement receptor enhancement as evidence of neutrophil activation after exercise-induced asthma. *Lancet* 1983; **ii:** 1220–1223.

140. Moqbel R, Durham SR, Shaw RJ *et al*. Enhancement of leukocyte cytotoxicity after exercise-induced asthma. *Am Rev Respir Dis* 1986; **133:** 609–613.
141. Carroll M, Durham SR, Walsh GM, Kay AB. Activation of neutrophils and monocytes after allergen- and histamine-induced bronchoconstriction. *J Allergy Clin Immunol* 1985; **75:** 290–296.
142. Durham SR, Carroll M, Walsh GM, Kay AB. Leukocyte activation in allergen-induced late-phase asthmatic reactions. *N Engl J Med* 1984; **311:** 1398–1402.
143. Boschetto P, Fabbri LM, Zocca E *et al*. Prednisone inhibits late asthmatic reactions and airway inflammation induced by toluene diisocyanate in sensitized subjects. *J Allergy Clin Immunol* 1987; **80:** 261–267.
144. Atkins PC, Norman M, Weiner H, Zweiman B. Release of neutrophil chemotactic activity during immediate hypersensitivity reactions in humans. *Ann Intern Med* 1977; **86:** 415–418.
145. Nagy L, Lee TH, Kay AB. Neutrophil chemotactic activity in antigen-induced late asthmatic reactions. *N Engl J Med* 1982; **306:** 497–501.
146. Lee TH, Nagy L, Nagakura T, Walport MJ, Kay AB. The identification and partial characterisation of an exercise-induced neutrophil chemotactic factor in bronchial asthma. *J Clin Invest* 1982; **69:** 889–899.
147. Lee TH, Nagakura T, Papageorgiou N, Iikura Y, Kay AB. Exercise-induced late asthmatic reactions with neutrophil chemotactic activity. *N Engl J Med* 1983; **308:** 1502–1505.
148. Buchanan DR, Cromwell O, Kay AB. Neutrophil chemotactic activity in acute severe asthma ('status asthmaticus'). *Am Rev Respir Dis* 1987; **136:** 1397–1402.
149. Corrigan CJ, Collard P, Nagy L, Kay AB. Cultured peripheral blood mononuclear cells derived from patients with acute severe asthma ('status asthmaticus') spontaneously elaborate a neutrophil chemotactic activity distinct from interleukin-8. *Am Rev Respir Dis* 1991; **143:** 538–544.
150. Yoshimura T, Matsushima K, Tanaka S *et al*. Purification of a human monocyte-derived neutrophil chemotactic factor that has peptide sequence similarity to other host defense cytokines. *Proc Natl Acad Sci USA* 1987; **84:** 9233–9237.
151. Gregory H, Young J, Schroder J-M, Mrowietz U, Christophers E. Structure determination of a human lymphocyte derived neutrophil activating peptide LYNAP. *Biochem Biophys Res Commun* 1988; **151:** 883–890.
152. Maestrelli P, O'Hehir RE, Lamb JR, Tsai J-J, Cromwell O, Kay AB. Antigen-induced neutrophil chemotactic factor from cloned human T lymphocytes. *Immunology* 1988; **65:** 605–609.
153. Maestrelli P, Tsai J-J, Cromwell O, Kay AB. The identification and partial characterization of a human mononuclear cell-derived neutrophil chemotactic factor apparently distinct from IL-1, IL-2, GM-CSF, TNF and IFN-gamma. *Immunology* 1988; **64:** 219–225.
154. Walz A, Dewald B, von Tscharner V, Baggiolini M. Effects of the neutrophil activating peptide NAP-2, platelet basic protein, connective tissue activating peptide III and platelet factor 4 on human neutrophils. *J Exp Med* 1989; **170:** 1745–1750.
155. Lee L-Y, Bleecker ER, Nadel JA. Effect of ozone on bronchomotor response to inhaled histamine aerosol in dogs. *J Appl Physiol* 1977; **43:** 626–631.
156. Chung KF, Becker AB, Lazarus SC, Frick OL, Nadel JA, Gold WM. Antigen-induced airway hyperresponsiveness and pulmonary inflammation in allergic dogs. *J Appl Physiol* 1985; **558:** 1347–1353.
157. Murphy KR, Wilson MC, Irvin CG *et al*. The requirement for polymorphonuclear leukocytes on the late asthmatic response and heightened airways reactivity in an animal model. *Am Rev Respir Dis* 1986; **134:** 62–68.
158. Holtzman MJ, Fabbri LM, O'Byrne PH *et al*. Importance of airway inflammation for hyperresponsiveness induced by ozone in dogs. *Am Rev Respir Dis* 1983; **127:** 686–690.
159. O'Byrne PH, Walters EH, Gold BD *et al*. Neutrophil depletion inhibits airway hyperresponsiveness induced by ozone exposure. *Am Rev Respir Dis* 1984; **130:** 214–219.
160. Marsh WR, Irvin CG, Murphy KR, Behrens BL, Larsen GL. Increases in airway reactivity to histamine and inflammatory cells in bronchoalveolar lavage after the late asthmatic response in an animal model. *Am Rev Respir Dis* 1985; **131:** 875–879.
161. Hutchinson AA, Hinson JM, Brigham KL, Snapper JR. Effect of endotoxin on airway responsiveness to aerosol histamine in sheep. *J Appl Physiol* 1983; **54:** 1463–1468.
162. Hinson JM, Hutchinson AA, Brigham KL, Meyrick BO, Snapper JR. Effect of granulocyte depletion on pulmonary responsiveness to aerosol histamine. *J Appl Physiol* 1984; **56:** 411–417.
163. Abraham WM, Perruchoud AP, Sielczak MW, Yerger LD, Stevenson JS. Airway inflammation during antigen-induced late bronchial obstruction. *Prog Respir Res* 1985; **19:** 48–88.
164. Irvin CG, Berend N, Henson PM. Airways hyperreactivity and inflammation produced by aerosolization of human C5a des Arg. *Am Rev Respir Dis* 1986; **134:** 777–783.
165. Hutson PA, Church MK, Clay TP, Miller P, Holgate ST. Early and late phase bronchoconstriction after allergen challenge of nonanesthetised guinea pigs. 1. The association of disordered airway

physiology to leukocyte infiltration. *Am Rev Respir Dis* 1988; **137:** 548–557.
166. Diaz P, Galleguillos FR, Gonzalez MC, Pantin C, Kay AB. Bronchoalveolar lavage in asthma: the effect of DSCG on leukocyte counts, immunoglobulins and complement. *J Allergy Clin Immunol* 1984; **74:** 41–48.
167. Martin RJ, Cicutto LC, Ballard RD, Szefler SJ. Airway inflammation in nocturnal asthma. *Am Rev Respir Dis* 1988; **137:** 284.
168. Otsuka H, Denburg J, Dolovich H *et al.* Heterogeneity of metachromatic cells in human nose: significance of mucosal mast cells. *J Allergy Clin Immunol* 1985; **76:** 695–702.
169. Okuda M, Sakaguchi Y, Suzuhi F, Ohtsuka H, Kawabori S. Ultrastructural heterogeneity of the basophilic cells in the allergic nasal mucosa. *Ann Allergy* 1985; **54:** 152–157.
170. Shanahan F, MacNiven I, Dyck N, Denburg J, Bienenstock J, Befus AD. Human lung mast cells: distribution and abundance of histochemically distinct subpopulations. *Int Arch Allergy Appl Immunol* 1987; **83:** 329–331.
171. Flint KC, Leung KBP, Pearce FL, Hudspith BN, Brostoff J, Johnson NM. Human mast cells recovered by bronchoalveolar lavage: their morphology, histamine release and the effects of sodium cromoglycate. *Clin Sci* 1985; **68:** 427–432.
172. Irani AA, Schechter NM, Craig SS, DeBlois G, Schwartz LB. Two types of human mast cells that have distinct neutral protease compositions. *Proc Natl Acad Sci USA* 1986; **83:** 4464–4468.
173. Schwartz LB, Irani AA, Roller K, Castells MC, Schechter NM. Quantitation of histamine, tryptase and chymase in dispersed human T and TC mast cells. *J Immunol* 1988; **139:** 2724–2729.
174. Peters SP, MacGlashan DW, Schulman ES *et al.* Arachidonic acid metabolism in purified human lung mast cells. *J Immunol* 1984; **131:** 1972–1979.
175. Lawrence ID, Warner JA, Cohan VL, Hubbard WC, Kagey-Sobotka A, Lichtenstein LM. Purification and characterization of human skin mast cells. Evidence for human mast cell heterogeneity. *J Immunol* 1987; **139:** 3062–3069.
176. Pearce CA, Greaves MW, Plummer VM, Yamamoto ES. Effect of disodium cromoglycate on antigen-evoked histamine release from human skin. *Clin Exp Immunol* 1974; **17:** 437–440.
177. Flint KC, Leung KBP, Hudspith BN, Brostoff J, Pearce FL, Johnson NMcI. Bronchoalveolar mast cells in extrinsic asthma: a mechanism for the initiation of allergen-specific bronchoconstriction. *BMJ* 1985; **291:** 923–926.
178. Wardlaw AJ, Cromwell O, Celestino D *et al.* Morphological and secretory properties of bronchoalveolar lavage mast cells in respiratory diseases. *Clin Allergy* 1986; **16:** 163–173.
179. Casale TB, Wood D, Richerson HB *et al.* Elevated bronchoalveolar lavage fluid histamine levels in allergic asthmatics are associated with methacholine bronchial hyperreactivity. *J Clin Invest* 1987; **79:** 1197–1203.
180. Howarth PH, Durham SR, Lee TH, Kay AB, Church MK, Holgate ST. Influence of albuterol, cromolyn sodium and ipratropium bromide on the airway and circulating mediator responses to allergen bronchial provocation in asthma. *Am Rev Respir Dis* 1985; **132:** 986–992.
181. Murray JJ, Tonnel AB, Brash AR *et al.* Release of prostaglandin D_2 into human airways during acute antigen challenge. *N Engl J Med* 1986; **315:** 800–804.
182. Holgate ST, Emanuel MB, Howarth PH. Astemizole and other H_1 antihistamine drug treatment of asthma. *J Allergy Clin Immunol* 1985; **76:** 375–382.
183. Beasley R, Varley J, Robinson C, Holgate ST. Cholinergic-mediated bronchoconstriction induced by prostaglandin D_2, its initial metabolite 9A,11β-prostaglandin F_2 and prostaglandin $F_{2\alpha}$ in asthma. *Am Rev Respir Dis* 1987; **136:** 1140–1144.
184. Baeza ML, Reddigari SR, Haak-Frendscho M, Kaplan AP. Purification and further characterisation of human mononuclear cell histamine releasing factor. *J Clin Invest* 1989; **83:** 1204–1212.
185. Lee TH, Assoufi BK, Kay AB. The link between exercise, respiratory heat exchange and the mast cell in bronchial asthma. *Lancet* 1983; **i:** 520–522.
186. Naclerio RM, Proud D, Togias AG *et al.* Inflammatory mediators in late antigen-induced rhinitis. *N Engl J Med* 1985; **313:** 65–79.
187. Shalit M, Schwartz LB, von Allmen BA *et al. In vivo* histamine and tryptase release during continuous and interrupted allergen challenge. *J Allergy Clin Immunol* 1988; **81:** 297–302.
188. Wodnar-Filipowicz A, Heusser CH, Moroni C. Production of the haemopoietic growth factors GM-CSF and interleukin-3 by mast cells in response to IgE receptor mediated activation. *Nature* 1989; **339:** 150–152.
189. Burd PR, Rogers HW, Gordon JR *et al.* Interleukin-3 dependent and independent mast cells stimulated with IgE and antigen express multiple cytokines. *J Exp Med* 1989; **170:** 245–257.
190. Holt PG, Schon-Hegrad MA, Oliver JJ. MHC class II antigen-bearing dendritic cells in pulmonary tissues of the rat: regulation of antigen presentation activity by endogenous macrophage populations. *J Exp Med* 1988; **167:** 262–274.

191. Holt PG, Schon-Hegrad MA, Phillips MJ, McMenamin PG. Ia-positive dendritic cells form a tightly meshed network within the human airway epithelium. *Clin Exp Allergy* 1989; **19:** 597–601.
192. Fokkens WJ, Vroom TM, Rijntjes E, Mulder PGH. CD-1 T6 HLA-DR expressing cells presumably Langerhans cells in nasal mucosa. *Allergy* 1989; **44:** 167–172.
193. Melewicz FM, Zeiger RS, Mellon MH, O'Connor RD, Spiegelberg HL. Increased IgE-dependent cytotoxicity by blood mononuclear cells of allergic patients. *Clin Exp Immunol* 1981; **43:** 526–533.
194. Joseph M, Tonnel AB, Torpier G, Capron A, Arnoux B, Benveniste J. Involvement of IgE in the secretory processes of alveolar macrophages from asthmatic patients. *J Clin Invest* 1983; **71:** 221–230.
195. Capron M, Jouault T, Prin L *et al.* Functional study of a monoclonal antibody to IgE Fc receptor (FcγRII) of eosinophils, platelets and macrophages. *J Exp Med* 1986; **164:** 72–89.
196. Holgate ST, Burns GB, Robinson C, Church MK. Anaphylactic- and calcium-dependent generation of prostaglandin D_2 (PGD_2), thromboxane B_2 and other cyclooxygenase products of arachidonic acid by dispersed human lung cells and relationship to histamine release. *J Immunol* 1984; **153:** 2138–2144.
197. Fuller RW, Morris PK, Richmond R *et al.* Immunoglobulin E-dependent stimulation of human alveolar macrophages: significance in type I hypersensitivity. *Clin Exp Immunol* 1986; **65:** 416–426.
198. Godard P, Chantreuil J, Damon M *et al.* Functional assessment of alveolar macrophages: comparison of cells from asthmatic and normal subjects. *J Allergy Clin Immunol* 1982; **70:** 88–95.
199. Arnoux B, Duval D, Benveniste J. Release of platelet activating factor PAF-acether from alveolar macrophages by the calcium ionophore A23187 and phagocytosis. *Eur J Clin Invest* 1980; **10:** 437–441.
200. MacDermot J, Kelsey CR, Waddell KA *et al.* Synthesis of leukotriene B4 and prostanoids by human alveolar macrophages: analysis by gas chromatography/mass spectrometry. *Prostaglandins* 1984; **27:** 163–179.
201. Tonnel AB, Joseph M, Gosset P, Fournier E, Capron A. Stimulation of alveolar macrophages in asthmatic patients after local provocation test. *Lancet* 1983; **i:** 1406–1408.
202. Mazingue C, Carriere V, Dessaint J-P *et al.* Regulation of IgE synthesis by macrophages expressing Fc epsilon receptors: role of interleukin-1. *Clin Exp Immunol* 1987; **67:** 587–593.
203. Haslett C, Henson PM. Resolution of inflammation. In: *The Molecular and Cellular Biology of Wound Repair.* Clark RAF, Henson PM eds. New York: Plenum, 1988; 185–211.
204. Boulet L-P, Cartier A, Thomson NC, Roberts RS, Dolovich J, Hargreave FE. Asthma and increases in nonallergic bronchial responsiveness from seasonal allergen exposure. *J Allergy Clin Immunol* 1983; **71:** 399–406.
205. Platts-Mills TAE, Chapman MD. Dust mites: immunology, allergic disease and environmental control. *J Allergy Clin Immunol* 1987; **80:** 755–775.
206. Platts-Mills TAE, Tovey ER, Mitchell EB, Moszoro H, Nock P, Wilkins SR. Reduction of bronchial hyperreactivity during prolonged allergen avoidance. *Lancet* 1982; **ii:** 675–677.
207. Schleimer RP. Effects of glucocorticosteroids on inflammatory cells relevant to their therapeutic applications in asthma. *Am Rev Respir Dis* 1990; **141:** S59–S69.
208. Burrows B, Martinez FD, Halonen M, Barbee RA, Cline MG. Association of asthma with serum IgE levels and skin-test reactivity to allergens. *N Engl J Med* 1989; **320:** 271–277.

2

Inflammatory mechanisms in asthma

K.F. Chung

Chronic inflammation in asthma

Recent studies of the bronchial mucosa of patients with mild asthma have firmly established asthma as a *chronic inflammatory disease* characterized by an airway submucosal infiltration of lymphocytes and eosinophils, epithelial shedding, subepithelial reticular fibrosis and oedema (Figure 2.1) [1–3]. The relationship between an acute inflammatory insult to the airways such as that induced by exposure to high ambient levels of ozone or to allergen in a sensitized animal and the induction of bronchial hyperresponsiveness has been the subject of earlier attention [4–6]. In some animal models, there was evidence for an involvement of inflammatory mechanisms in the induction of bronchial hyperresponsiveness [7]. However, the inflammatory process in asthma is of a chronic nature and without appropriate models of chronic airway inflammation, it has not been possible to

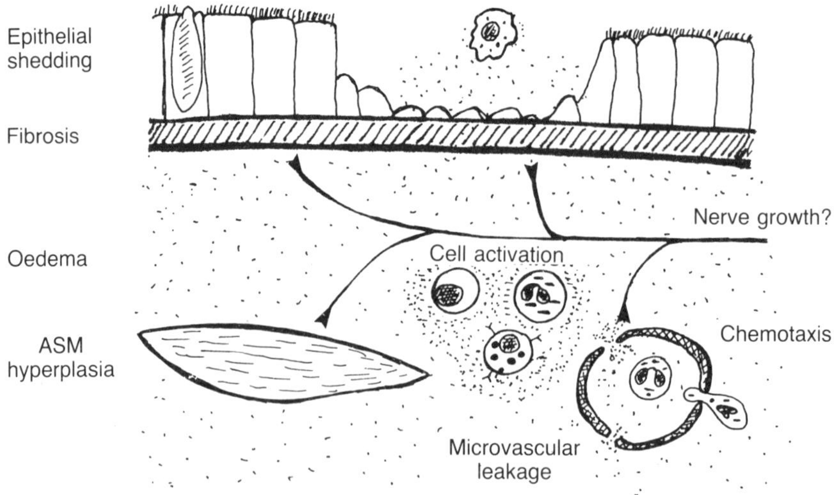

Figure 2.1 Schematic representation of the chronic inflammatory abnormalities found in the airway submucosa of patients with asthma. Inflammatory cells represented include lymphocytes, eosinophils and macrophages. ASM: Airway smooth muscle

study the potential of various chronic inflammatory mechanisms to contribute to the reversible airways obstruction and bronchial hyperresponsiveness characteristic of asthma.

From a clinical point of view, the contribution of inflammatory mechanisms to various stages of asthma remains to be defined. There appears to be an asymptomatic period of variable duration, the establishment of an 'allergic' state with bronchial hyperresponsiveness, followed by symptoms leading to the diagnosis of 'asthma' (Figure 2.2). Symptoms may disappear by adolescence in a significant proportion of asthmatic subjects, but bronchial hyperresponsiveness persists and symptoms may re-appear later in life [8]. Ongoing symptoms may indicate persistent, chronic and active inflammatory mechanisms that do not resolve and establish fibrosis, which may lead to chronic airways obstruction. Such a variable natural history coupled with a wide spectrum of clinical severity raises the question of heterogeneity of inflammatory mechanisms at various stages of the disease and for different types of presentation and evolutionary stages.

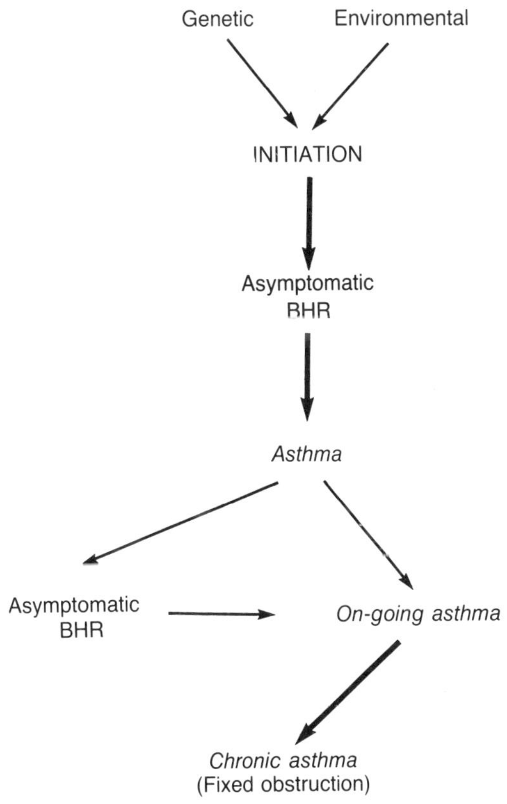

Figure 2.2 Natural history of asthma. Genetic and environmental factors may be important in the presymptomatic phase in switching on chronic inflammatory mechanisms and perhaps bronchial hyperresponsiveness. What underlies the onset of symptoms and the disappearance of symptoms in a subgroup of asthmatics is not clear. Ongoing symptoms and inflammation may indicate lack of resolution with progression to fibrosis

The important questions about the chronic inflammation of asthma may be listed as follows:

1. Why are asthmatics prone to developing this specific type of airway inflammation?
2. What factors trigger this inflammatory process?
3. What are the important mechanisms by which this inflammation perpetuates itself into chronicity?
4. How do chronic inflammatory mechanisms relate or lead to reversible airways obstruction and bronchial hyperresponsiveness, the physiological hallmarks of asthma?
5. Finally, how do drugs used to treat asthma modify chronic inflammation? This last area remains under-investigated because currently established drugs used to treat asthma were introduced into clinical practice well before the realization that inflammatory mechanisms are an important component of asthma.

Many of these important questions remain unanswered. In this chapter, several aspects of inflammatory mechanisms will be reviewed.

Initiating mechanisms

Asthma is very often associated with atopy as assessed by the presence of positive skin-prick tests, concomitant eczema and allergic rhinitis [9]. Some children and adults show none of these features, and these asthmatics are considered to have non-allergic or intrinsic asthma. The validity of this classification is now in doubt because the clinical course and pathologies of both types are similar. A recent study showed that the prevalence of asthma was closely related to serum IgE levels that have been standardized according to age and sex, even in the elderly population with negative skin-prick tests [10]. Those with low levels of IgE did not report any asthma but up to 28% of those with very high IgE levels did. A probable allergic basis for all asthma was proposed, including those patients with negative skin-prick tests. Even in children who have been asymptomatic throughout their lives and who have had no history of atopic diseases, airway hyperresponsiveness appears to be closely related to an allergic predisposition, as measured by total serum IgE levels [11].

Other factors, such as upper respiratory tract viral infections and environmental pollutants, may increase the production of specific IgE. An increased frequency of cell-bound IgE has been found in children with bronchiolitis or asthma following the onset of respiratory syncytial virus respiratory illness [12]. How virus-specific IgE contributes to asthma pathogenesis is not clear. Once increased production of serum IgE occurs, repeated prolonged exposures to common allergens such as house dust mite may increase the predisposition for development of asthma [13].

The regulation of IgE is controlled tightly by T lymphocytes. The production of interleukin-4 (IL-4) by T cells represents a crucial signal for B cells to switch towards IgE synthesis [14, 15]. Other cytokines such as IFN-γ, TGF-β and PGE_2 can inhibit IL-4 dependent IgE synthesis [14–16]. The mechanisms for the increased production of IgE in atopic subjects may involve an imbalance in T-cell subsets responsible for IL-4 secretion (a subset defined as the TH2 subset of lymphocytes) and IFN-γ (TH1 lymphocytes) secretion, with a predominance of lymphocytes able to secrete IL-4 [17]. The conditions that favour the expansion of TH2-type clones are not clear, but may involve interactions between dendritic cells of the respiratory mucosa, T cells and allergenic peptides, leading to maturation of various T-cell subsets. Once a TH2-subset of lymphocytes is activated, it preferentially expands with an increased cooperation between T and B cells leading to an IgE antibody response [18]. The susceptibility of particular individuals to develop the atopic status is probably under genetic control [19, 20] and the mechanisms by which these genes are switched on are not clear. It may be that chronic exposure to a particular allergen represents an important initialling step.

The acquisition of the allergic state may represent an important initiating step to the development of the airway inflammation characteristic of asthma. Many cell types within the airways of an allergic subject bear receptors for IgE – particularly mast cells, monocytes/macrophages and (probably) eosinophils – and may respond to specific stimuli such as allergen or to non-specific stimuli such as environmental pollutants and physical stimuli. These cells also appear to be primed and may release in addition to the lymphocyte an array of mediators and cytokines which amplify and maintain complex cellular and molecular interactions characteristic of asthma.

Cytokines in asthma

Cytokines include a group of polypeptide growth factors and differentiation factors (lymphokines and monokines), and glycoproteins such as the interleukins, which are important for interaction and coordination between cells in immune and inflammatory responses [21]. Most cytokines are pleiotropic and have multiple biological actions, and may act as a regulatory network between lymphoid cells, haematopoietic cells and endothelial cells. A single cytokine may act as a positive or negative signal, depending on the type of the target cells.

There is increasing evidence that cytokines are involved in the chronic airways inflammation of asthma and may play an important role in its perpetuation (Figure 2.3). Increased expression of particular cytokine proteins or their mRNA has been demonstrated in asthmatic airways and in experimental allergic models. Exposure of sensitized rat and human lung to allergen results in the expression of tumour necrosis factor-α (TNFα) in epithelial cells and macrophages [22, 23], suggesting that IgE-mediated mechanisms lead to increased synthesis of this cytokine. Airway epithelial cells express IL-8 [24] and granulocyte/macrophage colony-stimulating factor (GM-CSF) [25], with increased expression in asthmatic patients and after exposure to IL-1 [26]. Bronchial biopsies of asthmatic patients have shown increased gene expression of IL-3, IL-4 and IL-5, presumably in T lymphocytes [27]. Macrophages from asthmatic patients show an increased release of IL-1β [28], and both lymphocytes and alveolar macrophages from asthmatic patients

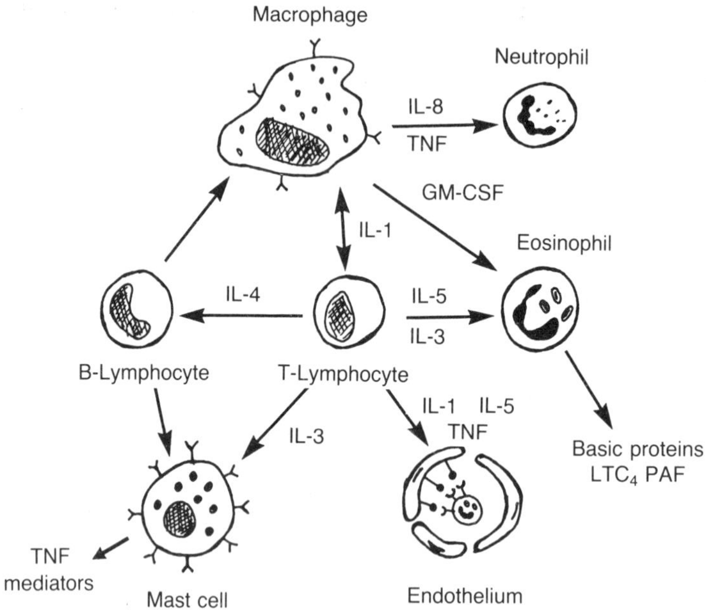

Figure 2.3 Potential role of cytokines in asthma. Cytokines are pleiotropic, have multiple biological actions and may act as a regulatory network between lymphocytes, eosinophils, neutrophils, macrophages, mast cells and endothelial cells. As such, they may play an important role in the initiation and modulation of inflammatory mechanism in asthma. IL: interleukin; GM-CSF: granulocyte/macrophage colony-stimulating factor; TNF: tumour necrosis factor

demonstrate an augmented expression of GM-CSF following allergen challenge [29]. Increased amounts of IL-1, IL-6 and GM-CSF have been measured in bronchoalveolar fluid of patients with symptomatic asthma [30], and the source of these cytokines appears to be epithelial cells and macrophages. Cytokines can generate other cytokines and therefore they can interact in a complex network: for example, IL-1 can stimulate GM-CSF synthesis in cultured airway epithelial cells [26] and TNFα increases IL-8 gene expression in human epithelial cells [24].

The contribution of these cytokines to the inflammatory process of asthma is not clear and availability of specific inhibitors or antagonists of these cytokines will help to define their role. Some cytokines appear to be important in the differentiation and survival of particular inflammatory cells: IL-3, IL-5 and GM-CSF act on eosinophil precursors to cause eosinophil differentiation [31, 32] and in addition may activate mature eosinophils and transform them into hypodense fractions, while increasing their survival *in vitro* [33, 34]. Factors identified as consisting of IL-5 and GM-CSF activities in sera of patients with asthma can prolong eosinophil survival [35]. These cytokines can also prime eosinophils such as to increase the release of granule-associated proteins such as eosinophil-derived neurotoxin (EDN) and eosinophil cationic protein (ECP) from stimulated eosinophils [36, 37]. GM-CSF can also enhance the production of leukotrienes from eosinophils [38, 39]. However, other cytokines (such as IL-4) can suppress IgG-mediated degranulation and antibody-dependent cytotoxicity of eosinophils [40].

Although the cytokine IL-2 has not yet been localized in the airways of patients with asthma, it is interesting that recombinant human (rh) IL-2 causes an increase in airway responsiveness in rats, associated with increased numbers of lymphocytes and eosinophils in bronchoalveolar lavage fluid [41]. IL-2 also is one of the most potent chemotactic agents for human eosinophils *in vitro* [42]: infusion of IL-2 in humans induces hypodense eosinophils in the circulation [43]. While rhGM-CSF and rhIL-5 can induce eosinophil accumulation in the lungs of guinea-pigs, they do not cause any increase in bronchial responsiveness [44].

Asthma is characterized by chronic structural changes in the airways such as airway smooth muscle hyperplasia and subepithelial fibrosis [45], which could result from the actions of cytokines or growth factors released from inflammatory cells in the airways. An increase in substance P-immunoreactive nerve profiles has also been reported in asthmatic airways [46]. It is possible that cytokines or nerve growth factors may be important in initiating this chronic change. We are only starting to unravel the complex interacting network of cytokines and growth factors in asthma.

Inflammatory mechanisms related to bronchial hyperresponsiveness and asthma symptoms

Bronchoalveolar lavage and bronchial biopsies

Many mechanisms have been suggested for bronchial hyperresponsiveness in asthma, including an imbalance of autonomic control of the airways, airway inflammatory changes and altered airways geometry [7, 47, 48]. The evidence that bronchial hyperresponsiveness can be provoked in animals in temporal association with airway inflammation has served as an impetus to investigate the inflammatory changes in the airways of patients with asthma. These studies have been made possible by the safe use of fibreoptic bronchoscopy in retrieving bronchoalveolar lavage fluid (BAL fluid) and bronchial mucosal biopsies from proximal airways. Several studies have reported significant increases in eosinophil, mast cell and epithelial cell counts in bronchoalveolar lavage fluid obtained from patients with asthma compared with normal control subjects [49, 50] with elevated concentrations of several mediators such as histamine and prostaglandin D_2 [49, 51]. Increased kallikrein activity has also been detected, which may lead to increased generation of bradykinin within the airways [52]. Cells recovered by lavage also demonstrate increased releasability of mediators such as the spontaneous release of histamine from mast cells and the generation of reactive oxygen metabolites from activated alveolar macrophages *ex vivo* [53, 54]. Significant inverse correlations have been observed between bronchial responsiveness to inhaled histamine and bronchoalveolar eosinophil and epithelial cell counts, and the concentration of major basic protein and histamine in lavage fluid [49, 50].

Bronchial biopsies obtained from patients with extrinsic asthma have been compared with those from healthy control subjects. Biopsies obtained via the rigid bronchoscope showed epithelial damage as a characteristic feature of asthma [1]. Thickening of the subepithelial basement membrane zone has been observed even in patients with mild disease and recently has been attributed to a subepithelial fibrotic process [45]. Immunostaining using the monoclonal antibody EG2 which specifically stains the cleaved, secreted form of eosinophil cationic protein has identified increased numbers of 'activated' eosinophils, within both the submucosal [3, 55] and the epithelial mucosal layers [3]. The numbers of activated eosinophils in the airways correlated significantly with asthma severity, as judged by a clinical score [3] and by the level of bronchial responsiveness to methacholine [56]. Mast cell numbers in the bronchial submucosa, as judged by conventional histology using a chloroacetate esterase stain were found to be increased in asthma [57], although this has not been confirmed by specific immunostaining for the mast cell granule proteins tryptase [58] and tryptase plus chymase [56]. Small increases in the T-lymphocyte numbers in the bronchial mucosa in asthma have been reported. A consistent increase in CD25+ (IL-2-receptor bearing) cells, probably representing 'activated' T lymphocytes in the bronchial submucosa of extrinsic asthmatics, has been shown; this was not present in allergic non-asthmatic subjects [55].

The observation of increased mRNA expression for the cytokine IL-5, a product of activated lymphocytes, was observed in asthmatic airways and this correlated with the number of EG2+ cells (representing activated eosinophils) determined by immunostaining [27]. This observation supports the hypothesis that the submucosal eosinophilia in asthma may be dependent on IL-5, which is known to increase eosinophil maturation. The precise source of IL-5 (T cells or mast cells) is yet to be determined. The specificity of these changes for asthma, compared with other bronchial diseases, and their modification following successful therapy have yet to be determined.

Sputum and blood constituents

Measurements performed in blood and sputum of asthmatic patients are, in general, representative of the findings in BAL fluid or in bronchial biopsies: for example, blood eosinophil counts are elevated in both extrinsic and intrinsic asthma, and eosinophil numbers correlate inversely with FEV_1, and with airway responsiveness to methacholine and histamine [59, 60]. Similarly, increases in bronchoalveolar eosinophils and eosinophil cationic proteins during allergen-induced late responses are mirrored by changes in blood eosinophils [19, 20, 60] and serum eosinophil cationic protein concentrations [61]. Acute severe asthma is accompanied by elevations in peripheral CD25+/CD4+ T-lymphocyte numbers as determined by flow cytometry [62]. CD25+ cell numbers were reduced following response to asthma therapy, with a time course that paralleled improvements in lung function [61]. Sputum cell counts are reproducible in the short term and consist of eosinophils and metachromatic cells [63]. Sputum eosinophilia and sputum and serum concentrations of eosinophil-derived major basic protein were increased in acute severe asthma and these levels decreased following successful treatment with corticosteroids [64]. Measurements in blood and sputum may provide information relevant to monitoring of day-to-day asthma and its response to treatment.

Experimental allergen exposure

In addition to spontaneous bronchial hyperresponsiveness occurring in patients with asthma, it may be provoked transiently under experimental conditions following exposure to allergens and to pollutants such as ozone. The increase in bronchial responsiveness occurs within a few hours of allergen exposure [19, 20, 59] usually preceding the onset of the late-phase response, and may last for several days [65]. Within minutes of exposure to allergen, release of histamine, several lipid mediators, such as thromboxane A_2, PGD_2 and the sulphidopeptide leukotrienes, have been demonstrated [49, 66, 67]. Within 2 h of allergen challenge, there is a significant increase in urinary leukotriene E_4 [68]. BAL fluid recovered following allergen provocation at the time of development of the late-phase response contains increased numbers of eosinophils and elevated concentrations of eosinophil cationic protein [69], both indices correlating with the size of the late-phase response as reflected in measurements of FEV_1. Increases in CD8+ T lymphocytes in BAL fluid were observed in asthmatic subjects who developed isolated early responses, as opposed to dual (early plus late) responses after allergen exposure [70]. In addition, CD4+ T lymphocyte numbers increased after allergen challenge [71], providing support for participation of T lymphocytes in the late-phase response. In asthmatic patients who developed histamine bronchial hyperresponsiveness after allergen challenge, an increase in circulating eosinophil, basophil and eosinophil/basophil progenitor cells has been observed [72], which may lead to the accumulation of eosinophils and basophils in the airway and contribute to airways inflammation in asthma. Local allergen challenge of the airways causes an influx of eosinophils and lymphocytes into bronchoalveolar lavage fluid, with release of GM-CSF. *In situ* hybridization reveals that lymphocytes mostly express GM-CSF mRNA following local allergen challenge [29].

Role of inflammatory cells

There is increasing evidence to support the general hypothesis that cells obtained from the airways of asthmatic patients are in an enhanced state of activation. Alveolar macrophages isolated from patients with asthma exhibit an augmented capacity to release mediators such as platelet-activating factor (PAF), leukotriene C_4 and reactive oxygen species when stimulated *ex vivo* [39, 73, 74]. This enhanced response may be caused by cytokines such as GM-CSF [75]. Circulating eosinophils from asthma patients release more superoxide anions on stimulation than those from atopic non-asthmatic subjects [75]. Alveolar macrophages obtained from asthmatic patients exhibit a suppressor influence on proliferation of circulating T lymphocytes to a greater degree than those obtained from normal subjects [76], but this suppression is abolished in the presence of specific allergen, leading to a marked augmentation of T-lymphocyte proliferation [77]. These observations suggest that chronic exposure to allergen may lead to a persistence and amplification of the inflammatory response. T lymphocytes may also be important for sustaining the chronic eosinophilic submucosal inflammation [78], which may lead to bronchial damage.

The eosinophil is likely to play a crucial role in the pathophysiology of asthma, and our concept of its participation in asthma has evolved with our increasing understanding of the biology of the eosinophil (Figure 2.4) [79]. The intercellular adhesion molecule 1 (ICAM-1) may play an important role in the adhesion and subsequent recruitment of eosinophils in asthma. A monoclonal antibody to ICAM-1 has been shown to block the functional activity of this adhesion molecule in primates, associated with a reduction in eosinophil recruitment into the airways and the inhibition of bronchial hyperresponsiveness following allergen challenge [80].

The precise mechanisms by which eosinophils are preferentially recruited to the airways in asthma are still unclear. It is possible that release of inflammatory mediators and cytokines such as PAF and TNFα within the airways may up-regulate the number of adhesion molecules such as ICAM-1. Release of chemotactic signals for the eosinophils is also likely to be important. Leukotriene B_4, PAF and IL-2

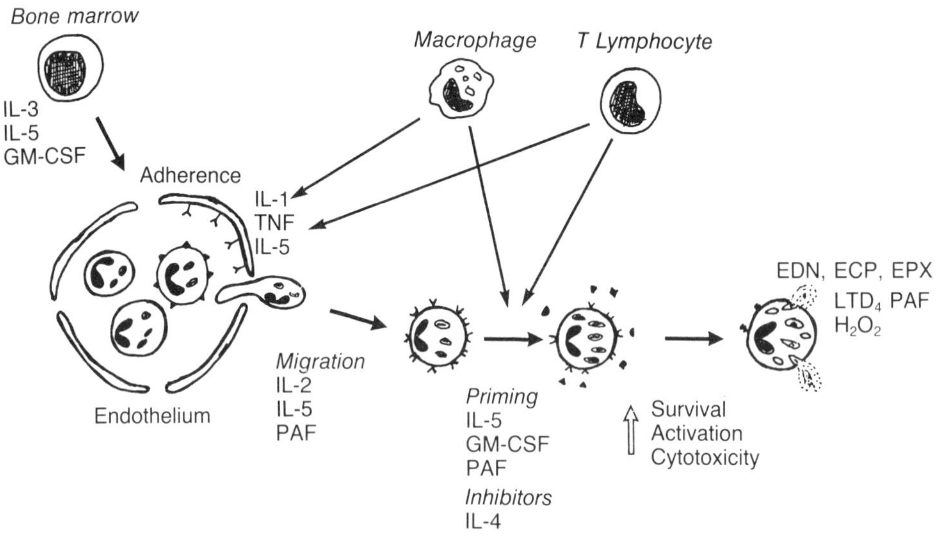

Figure 2.4 Involvement of eosinophils and cytokines in asthma. Increased production of eosinophils at the level of the bone marrow by the action of various cytokines may occur. Differential priming of eosinophils in the circulation may account for their selective migration into airway tissues. Priming of eosinophils with increasing survival, activation and cytotoxicity may also result in airway tissue through the action of cytokines released from macrophages and T lymphocytes. Release of various mediators or proteins from tissue eosinophils may contribute to bronchial oedema, airway hyperresponsiveness, bronchoconstriction and epithelial damage. IL: interleukin; GM-CSF: granulocyte/macrophage colony-stimulating factor; TNF: tumour necrosis factor; PAF: platelet-activating factor; EDN: eosinophil-derived neurotoxin; ECP: eosinophil cationic protein; EPX: eosinophil protein X; LTD_4: leukotriene D_4; H_2O_2: hydrogen peroxide

appear to be the most potent chemokinetic and chemotactic factors for the human eosinophil *in vitro* [42, 81]. Other cytokines such as IL-5 can produce selective hyperadherence of eosinophils, but not of neutrophils, to vascular endothelium. The eosinophil can secrete granule proteins such as major basic protein (MBP); the crystalloid core, eosinophilic cationic protein (ECP), eosinophil-derived neurotoxin (EDN) and eosinophil peroxidase in response to different stimuli (such as IgE or IgG-mediated stimuli) [82, 83]. Eosinophils can also generate newly formed lipid mediators such as PAF and sulphidopeptide leukotrienes [84, 85], and other lipid products include 15-lipoxygenase metabolites and lipoxins [86, 87]. The capacity for the eosinophil to release these mediators may be enhanced by various cytokines, as described above. It is likely that cytokines are also responsible for the presence of circulating hypodense eosinophils in asthma [35].

Eosinophils can therefore contribute to the pathogenesis of asthma by release of eosinophil cationic proteins that are cytotoxic to various cell types, particularly the airway epithelium. Damage to the airway epithelium leads to shedding of the mucosa and exposure of airway nerves, which may be directly stimulated by other mediators of inflammation such as bradykinin [88] to induce bronchoconstriction, mucus production and airway microvascular leakage. Proteins such as MBP may directly induce airway hyperresponsiveness [89], by mechanisms which are as yet unknown. The effects of the lipid mediators are described below.

Other cell types have also been implicated in the inflammatory process in asthmatic airways. Mast cells, which are increased in numbers in asthmatic tissue and are usually in a state of degranulation, are now known to produce cytokines such as TNFα under IgE-dependent activation. Therefore, rather than being considered as just a cell that releases histamine, the mast cell should be viewed as able to contribute to chronic inflammatory mechanisms. Airways epithelial cells have long been thought of as being only a physical protective barrier of the airway submucosa, but they also have the potential to generate lipid mediators such as PAF, products of the 15-lipoxygenase pathway and a whole array of cytokines.

Although much emphasis has been placed on the initiation of the chronic inflammatory process, the repair process and resolution of inflammation are very important. Subepithelial fibrosis, which has been described in asthma, is the result of a proliferation of myofibroblasts [45]. Fibrogenic cytokines such as TGFβ, PDGF or TNFα may be released by epithelial cells, alveolar macrophages and lymphocytes to induce airway wall fibrosis. Regeneration of denuded airway epithelium may also involve the release of fibronectin from adjacent epithelial cells. Finally, airway smooth muscle hyperplasia (which is a recognized feature in the airways of patients who have died of asthma) may result from the stimulated release of growth factors such as platelet-derived growth factors.

Mediators of asthma

A whole range of mediators is released into the airway wall of patients with asthma and may contribute to many of the features characteristic of asthma such as bronchoconstriction, airway hyperresponsiveness, airway wall oedema, mucus secretion and cell activation. Whether any particular mediator plays a prime role in these abnormalities is unlikely. As with the cytokines, these mediators should be considered as acting in concert to cause the characteristic features of asthma. Nevertheless, the study of specific mediators in asthma has given insight into potential inflammatory mechanisms and the effects of a few of these mediators (particularly the lipid mediators) are worth considering separately. The availability of potent and specific receptor antagonists or inhibition of synthesis of those mediators makes it possible to study their contribution to asthmatic inflammation.

Histamine

Histamine induces bronchospasm in asthmatics, and in normal subjects at higher concentrations, through histamine H_1 receptors. When instilled on the human nasal mucosa, histamine increases the recovery of albumin and bradykinin, indicating an increase in both vascular and epithelial permeabilities [90]. Histamine increases the secretion of mucus glycoproteins from human airways *in vitro*, an effect mediated by stimulation of H_2 receptors [91]. Histamine H_3 receptors may modulate neurotransmission in cholinergic nerves and inhibit the release of neuropeptides from airway sensory nerves, and may also be involved in autoinhibition of histamine release from mast cells [92]. Plasma histamine is detectable in the circulation of normal subjects, particularly in the early hours of the morning and is elevated in stable asthmatic subjects [93]. Increased amounts of histamine can be recovered from BAL fluid of asthmatic patients after allergen challenge or a hyperosmolar stimulus. Chlorpheniramine and clemastine, both potent H_1 antagonists, induce bronchodilation in asthmatic subjects. Exercise- and antigen-induced bronchoconstriction are partly mediated by the release of histamine [94–96]. The use of potent histamine antagonists such as terfenadine and astemizole has not proven to be beneficial in asthma [97].

Cyclo-oxygenase products

The cyclo-oxygenase products are formed from arachidonic acid and initiation of prostaglandin and thromboxane synthesis occurs by the action of phospholipase A_2 on membrane phospholipids. Arachidonic acid is oxidized by cyclo-oxygenase to cyclic endoperoxides, which gives rise to $PGF_{2\alpha}$, PGE_2, PGD_2 and thromboxane A_2 (TxA_2). These are potent bronchoconstrictor agents while PGE_1 and PGE_2 possess bronchodilator effects in asthmatic subjects, although bronchoconstrictor responses have also been reported, probably caused by stimulation of airway afferent vagal C-fibres. $PGF_{2\alpha}$ and PGD_2 can transiently increase the airway response to histamine and methacholine [98, 99]. Potentiation of cholinergic neurotransmission by $PGF_{2\alpha}$ and TxA_2-mimetic (U46619) occurs in canine airways *in vitro* [5, 6]. $PGF_{2\alpha}$ and PGE_2 are potent inducers of cough and of airway mucus secretion [100]. In addition, the TxA_2-mimetic (U46619) is a potent inducer of airway microvascular leakage [101].

The role of cyclo-oxygenase products in asthma, as determined by studies of inhibitors of the cyclo-oxygenese pathway, is not clear. For example, indomethacin or aspirin has no effect on the early acute response induced by inhaled allergen in asthmatic subjects, despite inhibition of the early rise in plasma TxB_2 [102]. However, flurbiprofen, another cyclo-oxygenase inhibitor, did reduce the early bronchoconstrictor response to allergen in atopic non-asthmatic subjects [103]. In addition, the late response appears to be inhibited by indomethacin, aspirin or benaxoprofen [102, 104]; in another study, indomethacin reduced only the associated increase in bronchial responsiveness of the late phase [105]. Inhibition of thromboxane synthase activity (which prevents TxA_2 generation) by OKY-046, and of the thromboxane receptor by AA-2414 significantly improved bronchial hyperresponsiveness in asthmatic patients [106], but this was not reproduced in another study using a different thromboxane receptor antagonist [107].

Lipoxygenase products

Arachidonic acid may be oxygenated at different sites by specific lipoxygenases, initiating the formation of leukotrienes. The enzyme 5-lipoxygenase converts arachidonic acid to the unstable leukotriene A_4 (LTA_4) which is hydrolysed to LTB_4. Alternatively, LTA_4 may be converted to the peptidolipid LTC_4, which can be metabolized to LTD_4 and LTE_4.

LTC_4 and LTD_4 are approximately 1000–5000 times more potent than histamine in causing bronchoconstriction in normal and asthmatic subjects [108]. LTE_4 is less potent than LTD_4, but has a longer duration of action [109]. Both LTC_4 and LTD_4 are potent *in vitro* stimulants of mucus release from human airways. LTC_4, LTD_4 and LTE_4 increase airway microvascular permeability in the guinea-pig [110], possibly by directly affecting postcapillary venular endothelial cells. LTB_4 is an extremely potent chemotactic and chemokinetic agent for neutrophils *in vitro* [111], but is less effective for eosinophils [81]. When instilled locally into human airways *in vivo*, LTB_4 increases recovery of neutrophils in BAL fluid. LTB_4 activates human neutrophils, to cause the release of lysosomal enzymes and superoxide anions, and enhances the expression of surface complement receptors on human neutrophils and eosinophils [112]. It increases bronchial responsiveness to acetylcholine in dogs, but not in humans. LTE_4 transiently enhances the constrictor effect of histamine [108, 113].

Sulphidopeptide leukotrienes such as LTE_4 have been recovered from BAL fluid of asthmatic subjects and, during allergen challenge, they are released into BAL fluid and urine [66, 114, 115]. Potent antagonists of LTD_4 such as ICI-204,219 and MK-571 inhibit both the early and late-phase responses to allergen and exercise-induced bronchoconstriction [116]. MK-571 and LY-171883 also induce a mild bronchodilation, with significant reduction in bronchodilator in patients with asthma [117, 118]. 5-lipoxygenase inhibitors, which prevent the formation of LTB_4 and sulphidopeptide leukotrienes, inhibit bronchoconstriction induced by cold dry air [119]. Overall, these studies demonstrate that the sulphidopeptide leukotrienes contribute significantly to bronchoconstrictor responses in asthma. Whether this represents a beneficial 'anti-inflammatory' effect is not clear.

Platelet-activating factor (PAF)

PAF is primarily synthesized from ether-linked phospholipids by the action of phospholipase A_2 to yield lyso-PAF, which is converted to PAF by the action of acetyltransferase enzyme. PAF can be generated from a wide range of inflammatory cells, including neutrophils, eosinophils, macrophages, epithelial cells, endothelial cells and mast cells. While some cytokines such as IL-1β, TNF and IFN-γ can induce the synthesis of PAF from human monocytes [120], PAF itself can increase the release of cytokines such as TNF and IL-1 from alveolar macrophages and monocytes respectively [121–123].

Inhaled PAF is a potent bronchoconstrictor agent in normal subjects [124, 125], but there is rapid tachyphylaxis to repeated inhalations of PAF. Asthmatic subjects who are hyperresponsive to methacholine show similar bronchoconstrictor responses to PAF to normal subjects [126]. PAF-induced bronchoconstriction is partly mediated by the release of bronchoconstrictor leukotrienes [127]. PAF is a potent inducer of airway microvascular leakage and may cause airway oedema [128, 129], and induces bronchial hyperresponsiveness in normal human subjects [124, 125, 130].

PAF also possesses several pro-inflammatory actions. It activates a wide range of inflammatory cells including eosinophils, platelets and macrophages. PAF is a potent chemokinetic and chemotactic agent for eosinophils *in vitro* [81] and induces pulmonary eosinophilia in guinea-pigs. In skin of atopic subjects, intradermal injection of PAF results in a selective accumulation of eosinophils [127], although inhalation in humans caused only an increased neutrophil recovery in BAL fluid [131]. Because PAF may also be generated by eosinophils [84] and eosinophil peroxidase may damage airway epithelium, interactions between PAF and eosinophils may represent a self-potentiating mechanism for inflammatory responses in the asthmatic airway [132].

Several potent PAF antagonists are now available for testing its role in asthmatic inflammation [133]. In animal models, PAF antagonists inhibit allergen-induced bronchial hyperresponsiveness and eosinophil infiltration of the airways of sensitized guinea-pigs [134, 135]. However, similar studies in patients with allergic asthma have yielded negative results [136].

Increased airway microvascular permeability

Airway oedema is a prominent feature of patients who have died in status asthmaticus [137]. An accompanying feature is the presence of exuded plasma in the interstitium of the airway wall and in the lumen, both of which may be responsible for the shedding of ciliated epithelial cells. Increased microvascular permeability is one of the cardinal signs of inflammation [138] and its importance in the pathophysiology of asthma has become increasingly apparent with the accumulation of new information on the physiological and pharmacological control of airway microvasculature [139, 140]. Although the bronchial circulation receives only 1–2% of total cardiac output, recent studies of the anatomical distribution of the bronchial microcirculation in casts of human airways reveal the presence of abundant capillary-venular plexuses in the submucosal layer [141] indicating the potential importance of the vascular network in the airways.

A wide range of inflammatory mediators induce airway microvascular leakage in animals, including histamine, leukotrienes, PAF and neurokinins such as substance P [142–144]. In asthmatic subjects, local instillation of antigen onto the bronchial mucosa causes acute swelling and narrowing of the airways which can be directly visualized through a bronchoscope [145, 146]. The response is rapid, resolves slowly and could represent airway mucosal oedema secondary to increased microvascular leakage. The duration of swelling may be dependent on the removal of exuded fluid by bronchial lymphatics, or its passage into the airway lumen. Very little information is available on the role of airway lymphatics in such circumstances because of the technical difficulties in studying their physiology. Re-entry of exuded fluid into the vascular compartment may occur, although there is no evidence for this. The precise degree to which measurements of airway resistance reflect smooth muscle contraction or acute inflammation after inhalation of a mediator is not known, although there is indirect evidence to suggest that oedema contributes significantly to increased resistance. Small increases in airway wall thickness due to oedema that do not lead to changes in base-line lung function may, theoretically, significantly increase airway responsiveness [48, 147].

The significance of transudation of plasma, in addition to inflammatory cells, into the airway lumen through the damaged epithelium is becoming increasingly apparent. Proteinaceous mucus plugs are found in the airways of asthmatics [137] and their sputum contains elevated levels of plasma proteins higher than in control subjects [146, 148]. Plasma proteins may increase the viscosity and quantity of airway mucus [149, 150], leading to decreased mucociliary clearance [151]. Indeed, increased airway microvascular permeability by agents such as PAF (administered via the trachea or intravenously) [152, 153], capsaicin (which stimulates the release of tachykinins such as substance P) and antigen in sensitized animals [152, 153] has been associated with an increase in luminal protein recovery, which is indicative of increased airway epithelial permeability.

Another potential effect of plasma exudation is the generation of plasma-derived mediators. Increased kallikrein activity, possibly secondary to plasma exudation, has been found in BAL fluid from asthmatics and may result in increased bradykinin generation [52]. Bradykinin has been shown to stimulate bronchial C-fibre sensory nerve endings in dogs [154] and to cause bronchoconstriction in asthmatic subjects [155]. Damage to the airway epithelium in asthma may result in exposure of these nerve terminals, which would then be stimulated by bradykinin to release sensory neuropeptides [88]. Consequent activation of local axon reflexes, with antidromic conduction down the collateral nerve fibres, has been proposed as a mechanism for development of neurogenic inflammation with plasma exudation [88]. Other mediators may also be generated from exuded plasma and inflammatory cells. Although complement activation has not been detected in the circulation of asthmatics during acute attacks or after allergen challenge [156], it may occur locally in airway tissue following increased bronchial microvascular permeability leading to a potentiation of airway inflammatory responses. However, there is no information as to whether significant amounts of both complement fragments and kinins are generated in the inflamed airway mucosa of asthmatic subjects.

Pharmacological modulation

Effect on airway responsiveness

The pharmacological modulation of bronchial responsiveness in asthma has been studied without concomitant examination of airway inflammatory changes. Chronic treatment with short-acting β_2-adrenergic agonists resulted in a small, but none the less significant, increase in the level of bronchial responsiveness [157, 158]. In contrast, inhaled corticosteroid improved airway responsiveness and, in some cases, restored responsiveness into the normal range [157–159]. Airway hyperresponsiveness was restored within 48 h of discontinuing steroid therapy [160]. In addition, inhaled corticosteroids may reduce the degree of maximal airway narrowing to methacholine [161]. The effect of several drugs used in the treatment of asthma has also been studied with reference to the increase in bronchial responsiveness and the induction of late-phase response following experimental allergen provocation [161, 162]. Short-acting β_2-agonists inhaled immediately before allergen challenge protect against the immediate bronchial response, but do not influence the late-phase response or associated increase in bronchial responsiveness. By contrast, drugs used in asthma prophylaxis and possessing anti-inflammatory properties, such as corticosteroids, sodium cromoglycate and nedocromil sodium, inhibit both the late-phase response and the accompanying increase in bronchial responsiveness [162, 163]. Sodium cromoglycate and nedocromil sodium also suppress the early response. Recent observations suggest that the inhibitory effect of asthma drugs on allergen-induced late responses may not be simply interpreted as representing an 'anti-inflammatory' effect. Theophylline, which has bronchodilator properties, inhibits allergen-induced late-phase response [164]. The long-acting β_2-agonist, salmeterol, inhibits both early- and late-phase responses and the associated increase in bronchial responsiveness [165]. The short-acting β_2-agonist, salbutamol, may possess a similar profile of inhibitory activity to salmeterol on the responses to allergen [166]. Examination of bronchial tissues will be necessary to determine the usefulness of late-phase responses or induced bronchial hyperresponsiveness as models of the inflammatory process in asthma.

Effect of corticosteroid therapy (Figure 2.5)

Corticosteroids are the most effective drugs currently available for the control of asthma. Recent studies have shown that inhaled steroids inhibit many of the features associated with asthmatic inflammation, including eosinophil and mast cell numbers, and improved epithelial cell integrity [167]. The mechanisms by which steroids inhibit asthmatic inflammation are not clear, but an understanding of these mechanisms may increase our concepts of inflammatory mechanisms in asthma. Corticosteroids may inhibit cytokine production (e.g. IL-1β, IL-2, IL-6, TNF, GM-CSF) at the level of gene transcription and translation and also by reducing tissue responsiveness [168]. In this way, they may prevent cell-to-cell interactions as illustrated by the effects of steroids on eosinophils. Steroids reduce the production of cytokines such as GM-CSF, IL-3 and probably IL-5 from lymphocytes or macrophages [169, 170], and therefore would prevent the increased survival and priming effects on eosinophils induced by these cytokines. In addition, steroids may have a direct effect on the eosinophil in preventing eosinophil priming and induction of hypodense eosinophils by GM-CSF [171].

At the more basic level, understanding of the regulation of transcription by corticosteroids is increasing [172, 173]. Corticosteroids bind to cytosolic receptors and the hormone–receptor complex interacts with glucocorticoid responsive elements on certain genes, which results in increased transcription of many proteins such as the β_2-receptor or lipocortin. Production of other proteins such as IL-1, IL-2 and TNF is inhibited by both transcriptional and post-transcriptional mechanisms. This effect may occur by the interference of the activated glucocorticoid receptor complex with transcription factors induced by cytokines such as the AP-1 complex which is made up of the proto-oncogenes c-jun and c-fos proteins. It is of interest that c-*fos* has been detected in epithelial cells of the bronchial mucosa of patients with asthma [174]

Clinical relevance of inflammatory mechanisms

A greater awareness of airway inflammatory mechanisms in asthma has greatly influenced our approach to therapy [175]. The mainstay of treatment hinges on the use of long-term anti-inflammatory agents for prophylaxis with intermittent use of inhaled β_2-agonists for symptomatic relief. The amount of β_2-agonist usage provides a useful clinical marker for the need or otherwise, to adjust regular prophylactic treatment. Other important clinical considerations are the time of initiation of anti-inflammatory therapy and how response to treatment is assessed: these currently rest on clinical symptomatic grading and on the frequency of use of bronchodilator drugs such as β_2-agonists to relieve symptoms.

There is little information as to whether different inflammatory mechanisms in asthma relate to the clinical presentation, severity, response to treatment and prognosis. One aspect would be to relate inflammatory mechanisms with the natural history of the disease (Figure 2.2). Very little information is available on the pathology of the airway inflammation in allergic, perhaps hyperresponsive, subjects with no symptoms of asthma but who may develop asthma later. Inflammatory mechanisms may differ depending on the duration of the disease process, and more evidence of fibrosis may be expected with long-standing asthma. Alternatively, in those whose disease symptoms remit, there may be evidence of resolution of the inflammatory process. It is possible that the inability of the inflammatory process to resolve may lead to chronic asthma with subsequent fibrosis. Certain markers of inflammation within the bronchial mucosa may be used to predict the clinical course of asthma in particular patients and this information may help in the management of the disease.

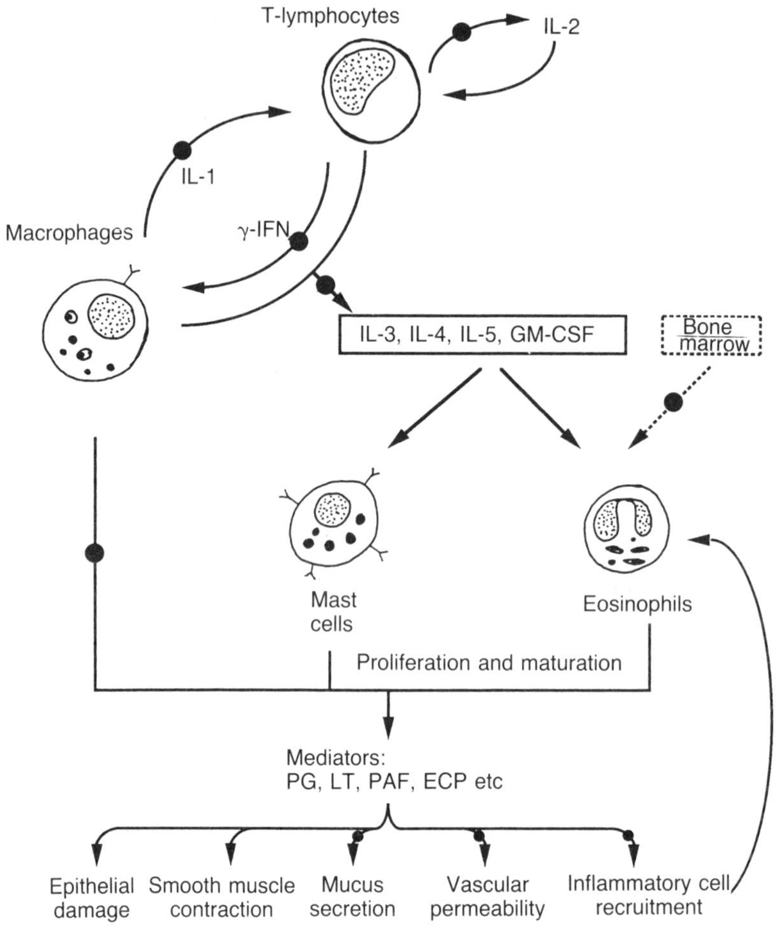

Figure 2.5 Schematic representation of potential inhibitory effects of glucocorticoids on several interactions between inflammatory cells, cytokines and inflammatory mediators (●). Glucocorticoids inhibit the release of IL-1, IL-2 and γ-interferon, preventing collaboration between macrophages and T lymphocytes. Release of other interleukins such as IL-3, IL-4 , IL-5 and granulocyte/macrophage colony-stimulating factor (GM-CSF) is also prevented, leading to inhibition of differentiation, proliferation and activation of mast cells and eosinophils. In addition, release of inflammatory mediators such as prostaglandins (PG), leukotrienes (LT), platelet-activating factor (PAF) or eosinophil-cationic protein (ECP) may be prevented by glucocorticoids

Although β_2-agonists, theophylline and inhaled steroids are the mainstay of asthma treatment, little is known about their effects on the various inflammatory mechanisms that occur in the asthmatic airway. The effects of those agents on various inflammatory markers in bronchial submucosal biopsies from asthmatic patients are currently being evaluated. This information may help to determine whether these different classes of drugs alter various inflammatory responses. For example, there is some controversy as to whether β_2-agonists may lead to an increase in severity of asthma or deaths from asthma, and so far there is little information on their effect on various inflammatory mechanisms in asthma. Perhaps of greater importance is to study whether corticosteroids are valuable at various stages of the disease, particularly at resolution: for example, they may not be beneficial for reversing fibreoptic processes [176]. The decision to initiate a particular line of therapy in asthma at present rests entirely on clinical grounds. An idea of the inflammatory mechanism underlying the symptoms of a particular asthmatic patient may determine which therapy is optimal.

Finally, a greater understanding of the inflammatory mechanisms in asthma increases the likelihood of providing strategies directed at preventing them. Many inflammatory cells, mediators and cytokines appear to be implicated in asthma but it is not known whether they all contribute equally or whether there is a hierarchy of mechanisms. Clearly, our approach to the problem would be different in the two situations. If there *is* an early, asymptomatic, phase that precedes the onset of asthma symptoms, during which the chronic inflammatory mechanisms become established, it would be important to prevent it, a step which may perhaps lead to a cure for this disease.

Acknowledgements

The expert assistance of Patricia Murphy in the preparation of this chapter is gratefully acknowledged.

References

1. Laitinen LA, Heino M, Laitinen A, Kava T, Haahtela T. Damage of the airway epithelium and bronchial reactivity in patients with asthma. *Am Rev Respir Dis* 1985; **131:** 599–606.
2. Beasley R, Roche WR, Roberts JA, Holgate ST. Cellular events in the bronchi in mild asthma and after bronchial provocation. *Am Rev Respir Dis* 1989; **139:** 806–817.
3. Bousquet J, Chanez P, Lacoste JY *et al*. Eosinophilic inflammation in asthma. *N Engl J Med* 1990; **323:** 1033–1039.
4. Holtzman MJ, Fabbri LM, O'Byrne PM, *et al*. Importance of airway inflammation for hyperresponsiveness induced by ozone. *Am Rev Respir Dis* 1983; **127:** 686–690.
5. Chung KF, Becker AB, Lazarus SC, Frick OL, Nadel JA, Gold WM. Antigen-induced airway hyperresponsiveness and pulmonary inflammation in allergic dogs. *J Appl Physiol* 1985; **558:** 1347–1353.
6. Chung KF, Evans TW, Graf PD, Nadel JA. Modulation of cholinergic neurotransmission in canine airways by thromboxane-mimetic U 46619. *Eur J Pharmacol* 1985; **117:** 373–375.
7. Chung KF. Role played by inflammation in the hyperreactivity of the airways in asthma. *Thorax* 1986; **41:** 657–662.
8. Nelson HS. The natural history of asthma. *Ann Allergy* 1991; **66:** 196–203.
9. Zimmerman B, Feanny S, Reisman J *et al*. Allergy in asthma. I. The dose relationship of allergy to severity of childhood asthma. *J Allergy Clin Immunol* 1988; **81:** 63–70.
10. Burrows B, Martinez FD, Halonen M. Association of asthma with serum IgE levels and skin-test reactivity to allergens. *N Engl J Med* 1989; **320:** 71–272.
11. Sears MR, Burrows B, Flannery EM, Herbison GP, Hewitt CJ, Holloway MD. Relation between airway responsiveness and serum IgE in children with asthma and in apparently normal children. *N Engl J Med* 1991; **325:** 1067–1071.
12. Welliver RC, Sun M, Rinaldo D, Ogra PL. Predictive value of respiratory syncytial virus-specific IgE responses for recurrent wheezing following bronchiolitis. *J Pediatr* 1986; **109:** 776–780.
13. Sporik R, Holgate ST, Platts-Mills TAE, Cogswell JJ. Exposure to house-dust mite allergen (Der pl) and the development of asthma in childhood. *N Engl J Med* 1990; **323:** 502–507.
14. Del Prete GF, Maggi E, Parronchi P *et al*. IL-4 is an essential factor for the IgE synthesis induced *in vitro* by human T cell clones and their supernatants. *J Immunol* 1988; **140:** 4193–4198.
15. Mosmann TR, Coffman RL. Heterogeneity of cytokine secretion patterns and function of helper T cells. *Adv Immunol* 1989; **46:** 111–147.

16. Pene J, Rouset F, Briere F *et al.* IgE production by normal human B cells induced by alloreactive T cell clones is mediated by IL-4 and suppressed by IFN-γ. *J Immunol* 1988; **141:** 1218–1224.
17. Snapper CM, Finkelman FD, Paul WE. Regulation of IgG1 and IgE production by interleukin-4. *Immunol Rev* 1988; **102:** 51–75.
18. Aiello FB, Longo DL, Overton R, Takacs L, Durum SK. A role for cytokines in antigen presentation: IL-4 induces accessory functions of antigen-presenting cells. *J Immunol* 1990; **144:** 2572–2581.
19. Cookson WOCM, Craddock CF, Benson MK, Durham SR. Falls in blood eosinophils parallel the late asthmatic response. *Am Rev Respir Dis* 1989; **139:** 458–462.
20. Cookson WOCM, Sharp RA, Faux JA, Hopkins JM. Linkage between immunoglobulin E responses underlying asthma and rhinitis and chromosome 11q. *Lancet* 1989; **i:** 1292–1295.
21. Arai K, Lee F, Miyajima A, Miyatake S, Arai N, Yokota T. Cytokines: coordinators of immune and inflammatory responses. *Ann Rev Biochem* 1990; **59:** 783–836.
22. Ohno I, Ohkawara Y, Yamauchi K, Tanno Y, Akishime T. Production of tumour necrosis factor with IgE receptor triggering from sensitized lung tissue. *Am J Respir Cell Mol Biol* 1990; **3:** 285–289.
23. Ohkawara Y, Yamauchi K, Tanno Y *et al.* Identification of TNF producing cells in sensitised human lung after IgE receptor triggering. *Am Rev Respir Dis* 1991; **143:** A201.
24. Nakamura H, Yoshimura K, Jaffe HA, Crystal RG. Transcriptional regulation of interleukin-8 gene expression by tumour necrosis factor-α in bronchial epithelial cells. *Am Rev Respir Dis* 1991; **143:** A201.
25. Ohtoshi T, Vancheri C, Cox G *et al.* Monocyte-macrophage differentiation induced by human upper airway epithelial cells. *Am J Respir Cell Mol Biol* 1991; **4:** 255–263.
26. Marini M, Soloperto M, Mezzetti M, Fasoli A, Mattoli S. Interleukin-1 binds to specific receptors on human bronchial epithelial cells and upregulates granulocyte/macrophage colony-stimulating factor synthesis and release. *Am J Respir Cell Mol Biol* 1991; **4:** 519–524.
27. Hamid Q, Azzawi M, Ying S *et al.* Expression of mRNA for interleukins in mucosal bronchial biopsies from asthma. *J Clin Invest* 1991; **87:** 1541–1546.
28. Pujol JL, Cosso B, Pauvres J-P, Clot J, Michel J B, Godard P. Interleukin-1 release by alveolar macrophages in asthmatic patients and healthy subjects. *Int Arch Allergy Appl Immunol* 1990; **91:** 207–210.
29. Broide DH, Firestein GS. Endobronchial allergen challenge: demonstration of cellular source of granulocyte macrophage colony-stimulating factor by *in situ* hybridization. *J Clin Invest* 1991; **88:** 1048–1053.
30. Mattoli S, Mattoso VL, Soloperto M, Allegra L, Fasoli A. Cellular and biochemical characteristics of bronchoalveolar lavage fluid in symptomatic nonallergic asthma. *J Allergy Clin Immunol* 1991; **87:** 794–802.
31. Sanderson CJ, Warren DJ, Strath M. Identification of a lymphokine that stimulates eosinophil differentiation in vitro. Its relationship to interleukin 3, and functional properties of eosinophils produced in cultures. *J Exp Med* 1985; **162:** 60–74.
32. Owen WF, Rothenberg ME, Silberstein DS *et al.* Regulation of human eosinophil viability, density and function by granulocyte/macrophage colony-stimulating factor in the presence of 3T3 fibroblasts. *J Exp Med* 1987; **166:** 129–141.
33. Rothenberg ME, Petersen J, Stevens RL. IL5-dependent conversion of normodense human eosinophils to the hypodense phenotype use s 3T3 fibroblasts for enhanced viability, accelerated hypodensity and sustained antibody-dependent cytotoxicity. *J Immunol* 1989; **143:** 2311–2316.
34. Tai PC, Sun L, Spry CJF. Effects of IL-5, granulocyte/macrophage colony-stimulating factor (GM-CSF) and IL-3 on the survival of human blood eosinophils in vitro. *Clin Exp Immunol* 1991; **85:** 312–316.
35. Walker C, Virchow JC, Bruijnzeel PLB, Blaser K. T Cell subsets and their soluble products regulate eosinophilia in allergic and non allergic asthma. *J Immunol* 1991; **146:** 1829–1835.
36. Fujisawa T, Abu-Ghazaleh R, Kita H, Sanderson CJ, Gleich GJ. Regulatory effect of cytokines on eosinophil degranulation. *J Immunol* 1990; **144:** 642–646.
37. Tai PC, Spry CJ. The effects of recombinant granulocyte-macrophage colony-stimulating factor (GM-CSF) and interleukin-3 on the secretory capacity of human blood eosinophils. *Clin Exp Immunol* 1990; **80:** 426–434.
38. Silberstein DS, Owen WF, Gasson JC *et al.* Enhancement of human eosinophil cytotoxicity and leukotriene synthesis by biosynthetic (recombinant) granulocyte-macrophage colony-stimulating factor. *J Immunol* 1986; **137:** 3290–3294.
39. Howell CJ, Pujol J-L, Crea AEG *et al.* Identification of an alveolar macrophage-derived activity in bronchial asthma that enhances leukotriene C4 generation by human eosinophils stimulated by ionophore A23187 as a granulocyte-macrophage colony-stimulating factor. *Am Rev Respir Dis* 1989; **140:** 1340–1347.

40. Baskar P, Silberstein DS, Pincus SH. Inhibition of IgG-triggered human eosinophil function by IL-4. *J Immunol* 1990; **144:** 2321–2326.
41. Renzi PM, Sapienza S, Du T, Wang NS, Martin JG. Lymphokine-induced airway hyperresponsiveness in the rat. *Am Rev Respir Dis* 1991; **143:** 375–379.
42. Rand TH, Silberstein DS, Kornfeld H, Weller PF. Human eosinophils express functional interleukin 2 receptors. *J Clin Invest* 1991; **88:** 825–832.
43. Sedgwick JB, Frick WE, Sandel PM, Hawk JA, Borden E, Busse WW. The appearance of hypodense eosinophils during interleukin-2 treatment. *J Allergy Clin Immunol* 1990; **85:** 557–566.
44. Sanjar S, Smith D, Kings MA, Morley J. Pretreatment with rh-GMCSF, but not rh-IL3, enhances PAF-induced eosinophil accumulation in guinea-pig airways. *Br J Pharmacol* 1990; **100:** 399–400.
45. Roche WR, Beasley R, Williams JH, Holgate ST. Subepithelial fibrosis in the bronchi of asthmatics. *Lancet* 1989; **i:** 520–524.
46. Ollerenshaw SL, Jarvis D, Sullivan CE, Woolcock AJ. Substance P immunoreactive nerves in airways from asthmatics and non-asthmatics. *Eur Respir J* 1991; **4:** 673–682.
47. Boushey HA, Holtzman MJ, Sheller JR, Nadel JA. Bronchial hyperreactivity. *Am Rev Respir Dis* 1980; **121:** 389–413.
48. Moreno RH, Hogg JC, Pare PD. Mechanics of airway narrowing. *Am Rev Respir Dis* 1986; **133:** 1171–1180.
49. Casale TB, Wood D, Richardson HB *et al.* Elevated bronchoalveolar lavage fluid histamine levels in allergic asthmatics are associated with methacholine bronchial hyperresponsiveness. *J Clin Invest* 1987; **79:** 1197–1203.
50. Wardlaw AJ, Dunnette S, Gleich GJ, Collins JV, Kay AB. Eosinophils and mast cells in bronchoalveolar lavage in subjects with mild asthma: relationship to bronchial hyperreactivity. *Am Rev Respir Dis* 1988; **137:** 62–69.
51. Lin MC, Blacker ER, Lichtenstein LM *et al.* Evidence for elevated levels of histamine, prostaglandin D_2 and other bronchoconstricting prostaglandins in the airways of subjects with mild asthma. *Am Rev Respir Dis* 1990; **142:** 126–132.
52. Christiansen SC, Proud D, Cochrane CG. Detection of tissue kallikrein in the bronchoalveolar lavage fluid of asthmatic patients. *J Clin Invest* 1987; **79:** 188–197.
53. Flint KC, Leung KBP, Huspith BN, Brostoff J, Pearce FL, Johnson NMcl. Bronchoalveolar mast cells in extrinsic asthma: mechanism for the initiation of antigen specific bronchoconstriction. *BMJ* 1985; **291:** 923–927.
54. Kelly CJ, Stenton CS, Bird E, Hendrick DJ, Walters EH. Number and activity of inflammatory cells in bronchoalveolar lavage fluid in asthma and their relation to airway responsiveness. *Thorax* 1988; **43:** 684–692.
55. Azzawi M, Bradley B, Jeffrey PK *et al.* Identification of activated T lymphocytes and eosinophils in bronchial biopsies in stable atopic asthmatics. *Am Rev Respir Dis* 1990; **142:** 1407–1411.
56. Bradley B, Azzawi M, Jacobsen M *et al.* Eosinophils, T-lymphocytes, mast cells, neutrophils and macrophages in bronchial biopsy specimens from atopic subjects with asthma. *J Allergy Clin Immunol* 1991; **88:** 661–674.
57. Lozwmicz S, Gomez E, Ferguson H, Davies RJ. Inflammatory cells in the airways in mild asthma. *BMJ* 1988; **297:** 1515–1516.
58. Djukanovic R, Wilson JW, Britton KM *et al.* Quantitation of mast cells and eosinophils in the bronchial mucosa of symptomatic atopic asthmatics and healthy control subjects using immunohistochemistry. *Am Rev Respir Dis* 1990; **142:** 863–871.
59. Durham SR, Kay AB. Eosinophils, bronchial hyperreactivity and late-phase asthmatic reactions. *Clin Allergy* 1985; **15:** 411–418.
60. Taylor KJ, Luksza AR. Peripheral blood eosinophil counts and bronchial responsiveness. *Thorax* 1987; **42:** 452–456.
61. Rak S, Lowhagen O, Venge P. The effect of immunotherapy on bronchial hyperresponsiveness and eosinophil cationic protein in pollen allergic patients. *J Allergy Clin Immunol* 1988; **82:** 470–480.
62. Corrigan CJ, Hartnell A, Kay AB. T-lymphocyte activation in acute severe asthma. *Lancet* 1988; **i:** 1129–1132.
63. Gibson PG, Girgis-Gabardo A, Morris MM *et al.* Cellular characteristics of sputum from patients with asthma and chronic bronchitis. *Thorax* 1989; **44:** 693–699.
64. Frigas E, Loegering D, Solley G, Farrow E, Gleich GJ. Elevated levels of eosinophil major basic protein in the sputum of patients with bronchial asthma. *Mayo Clin Proc* 1981; **56:** 345–353.
65. Cartier A, Thomson NC, Frith PA, Roberts R, Hargreave FE. Allergen-induced increase in bronchial responsiveness to histamine: relationship to the late asthmatic response and change in airway caliber. *J Allergy Clin Immunol* 1982; **70:** 170–177.
66. Wenzel SE, Larsen GL, Johnston G, Voelkel NF, Westcott JY. Elevated levels of leukotriene C4 in

bronchoalveolar lavage fluid from atopic asthmatics after endobronchial allergen challenge. *Am Rev Respir Dis* 1990; **142:** 112–119.
67. Murray JJ, Tonnel AG, Brash AR *et al.* Release of prostaglandin D_2 into human airways during acute allergen challenge. *N Engl J Med* 1986; **315:** 800–804.
68. Manning PJ, Rokach J, Malo JL *et al.* Urinary leukotriene E_4 levels during early and late asthmatic responses. *J Allergy Clin Immunol* 1990; **86:** 211–220.
69. De Monchy JGR, Kauffman HK, Venge P. Bronchoalveolar eosinophilic during allergen-induced late asthmatic reactions. *Am Rev Respir Dis* 1985; **131:** 373–376.
70. Gonzalez MC, Diaz P, Galteguillos FR, Ancic P, Cromwell O, Kay AB. Allergen-induced recruitment of bronchoalveolar OKT_4 and suppressor OKT8 cells in asthma. Relative increases in OKT8 cells in single early responders compared with those in late-phase responders. *Am Rev Respir Dis* 1987; **136:** 600–604.
71. Metzger WJ, Zavala D, Richerson HB *et al.* Local allergen challenge and bronchoalveolar lavage of allergic asthmatic lungs. *Am Rev Respir Dis* 1987; **135:** 433–440.
72. Gibson PG, Manning PJ, O'Byrne PM *et al.* Allergen-induced asthmatic responses: relationship between increases in airway responsiveness and increases in circulating eosinophils, basophils and their progenitors. *Am Rev Respir Dis* 1991; **143:** 331–335.
73. Arnoux B, Joeph M, Simoes AH *et al.* Antigenic release of PAF-acether and beta-glucuronidase from alveolar macrophages of asthmatics. *Bull Eur Physiopathol Respir Dis* 1987; **23:** 119–124.
74. Cluzel M, Damon M, Chanez P *et al.* Enhanced alveolar cell luminol-dependent chemiluminescence in asthma. *J Allergy Clin Immunol* 1987; **80:** 195–201.
75. Chanez P, Yukawa T, Dent G, Barnes PJ, Chung KF. Generation of oxygen free radicals from blood eosinophils from asthma patients after stimulation with platelet-activating factor and pharbolester. *Eur Respir J* 1990; **3:** 1002–1007.
76. Spiteri M, Knight RA, Worsdell M, Barnes PJ, Chung KF. Alveolar macrophage (AM)-driven mixed lymphocyte cultures (MLC) in bronchial asthma. *Am Rev Respir Dis* 1991; **143:** A435.
77. Spiteri MA, Knight RA, Worsdell M, Barnes PJ, Chung KF. Alveolar macrophage (AM)-induced suppression of T-cell hyperresponsiveness in asthma is reversed following allergen exposure *in vitro*. *Am Rev Respir Dis* 1991; **143:** A801.
78. Kay AB. Lymphocytes in asthma. *Respir Med* 1991; **85:** 87–90.
79. Frigas E, Gleich GJ. The eosinophil and pathophysiology of asthma. *J Allergy Clin Immunol* 1986; **77:** 527–537.
80. Wegner CD, Gundel RH, Reilly P, Haynes N, Letts LG, Rothlein R. Intercellular adhesion molecule-1 ICAM-1 in the pathogenesis of asthma. *Science* 1990; **247:** 456–459.
81. Wardlaw AJ, Moqbel R, Cromwell O, Kay AB. PAF-acether is a potent chemotactic and chemokinetic factor for human eosinophils. *J Clin Invest* 1986; **78:** 1701–1706.
82. Capron M, Leprevost C, Prin L. Immunoglobulin-mediated activation of eosinophils. In: *Eosinophils in Asthma.* (Morley J, Colditz I, eds). London: Academic Press, 1989; 49–60.
83. Kita H, Abu-Ghazaleh RI, Gleich GJ, Abraham RT. Regulation of Ig-induced eosinophil degranulation by adenosine 3', 5'-cyclic monophosphate. *J Immunol* 1991; **146:** 2712–2718.
84. Lee TC, Lenihan DJ, Malone B, Roddy LL, Wasserman SI. Increased biosynthesis of platelet activating factor in activated human eosinophils. *J Biol Chem* 1984; **259:** 5526–5530.
85. Weller PF, Lee CW, Foster DW, Corey EJ, Austen KF, Lewis RA. Generation and metabolism of 5-lipoxygenase pathway leukotrienes by human eosinophils: predominant production of leukotriene C_4. *Proc Natl Acad Sci USA* 1983; **80:** 7626–7630.
86. Sigal E, Grumberger D, Cashman JR, Craik CS, Caughey GH, Nadel JA. Arachidonate 15-lipoxygenase from human eosinophil enriched leukocytes: partial purification and properties. *Biochem Biophys Res Commun* 1988; **150:** 376–383.
87. Serban CN, Hirsch U, Palmblad J, Samuelsson B. Formation of lipoxin A by granulocytes from eosinophilic donors. *FEBS Lett* 1987; **217:** 242–246.
88. Barnes PJ. Asthma as an axon reflex. *Lancet* 1986; **i:** 242–244.
89. Gundel RH, Gordon Letts L, Gleich GJ. Human eosinophil major basic protein induces airway constriction and airway hyperresponsiveness in primates. *J Clin Invest* 1991; **87:** 1470–1473.
90. Baumgarten CR, Nichol RC, Naclerio RM, Lichtenstein LM, Norman PS, Proud D. Plasma kallikrein during experimentally-induced allergic rhinitis: Role in kinin formation and contribution to TAME-esterase activity in nasal secretions. *J Immunol* 1986; **137:** 977–982.
91. Shelhamer J, Marom Z, Kaliner M. Immunologic and neuropharmacologic stimulation of mucous glycoprotein release from human airways *in vitro*. *J Clin Invest* 1980; **66:** 1400–1408.
92. Barnes PJ. Histamine receptors in the lung. *Agents Actions* 1991; (Suppl. 33): 103–122.
93. Barnes PJ, Ind PW, Brown MJ. Plasma histamine and catecholamines in stable asthmatics subjects. *Clin Sci* 1982; **62:** 661–665.

94. Doward AJ, Patel KR. A comparison of Ketotifen with clemastine, ipratropium bromide and sodium cromoglycate in exercise-induced asthma. *Clin Allergy* 1982; **12:** 355–361.
95. Phillips MJ, Ollier S, Gould C, Davies RJ. Effect of antihistamines and antiallergic drugs on responses to allergen and histamine provocation tests in asthma. *Thorax* 1984; **39:** 345–351.
96. Chan TB, Shelton DM, Eiser NM. Effect of an oral H_1-receptor antagonist, terfenadine, on antigen-induced asthma. *Br J Dis Chest* 1986; **80:** 375–384.
97. Taytard A, Beaumont D, Pujet JC, Sapene M, Lewis PJ. Treatment of bronchial asthma with terfenadine: a randomized controlled trial. *Br J Clin Pharmacol* 1987; **24:** 743–746.
98. Walters EH, Parrish RW, Bevan C, Smith AP. Induction of bronchial hypersensitivity: evidence for a role of prostaglandins. *Thorax* 1981; **36:** 571–574.
99. Fuller RW, Dixon CMS, Dollery CT, Barnes PJ. Prostaglandin D_2 potentiates airway responses to histamine and methacholine. *Am Rev Respir Dis* 1986; **133:** 252–254.
100. Lopez-Vidriero MI, Das I, Smith AP, Picot R, Reid L. Bronchial secretion from normal human airways after inhalation of prostaglandin F_2 alpha, acetylcholine, histamine and citric acid. *Thorax* 1977; **32:** 734–739.
101. Lotvall JO, Elwood W, Tokuyama K, Barnes PJ, Chung KF. A thromboxane-mimetic, U46615, increases airway microvascular leakage. *J Appl Physiol* 1993 (In press).
102. Shephard EG, Malon L, MacFarlane CM, Mouton W, Joubert JR. Lung function and plasma levels of thromboxane B_2, 6-keto-prostaglandin F_1 alpha, beta-thromboglobulin in antigen-induced asthma before and after indomethacin pretreatment. *Br J Clin Pharmacol* 1985; **19:** 459–470.
103. Curzen N, Rafferty P, Holgate ST. Effects of cyclo-oxygenase inhibitor, flurbiprofen and on H1 histamine receptor antagonist, terfenadine alone and in combination on allergen induced immediate bronchoconstriction in man. *Thorax* 1987; **42:** 946–952.
104. Fairfax AJ, Hanson JM, Morley J. The late reaction following bronchial provocation with house dust mite allergen: Dependence on arachidonic acid metabolism. *Clin Exp Immunol* 1983; **52:** 393–398.
105. Kirby JG, Hargreave FE, Cockcroft DW, O'Byrne PM. Effect of indomethacin on allergen-induced asthmatic responses. *J Appl Physiol* 1989; **66:** 578–583.
106. Fujimura M, Sasaki F, Nakatsumi Y *et al.* Effects of thromboxane synthetase inhibitor (OKY-046) and α lipoxygenase inhibitor (AA-861) on bronchial responsiveness to acetylcholine in asthmatic subjects. *Thorax* 1986; **41:** 955–959.
107. Stenton SC, Ward C, Duddridge M *et al.* Actions of GR 32191 B, a thromboxane receptor antagonist, on the effects of inhaled PAF in human airways. *Clin Exp Allergy* 1990; **20:** 311–317.
108. Barnes NC, Piper PJ, Costello JF. Comparative effects of inhaled leukotriene C4, leukotriene D4, and histamine in normal human subjects. *Thorax* 1984; **39:** 500–504.
109. Davidson AB, Lee TH, Scanlon PD *et al.* Bronchoconstrictor effects of leukotriene E4 in normal and asthmatic subjects. *Am Rev Respir Dis* 1987; **135:** 500–504.
110. Hua XY, Dahlen SE, Lundberg JM, Hammerstrom S, Hedqvist P. Leukotrienes C4 and E4 cause widespread and extensive plasma extravasation in the guinea-pig. *Naunyn-Schmiedeberg's Arch Pharmacol* 1985; **330:** 136–141.
111. Ford-Hutchinson AW, Bray MA, Doig MV, Shipley ME, Smith MJH. Leukotriene B4, a potent chemokinetic and aggregating substance released from polymorphonuclear leukocytes. *Nature* 1981; **286:** 264–265.
112. Nagy L, Lee TH, Goetzl EJ, Pickett W, Kay AB. Complement receptor enhancement and chemotaxis of human neutrophils and eosinophils by leukotrienes and other lipoxygenase products. *Clin Exp Immunol* 1982; **47:** 541–547.
113. Arm JP, Spur BW, Lee TH. The effects of inhaled leukotriene E_4 on the airway responsiveness to histamine in subjects with asthma and normal subjects. *J Allergy Clin Immunol* 1988; **82:** 654-660.
114. Taylor GW, Taylor IK, Black P *et al.* Urinary leukotriene E4 after antigen challenge and in acute asthma and allergic rhinitis. *Lancet* 1989; **i:** 584–587.
115. Lam S, Chan H, Leriche JC, Chan Yeung M, Salari H. Release of leukotrienes in patients with bronchial asthma. *J Allergy Clin Immunol* 1988; **81:** 711–717.
116. Taylor IK, O'Shaughnessy KM, Fuller RW, Dollery CT. Effect of cysteinyl-leukotriene receptor antagonist ICI 204-219 on allergen-induced bronchoconstriction and airway hyperreactivity in atopic subjects. *Lancet* 1991; **337:** 690–694.
117. Gaddy J, Bush RK, Margolskee D, Williams VC, Busse W. The effects of a leukotriene D_4 (LTD_4) antagonist MK-571 in mild to moderate asthma. *J Allergy Clin Immunol* 1990; 85: 197A.
118. Cloud ML, Enas GC, Kemp J *et al.* A specific LTD_4/LTE_4-receptor antagonist improves pulmonary function in patients with mild, chronic asthma. *Am Rev Respir Dis* 1989; **140:** 1336–1339.
119. Israel E, Dermarkarian R, Rosenberg M *et al.* The effects of a 5-lipoxygenase inhibitor on asthma induced by cold, dry air. *N Engl J Med* 1990; **323:** 1740–1744.

120. Valone FH, Epstein LB. Biphasic platelet-activating factor synthesis by human monocytes stimulated with IL-1β, tumour necrosis factor, or IFNα. *J Immunol* 1988; **141:** 3945–3956.
121. Dubois C, Bissonette E, Rola-Pleszczyski M. Platelet-activating factor (PAF) enhances tumor necrosis factor production by alveolar macrophages. *J Immunol* 1989; **143:** 964–970.
122. Salem P, Deryckx A, Vivier E *et al.* Immunoregulatory function of PAF acether IV. Enhancement of IL1-production by muramyl dipeptide stimulated monocytes. *J Immunol* 1990; **144:** 1338.
123. Bonavida B, Mencia-Huerta JM, Braquet P. Effect of platelet activating factor on monocyte activation and production of tumor necrosis factor. *Int Arch Allergy Appl Immunol* 1989; **88:** 57–160.
124. Cuss FM, Dixon CMS, Barnes PJ. Effects of inhaled platelet activating factor on pulmonary function and bronchial responsiveness in man. *Lancet* 1986; **ii:** 189–192.
125. Rubin AH, Smith LJ, Patterson R. The bronchoconstrictor properties of platelet-activating factor in humans. *Am Rev Respir Dis* 1987; **136:** 1145–1151.
126. Chung KF, Barnes PJ. Effect of inhaled platelet-activating factor on airway calibre, bronchial responsiveness and circulating cells in asthmatic subjects. *Thorax* 1989; **44:** 108–115.
127. Henocq E, Vargaftig BB. Skin eosinophilia in atopic patients. *J Allergy Clin Immunol* 1988; **81:** 691–695.
128. Evans TW, Chung KF, Rogers DF, Barnes PJ. Increased vascular permeability of the airways induced by platelet-activating factor : possible mechanisms. *J Appl Physiol* 1987; **63:** 479–484.
129. Tokuyama K, Lotvall J, Barnes PJ, Chung KF. Airway narrowing after inhalation of platelet-activating factor in guinea-pig: contribution of airway microvascular leakage and edema. *Am Rev Respir Dis* 1991; **143:** 1345–1349.
130. Kaye MG, Smith LJ. Effects of inhaled leukotriene D_4 and platelet-activating factor on airway reactivity in normal subjects. *Am Rev Respir Dis* 1990; **141:** 993–997.
131. Wardlaw A, Chung KF, Moqbel R *et al.* Effect of inhaled platelet-activating factor in humans and bronchoalveolar lavage fluid neutrophils. *Am Rev Respir Dis* 1990; **141:** 386–392.
132. Barnes PJ, Chung KF, Page CP. Platelet-activating factor: A mediator of inflammation and allergic disorders. *J Allergy Clin Immunol* 1988; **81:** 919–934.
133. Chung KF. PAF antagonists as asthma therapy. In: *New Drugs for Asthma.* (Barnes PJ ed.) IBC Technical Services Ltd, London, 1989; 103–116.
134. Lelouch-Tubiana A, Lefart J, Simon MT, Pfister A, Vargaftig BB. Eosinophil recruitment into guinea-pig lungs after PAF-acether and allergen administration: modulation by prostacyclin, platelet depletion and selective antagonists. *Am Rev Respir Dis* 1988; **137:** 948–954.
135. Coyle AJ, Unwin SC, Page CP, Touvay C, Villain B, Braquet P. The effect of selective antagonist BNS2021 on PAF and antigen-induced bronchi hyperreactivity and eosinophil accumulation. *Eur J Pharmacol* 1988; **148:** 51–58.
136. Bel EH, Desmet M, Rossing TH, Timmers MC, Dijkman JH, Sterk PJ. The effect of specific oral PAF-antagonist, MK-287, on antigen -induced early and late asthmatic reactions in man. *Am Rev Respir Dis* 1991; **143:** A811.
137. Dunnill MS. The pathology of asthma with special reference to changes in the bronchial mucosa. *J Clin Pathol* 1960; **13:** 27–33.
138. Ryan GB, Majno. Acute inflammation: a review. *Am J Pathol* 1977; **86:** 185–276.
139. Chung KF, Rogers DF, Barnes PJ, Evans TW. the role of increased microvascular permeability and plasma exudation in asthma. *Eur Respir J* 1990; **3:** 329–337.
140. Persson CGA. Role of plasma exudation in asthmatic airways. *Lancet* 1986; **ii:** 1126–1129.
141. Laitinen LA, Laitinen A, Widdicombe J. Effects of inflammatory and other mediators on airways vascular beds. *Am Rev Respir Dis* 1987; **135:** S67–S70.
142. Evans TW, Rogers DF, Aursudkij B, Chung KF, Barnes PJ. Regional and time-dependent effects of airway inflammatory mediators on microvascular permeability in the guinea-pig. *Clin Sci* 1989; **76:** 479–485.
143. O'Donnell S, Barnett CJK. Microvascular leakage due to platelet-activating factor in guinea-pig trachea and bronchi. *Eur J Pharmacol* 1987; **138:** 385–396.
144. Rogers DF, Belvisi MG, Aursudkij B, Evans TW, Barnes PJ. Effects and interactions of sensory neuropeptides on airway microvascular leakage in guinea-pigs. *Br J Pharmacol* 1988; **95:** 1109–1116.
145. Hutchcroft BJ. In: *Asthma: Physiology, Immunopharmacology and Treatment.* (Lichtenstein L, Austen KF, eds). New York: Academic Press, 1977; 14–16.
146. Fick RB, Richerson HB, Zavala DC, Hunninghake GW. Bronchoalveolar lavage in allergic asthmatics. *Am Rev Respir Dis* 1987; **135:** 1204–1209.
147. Freedman BJ. The functional geometry of the bronchi: the relationship between changes in external diameter and calibre, and a consideration of the passive role played by the mucosa in bronchoconstriction. *Bull Physiopathol Respir* 1972; **8:** 545–551.
148. Brogan TD, Ryley HC, Neale L, Yassa J. Soluble proteins of bronchopulmonary secretions from patients with cystic fibrosis, asthma, and bronchitis. *Thorax* 1975; **30:** 72–79.

149. List SJ, Findlay BP, Forstner GG, Forstner JF. Enhancement of the viscosity of mucin by serum albumin. *Biochem J* 1978; **175:** 565–571.
150. Peatfield AC, Hall RL, Richardson PS, Jeffrey PK. The effect of serum on the secretion of radio-labelled mucous macromolecules into the lumen of the cat trachea. *Am Rev Respir Dis* 1982; **125:** 210–215.
151. Wilson GB, Fridenberg HH. Ciliary diskinesia factors in cystic fibrosis and asthma. *Nature* 1977; **266:** 463–464.
152. Persson CGA, Erjefalt I. Inflammatory leakage of macromolecules from the vascular compartment of the tracheal lumen. *Acta Physiol Scand* 1986; **126:** 615–616.
153. Tokuyama K, Lotvall JO, Barnes PJ, Chung KF. Mechanism of airway narrowing caused by inhaled platelet-activating factor: role of airway microvascular leakage. *Am Rev Respir Dis* 1991; **143:** 1345–1349.
154. Kaufman MP, Coleridge HM, Coleridge JCG, Baker DG. Bradykinin stimulates afferent vagal C-fibers in intrapulmonary airways of dogs. *J Appl Physiol* 1980; **48:** 511–517.
155. Fuller RW, Dixon CMS, Cuss FMC, Barnes PJ. Bradykinin-induced bronchoconstriction in man: mode of action. *Am Rev Respir Dis* 1987; **135:** 176–180.
156. Hutchcroft BJ, Guz A. Levels of complement component during allergen-induced asthma. *Clin Allergy* 1978; **8:** 59–64.
157. Kerrebijn KF, Von Essen-Zandvliet EEM, Neijens HJ. Effect of long-term treatment with inhaled corticosteroids and beta-agonists on bronchial responsiveness in asthmatic children. *J Allergy Clin Immunol* 1987; **79:** 653–659.
158. Kraan J, Koeter GH, Van der Mark TW, Sluiter HJ, De Vries K. Changes in bronchial hyperreactivity induced by 4 weeks of treatment with antiasthmatic drugs in patients with allergic asthma: a comparison between budesonide and terbutaline. *J Allergy Clin Immunol* 1985; **76:** 628–636.
159. Juniper EF, Kline PA, Vanzileghen MA, Ramsdale EH, O'Byrne PM, Hargreave FE. Effect of long-term treatment with an inhaled corticosteroid Budesonide on airway hyperresponsiveness and clinical asthma in nonsteroid-dependent asthmatics. *Am Rev Respir Dis* 1990; **142:** 832–836.
160. Varthenen AS, Knox AJ, Wisniewski A, Tattersfield AE. Time course of change in bronchial reactivity with an inhaled corticosteroid in asthma. *Am Rev Respir Dis* 1991; **143:** 1317–1321.
161. Bel EH, Timmers MC, Zwinderman AH, Dijkman JH, Sterk PJ. The effect of inhaled corticosteroids on the maximal degree of airway narrowing to methacholine in asthmatic subjects. *Am Rev Respir Dis* 1991; **143:** 109–113.
162. Cockroft DW, Murdoch KY. Comparative effects of inhaled salbutamol, sodium cromoglycate and BDP on allergen-induced early asthmatic responses, late asthmatic responses and increased bronchial responsiveness to histamine. *J Allergy Clin Immunol* 1987; **79:** 734 710.
163. Matolli S, Forest A, Corbo GM, Pollidori G, Giappi G. Effects of two doses of cromolyn on allergen-induced late asthmatic response and increased responsiveness. *J Allergy Clin Immunol* 1987; **79:** 747–754.
164. Pauwels R, van Renterghem D, van der Straeten M, Johannsson N, Persson CGA. The effect of theophylline and enprofylline on allergen-induced bronchoconstriction. *J Allergy Clin Immunol* 1985; **76:** 583–590.
165. Twentyman OP, Finnerty JP, Harris A, Palmer J, Holgate ST. Protection against allergen-induced asthma by salmeterol. *Lancet* 1990; **336:** 1338 1342.
166. Twentyman OP, Finnerty JP, Holgate ST. The inhibitory effect of nebulized albuterol on the early and late asthmatic reactions and increase in airway responsiveness provoked by inhaled allergen in asthma. *Am Rev Respir Dis* 1991; **144:** 782–787.
167. Laitinen LA, Laitinen A, Haahtela T. Treatment of eosinophilic airway inflammation with inhaled corticosteroid, budesonide, in newly diagnosed asthmatic subjects. *Eur Respir J* 1991; **4:** 342(s).
168. Kern JA, Lamb RJ, Reed JC, Daniele RP, Nowell PC. Dexamethasone inhibition of interleukin 1 beta production by human monocytes: posttranscriptional mechanisms. *J Clin Invest* 1988; **81:** 237–244.
169. Gillis S, Crabtree GR, Smith KA. Glucocorticoid-induced inhibition of T-cell growth factor production. I The effect on mitogen-induced lymphocyte proliferation. *J Immunol* 1979; **123:** 1624–1631.
170. Raghavachar A, Fleischer S, Frickhofen N, Heimpel H, Fleischer B. T lymphocyte control of human eosinophilic granulopoiesis. *J Immunol* 1987; **139:** 3753–3758.
171. Lamas AM, Leon OG, Schleimer RP. Glucocorticoids inhibit eosinophil responses to granulocyte macrophage colony-stimulating factor. *J Immunol* 1991; **147:** 254–259.
172. Munck A, Mendel DB, Smith LI, Orti E. Glucocorticoid receptors and actions. *Am Rev Respir Dis* 1990; **141:** S2–S10.
173. Beato M. Gene regulation by steroid hormones. *Cell* 1989; **56:** 335–344.
174. Demoly P, Basset-Seguin N, Chanez P *et al.* C-fos proto-oncogene expression in bronchial biopsies of asthmatics. *Am J Resp Cell Mol Biol* 1992; **7:** 128–133.

175. British Thoracic Society. Guidelines for management of asthma in adults: I – chronic persistent asthma. *BMJ* 1990; **301:** 651–653.
176. Lacronique JG, Rennard SI, Bitterman PB, Ozaki T , Crystal RG. Alveolar macrophages in idiopathic pulmonary fibrosis have glucocorticoid receptors, but glucocorticoid therapy does not suppress alveolar macrophage release of fibroreaction and alveolar macrophage derived growth factor. *Am Rev Respir Dis* 1984; **130:** 450–456.

3

Asthma and the environment

A.J. Newman Taylor

The environment 'everything that isn't me' – Albert Einstein

Introduction

Asthma is most commonly defined as airway narrowing which varies over short periods of time, either spontaneously or as a result of treatment. This defining criterion of asthma seems to be the manifestation of a characteristic pattern of airway inflammation and asthma could equally (and probably more properly) be described as a chronic desquamative eosinophilic bronchitis. In considering the causes of asthma it is useful to distinguish those factors which initiate asthma, the so-called 'inducers', which will influence its incidence, from those which provoke airway narrowing in cases of asthma, the so-called 'inciters'.

Interest in the environmental factors which may influence the initiation and provocation of asthma is based on the principle that to reduce the incidence or severity of disease requires identification of, and subsequent avoidance of exposure to, its causes. Strong evidence for environmental determinants of asthma has come from studies of asthma epidemics, of occupational asthma and, by inference, from differences in the frequency of asthma between different populations, particularly between migrants and their community of origin, and secular changes in the incidence of asthma. Paradoxically, while there is increasing evidence in Western Europe and Australasia of an increase in the prevalence, and probably incidence, of asthma that is too rapid to be explained by changes in the gene pool, understanding of the genetic basis of atopy has increased more substantially than knowledge of the important environmental determinants of asthma. Both genetic and environmental factors are important and interact, but environmental influences probably predominate in the development of asthma, seem currently to be increasing in importance and are more likely to be directly amenable to intervention. Interactions between different environmental factors are also probably important influences in determining the initiation and provocation of asthma.

Asthma and atopy

Asthma is associated with atopy – the tendency to produce IgE antibody to allergens commonly encountered in the general environment – which is usually identified by the provocation of immediate 'wheal and flare' responses in the skin by extracts of common inhalant allergens. In a sample of more than 3000 persons randomly selected from the general population in the south-west USA Burrows *et al.* [1] found a close relationship at all ages between the prevalence of asthma and an index of skin-test reactivity which incorporated both the number and size of skin-test responses to local inhalant aero-allergens. Among college students Cockroft *et al.* [2] found the prevalence of airway hyperresponsiveness to inhaled histamine to correlate significantly with the degree of atopy. Burrows *et al.* [3] found asthma to be associated with a significantly increased level of total IgE in serum. The prevalence of asthma increased in each age group with rising total IgE level. On the basis of these findings they suggested that asthma was an IgE-associated disease at all ages.

Genetic influences on atopy

The familial nature of atopic diseases – eczema, hay fever and asthma – and the heterogeneity within families, both of the clinical manifestations and the allergens relevant in particular individuals, has long been appreciated. Identification of IgE as the reaginic antibody provided a more stable phenotype for investigation than clinical manifestations. Two major genetic influences on IgE production have been identified, one which controls basal levels of IgE, the other, probably a major histocompatibility complex (MHC) gene, determines IgE specificity.

Using a broad definition of atopy as a high serum total IgE, or the presence of either specific IgE in serum or a skin prick test response to common inhalant allergens, atopy has been associated with a gene on the long arm of chromosome 11 inherited in a dominant fashion [4, 5]. A single dominant gene would seem to determine total IgE, specific IgE and associated skin-test responses.

Evidence that the specificity of the IgE response is determined by MHC genes is stronger in rodents than humans. Nevertheless, studies on skin-test responses to highly purified low molecular weight allergens have identified an association with specific HLA phenotypes. Marsh *et al.* [6] found an association between the minor ragweed allergen Ra5 and the HLA DW2 phenotype. Relationships of specific IgE to other allergens with HLA phenotype have been weaker and less consistent, possibly because any MHC relationship is likely to be with single epitopes.

Environmental influences on asthma

General evidence for the importance of environmental influences in asthma comes from three major sources: family studies, studies of migrants, and evidence for a secular change.

Family studies

Studies of twins have confirmed the importance of genetic control of IgE production but have identified less genetic influence on the development of asthma.

Monozygotic twins have a high concordance for atopy but a lower concordance for asthma [7]. Schade [8] found that 59% of monozygotic twins, but only 12% of dizygotic twins, were concordant for atopy. In a survey of 700 twin pairs in Sweden Lubs [9] found that 19% of monozygotic twins and 4.8% of dizygotic twins were concordant for asthma. A more recent segregation analysis of airway responsiveness in families found that the environmental influence on airway responsiveness was large in relation to the genetic component [10].

Geographical variation: migrant studies

Studies of migrant populations living in different environments from their place of origin have consistently found more asthma in those living in urbanized Western communities than in those who have remained in poorer rural areas, where the prevalence has usually been very low. Although in some studies this may have reflected differences in diagnostic criteria, ascertainment and access to medical facilities, two studies which identified large differences in prevalence used identical diagnostic criteria in both the migrant population and in those in their place of origin.

Waites *et al.* [11] compared the prevalence of asthmatic symptoms (elicited by questionnaire) in Tokelauan children who were the offspring of migrants to New Zealand with children in Tokelau: 25% of 11–14-year-old children in Tokelau had symptoms of asthma compared with 25.3% of children in New Zealand. van Niererk *et al.* [12] compared the prevalence of asthma in Xhosa children who were living in Cape Town with those remaining in their homeland, and used asthma provoked by exercise as an objective measure of asthma. They found the prevalence of asthma to be some 20 times greater among those living in Cape Town; only 0.15% of Xhosa children living in rural homeland had asthma compared with 3.2% of the children living in Cape Town.

Time trends: secular trends

There is consistent and striking evidence from several countries (which include England, Finland, Sweden and New Zealand) that the prevalence of asthma has been rising. Morrison Smith *et al.* [13] reported an increase among Birmingham schoolchildren and Mitchell [14] reported a similar increase among schoolchildren in Lower Hutt, New Zealand. These increases may have reflected changes in diagnostic labelling and an increase in the frequency of diagnosing asthma, or a change in the local population between the times of surveys, particularly in Birmingham, which was being rebuilt during this period. However, Fleming and Crombie [15] found an increase in the prevalence of asthma and hay fever in a survey of general practices in England and Wales without evidence of a diagnostic shift from acute bronchitis to asthma. Increases in asthma prevalence have also been reported in national samples in England [16] and service recruits in Finland [17] and Sweden [18]. Burr *et al.* [19] found an increase in both reported asthma and exercise-induced asthma between two surveys of schoolchildren undertaken 15 years apart in Caerphilly, South Wales.

The consistent differences reported in prevalence of asthma between migrants and their community of origin, and the secular increase in the prevalence (and probably incidence) of asthma in several countries, although identifying the influence of important environmental determinants of asthma, are largely unexplained. There is, however. considerable evidence for the importance of environmental determinants of asthma, and plausible hypotheses have been advanced to explain the secular increase in asthma incidence and, although less convincingly, the increased prevalence in migrant populations. The major environmental influences examined are shown in Table 3.1. Although these will be considered separately in this chapter, there is increasing evidence for interaction of different factors, such as tobacco smoking, with environmental and occupational allergens in the development of asthma. Inhaled allergen dose is likely to be important, but the timing of allergen exposure may be as important as dose in determining the development of asthma, the risk of sensitization being greatest during the initial period of exposure to novel antigen; in infancy with general environmental allergens and in the first year after starting a new job with occupational allergens.

Table 3.1 Potential environmental determinants of asthma

- Environmental allergens
- Occupational allergens
- Tobacco smoking
- Air pollution
- Diet
- Respiratory infection

Environmental allergens

The major environmental allergens, although varying considerably in character in different parts of the world fall into four major groups – pollen, grains and mould spores outdoors and mites and animal products indoors (Table 3.2). Of these the most important allergen world-wide is the house-dust mite *Dermatophagoides pteronyssinus*, although domestic cats in more affluent, and cockroaches in less affluent, communities can also be major causes of allergy and asthma.

Convincing direct evidence for specific environmental allergens as causes of asthma comes from three major sources – studies of asthma epidemics, experimental studies with allergens in humans, and observations in sensitized individuals both of natural allergen exposure and the effects of allergen avoidance.

Several asthma epidemics have followed the introduction of a new allergen into a community: for example, the increase in asthma in Kuwait following the introduction of *Prosopsis* trees [20] and in Papua New Guinea, where the prevalence in 1972 was 0.01% and in 1980 7.3%, an increase attributed to the introduction of cotton

Table 3.2 Important environmental allergens

Outdoors	**Indoors**
Pollens:	House-dust mites:
Grasses	*D. pteronyssinus*
Ragweed	*D. farinae*
Trees, e.g.	Domestic animals:
Birch	Wanted (cat, dog, guinea-pig, etc.)
Mould spores:	Unwanted (cockroach)
Alternaria alternata	
Cladosporium herbarum	
Aspergillus fumigatus	

blankets contaminated by *D. pteronyssinus* into their homes [21, 22]. The best-studied epidemics of asthma, in which a specific cause has been identified and effective remedial action subsequently taken, have been the outbreaks of asthma which occurred in Barcelona between 1981 and 1988. These have been clearly attributed to pollution of the city air by soya bean dust which was dispersed during unloading in the harbour in climactic conditions that favoured its accumulation in high concentrations [23]. Measurement of soya bean antigen in the city air demonstrated high concentrations during unloading days and particularly high concentrations during asthma epidemic days [24]. A case referent study of 86 cases of asthma seen in hospital emergency rooms during 2 epidemic days in September 1987 found that 75% had specific IgE to soya bean antigen, compared with only 5% of asthma cases admitted on non-epidemic days [25]. No further outbreaks have occurred since remedial action was undertaken to prevent the escape of soya bean dust from silos during unloading [26].

Exposure under experimental conditions of individuals to allergens to which they are sensitized provokes both a reduction in airway calibre – which may occur within minutes and be short lived (early asthmatic response), or after 1 or more hours (late asthmatic response) and be longer lasting – and an increase in airway responsiveness, which is usually associated with, but persists longer than, the late asthmatic response [27]. An increase in airway responsiveness in sensitized individuals has also been reported during the ragweed pollen season [28]. There is less direct evidence of an association between airway hyperresponsiveness and indoor air pollution, but a study of patients seen in hospital emergency rooms with acute asthma found that the association with IgE specific to the indoor allergens house-dust mite, cat and cockroach was stronger than IgE specific to outdoor allergens such as grass and ragweed [29].

The most convincing evidence for the importance of house-dust mites as causes of asthma comes from intervention studies which have demonstrated both symptomatic and objective improvement after avoidance of exposure. Kerrebijn *et al.*

[30] reported considerable clinical improvement and progressive reduction in airway responsiveness to inhaled histamine in children who moved from their homes to a mite-free environment in a sanatorium at 2000 m in Davos, Switzerland over a 12-month period. Similarly, Platts Mills *et al.* [31] observed a progressive reduction in airway responsiveness to inhaled histamine in five of seven patients admitted from home to a modified hospital room for 6 or more weeks. The mite antigen concentration in dust from the patients' homes was on average 13.6 μg house-dust mite allergen/g dust compared with 0.2 μg/g in the hospital room.

Few studies have examined the relationship between measured allergen exposure and risk of allergy and asthma. Sporik *et al.* [32], in a prospective study of children, one of whose parents had asthma or hay fever, examined the relationship between exposure to house-dust mite allergen in their homes during their first year of life and the prevalence of reported asthma, treatment consumption, specific IgE and skin-test reactions to house-dust mite at age 11 years. They found a close association between current asthma and skin-test response to *D. pteronyssinus* and a gradient in the proportion of children with a positive skin-test reaction and current asthma in relation to the measured concentration of house-dust mite allergen in the children's home during the first year of life. Those children who had been exposed to more than 10 μg house-dust mite allergen/g dust in infancy had an almost fivefold greater prevalence of asthma at age 11 years, and the higher the concentration of house-dust mite allergen in the home, the earlier the onset of asthma.

Occupational allergens

Allergens and low molecular weight chemicals encountered at work provide an important potential source of information for the contribution of allergy to the development of asthma in adult life. The annual incidence of new cases of occupational asthma in the UK has been estimated to be between 500 and 1500 [33], but this is almost certainly an underestimate because the cases include only those reported by chest and occupational physicians to a voluntary reporting scheme – survey of work and occupational related disease (SWORD). Occupational asthma is important because it is usually caused by a single identifiable agent, the avoidance of which can lead to improvement (and in some cases resolution) of disease and adequate control of which in the workplace can reduce disease incidence. Furthermore, the well-defined circumstances of exposure and of the populations exposed provide a unique opportunity to examine exposure–response relationships for specific environmental causes of asthma. To date, this opportunity has been insufficiently exploited.

The number of reported causes of occupational asthma is now very considerable: some of the more important are listed in Table 3.3. Asthma caused by both proteins and low molecular weight chemicals fulfils the criteria for an acquired hypersensitivity response:

Table 3.3 Causes of occupational asthma

	Proteins	*Low molecular-weight chemicals*
Animal	Excreta of rats, mice etc.; locusts, grain mites	
Vegetable	Grain/flour Castor bean Green coffee bean Ispaghula	Plicatic acid (western red cedar) Colophony (pinewood resin)
Microbial	Harvest moulds *Bacillus subtilis* enzyme	Antibiotics, e.g. penicillins, cephalosporins
'Minerals'		Acid anhydrides Isocyanates Complex platinum salts Polyamines Reactive dyes

1. It occurs in only a proportion – usually a minority – of those exposed to its cause.
2. It develops only after an initial symptom-free period of exposure which is usually months, but may be years.
3. In those who develop asthma, airway responses – both reduction in airway calibre and increase in non-specific airway responsiveness – are provoked by inhalation of the specific agent in concentrations which were previously tolerable and which do not provoke similar responses in others equally exposed (i.e. in concentrations not toxic to mucosal surfaces).

That occupational asthma is the outcome of an allergic response to a specific agent inhaled at work has been inferred from the finding of specific IgE in serum, or the demonstration of an immediate skin-test reaction, to the specific cause. While such evidence has been reported for the majority of protein causes, similar evidence for low molecular weight chemicals is restricted to acid anhydrides, platinum salts and reactive dyes.

As with environmental allergens, evidence that occupational agents can cause asthma comes from three major sources: epidemiological studies – particularly studies of outbreaks of asthma; inhalation tests in humans; and the effects of avoidance of exposure.

Several studies have reported outbreaks of asthma following the introduction of a new agent into a place or places of work. Probably the best studied were the outbreaks of asthma in the late 1960s in work forces in the UK [34, 35], the USA [36] and Australia [37] which followed the introduction of proteolytic enzymes in uncontrolled conditions into the detergent manufacturing industry. In a 7-year follow-up study of a detergent enzyme workforce exposed to the *B. subtilis* enzyme alcalase Juniper *et al.* [33] showed a clear relationship between the incidence of skin-test reactions to alcalase and increasing category of intensity of exposure to the enzyme. Similar, but less widespread epidemics of asthma have followed the introduction of new chemicals into factories; toluene diisocyanate (TDI) into one [39] and the acid anhydride tetrachlorophthalic anhydride (TCPA) into another [40].

Inhalation of specific agents by sensitized individuals can reproducibly provoke asthmatic responses associated with an increase in non-specific airway responsiveness [41]. Studies of cases of occupational asthma have also demonstrated falls in peak expiratory flow rates [42] and increased airway responsiveness [43].

Several studies of the outcome of occupationally induced asthma after avoidance of exposure to the initiating cause have been reported. In general these have shown that, while improvement is usual, symptomatic asthma and airway hyperresponsiveness can persist in many (in some reports in the majority of) cases. While such follow-up studies are liable to be biased by only the more severe cases being investigated and only those with continuing symptoms being followed up, continuing asthma has also been reported in those studies where all cases were believed to have been seen and followed up. Malo *et al.* [44] investigated 31 snow crab workers with occupational asthma, diagnosed by inhalation testing, up to 5 years from avoidance of exposure. All denied exposure to crab meat, by either inhalation or ingestion. Respiratory symptoms persisted in all 31, of whom 26 had a measurable histamine PC_{20}. Venables *et al.* [45] followed up six cases of asthma caused by TCPA after more than 4 years of avoidance of exposure: five had continuing respiratory symptoms and airway responsiveness to inhaled histamine was present in the five in whom it was measured. IgE specific to TCPA – human serum albumin (HSA) declined in parallel in all six with a half-life of 1 year, making it very unlikely that their persisting asthma was caused by continuing inadvertent exposure.

The reason for the persistence of asthma despite avoidance of exposure to its initiating cause is not known. Cases of TDI-induced asthma with continuing symptoms and airway responsiveness 4–40 months from last exposure were found to have eosinophilic and lymphocytic infiltration of the bronchial mucosa and an increased proportion of eosinophils in fluid recovered at bronchoalveolar lavage, identifying persistent airway inflammation [46]. These observations have considerable potential relevance to bronchial asthma without identifiable cause, as they show that respiratory symptoms and airway hyperresponsiveness can persist for years, if not indefinitely, after exposure to its specific initiating cause has ceased.

Tobacco smoking

Several studies have reported an increase in total IgE concentration in the serum of cigarette smokers [47, 48]. Furthermore, the proportion of cigarette smokers with mucus hypersecretion with a reduced FEV_1 has been found to increase progressively with increasing total IgE [48]. The basis for these relationships is unclear. Cigarette smokers do not have higher response rates to skin tests with common inhalant allergens than non-smokers [49]. There is, however, consistent evidence that cigarette smokers are at increased risk of developing specific IgE and asthma when exposed to several agents which cause asthma at work. Venables *et al.* [50] found that cigarette smokers in a factory using TCPA in plastic manufacture were five times more likely than non-smokers to develop IgE specific to a TCPA–HSA conjugate. All seven cases of asthma induced by TCPA in this work force were cigarette smokers [40]. Similarly, in a cohort study of platinum refinery workers, Venables *et al.* [51] found that cigarette smokers were five times more likely to develop a skin-test reaction to ammonium hexachloroplatinate, an essential intermediate in platinum refinery, and two to three times more likely to have developed respiratory symptoms. An increased frequency of immediate skin-test responses to snow crab antigen has also been found among cigarette smokers [52].

The explanation for this effect is not clear, but airway epithelial damage caused by inhaled tobacco smoke may enhance the risk of IgE production and asthma among those exposed to novel antigen. Some support for this concept of a local non-specific effect of inhaled tobacco smoke comes from studies in animals, which have shown that respiratory irritants such as ozone (O_3) and sulphur dioxide (SO_2) exert a similar effect. Biagini and colleagues [53] found that O_3 inhaled concurrently with ammonium hexachloroplatinate by cynomolgus monkeys increased their risk of developing specific IgE and airway responsiveness to inhaled platinum salt and methacholine. Similarly, concurrent inhalation of SO_2 and ovalbumin by guinea-pigs was associated with a dose-dependent increase in production of IgG and IgG1 to ovalbumin, and a reduction in airway calibre provoked by subsequent inhalation of ovalbumin [54].

Maternal cigarette smoking has also been associated with an increased frequency of allergy in their offspring. Burr *et al.* [55] found that maternal smoking was significantly associated with an increased frequency of wheezing during the first year of life, but smoking by other household members had no effect. Whether tobacco smoke exerts its effects during fetal or infant life is unclear. Magnusson [56] found that maternal smoking, particularly when both parents were non-atopic, was associated with an increase in infant allergy and cord IgE, suggesting an effect in fetal life. However, a subsequent study [57] has failed to confirm these findings.

These observations suggest an interaction between allergen inhalation and tobacco smoke inhaled (actively by adults and passively in fetal and infant life) and allergen exposure in increasing the risk of IgE production, allergy and asthma. It is therefore of considerable interest that the reported rise in the prevalence of asthma, at least in the UK, parallels the marked increase in smoking by women of childbearing age in the late 1940s which continued until the mid 1970s. It is at least plausible on current evidence that maternal smoking during and following pregnancy may be an important contributory factor in the rising prevalence of asthma observed in Northern Europe and Australia.

Air pollution

Although intuitively it seems likely that air pollutants such as SO_2 and O_3 exert an influence on the development and provocation of asthma, convincing evidence for an important effect of air pollution on asthma in humans remains hard to obtain. In part this reflects the difficulties inherent in obtaining evidence. Concentrations of air pollutants can vary considerably over short distances and air sampling can be undertaken only in a limited number of locations; the measurements obtained may therefore not necessarily be representative of the exposures experienced by asthmatics (and others) in the area around the sampler. Furthermore, exposure to a mixture of pollutants occurs and other causes of respiratory ill health, which include cold air and respiratory viruses. Changes in behaviour, such as remaining indoors and increased treatment consumption by asthmatics, at times of 'poor quality' air (particularly with the widespread publicity this now attracts) may also confound any effects in asthmatics.

Notwithstanding these caveats, a study by Anderson [58] found a virtual absence of asthma among New-Guinea highlanders despite exposure to high levels of particulate indoor air pollution, suggesting that air pollution alone was not sufficient to cause asthma. The subsequent increased frequency of asthma followed the introduction of *D. pteronyssinus* into the environment and was associated with evidence of allergy to it.

If air pollution alone is unlikely to cause asthma, evidence suggests that air pollutants may interact with allergens to increase the risk of allergic disease. The Japanese have observed a marked increase in allergy to Japanese cedar pollen during the past 30 years, which they have associated with the increasing number of diesel fuel burning vehicles and pollution by diesel fuel exhaust particulates. Miyamoto *et al.* [59] reported the results of a prevalence survey of symptoms during the cedar pollen season (March and April) in relation to exposure to cedar pollen and air pollution: they found the prevalence of symptoms to be highest in those living within 200 m of intercity roads lined by cedar trees (13.2%), lower in areas of heavy traffic with little cedar (9.6%) and in cedar forests with little traffic (5.1%), and least at altitude, where there were few Japanese cedar trees. These observations were based only on questionnaire results. In other studies reported by the same workers [59], the adjuvant properties of diesel exhaust particles and suspended airborne particulates from air samples taken from the roadside have been examined in animal studies and found to enhance IgE sensitization to ovalbumin to a similar degree to *Bordetella pertussis*.

The capacity of air pollutants to provoke asthma in humans and their importance in contributing to episodes of asthma in the community has been investigated in experimental studies by examining the relationship of use of health services to the concentration of pollutants in the air.

Increased airway responsiveness to inhaled respiratory irritants such as SO_2 is a characteristic of asthma, and respiratory irritants such as SO_2 would be expected to provoke asthma. Inhalation of SO_2 during exercise provoked a dose-related fall in FEV_1 in asthmatic patients, but not normal subjects [60]; O_3 also provoked a dose-related fall in lung function, but this is no greater in asthmatics than in non-asthmatics [61]; SO_2 and O_3 inhaled concurrently during exercise interact to provoke a greater fall in FEV_1 than either alone [62]; inhalation of oxides of nitrogen (NOX) appears to have no effect on asthmatics when inhaled in ambient concentrations [61].

In a recent study [63], previous inhalation of O_3 in a concentration of 0.35 ppm, insufficient in itself to provoke a fall in FEV_1, reduced on average by one-half the concentration of ragweed pollen antigen in 11 asthmatic patients required to provoke a 20% fall in FEV_1.

Bates and colleagues have studied the relationship between air pollution and hospital admission rates for asthma in Ontario [64–66]. Temperature alone seemed important in the winter months and only O_3 concentration 24 h before admission in the summer months was particularly related to asthma admissions. A similar study in Vancouver identified no relation between air pollution and asthma in the winter and no specific relationship with asthma admissions with levels of SO_2, NOX or O_3 in the summer months [67].

The importance of air pollution in asthma remains to be properly defined. It seems insufficient alone to induce asthma and, although SO_2 and O_3 in experimental studies can provoke falls in FEV_1, evidence that air pollutants exert a significant effect in exacerbating asthma is difficult to obtain. However, evidence that air pollutants may interact with inhaled allergens to induce allergy and provoke asthma is emerging and their contribution to asthma may be more important than is at present appreciated.

Diet

The contribution of diet to asthma has been debated for most of this century and opinion remains divided. It is clear that certain drugs when ingested can provoke asthma, the most important of which are non-steroidal anti-inflammatory drugs such as aspirin and β-adrenoreceptor inhibitors such as propranolol. Many studies have examined the influence of maternal and infant diet on the risk of developing allergic disease with little consistency in their results, possibly because of the difficulty in controlling for potential confounding factors. On balance there seems little evidence of benefit from dietary restrictions during pregnancy (and considerable potential for harm) but some evidence that breast feeding and dietary intervention during lactation can provide some benefit. Magnusson *et al.* [68] observed no effect of a maternal avoidance diet during pregnancy, but a subsequent study found that maternal avoidance of eggs, cows' milk and fish during lactation inhibited the development of eczema, but not asthma or rhinitis, during the first 18 months of the child's life [69]. A large study of dietary intervention in infants at high risk of developing allergic disease because of their family history found no benefit from withholding cows' milk, but infants who were breast fed experienced a lower incidence of wheeze, prolonged colds, vomiting and diarrhoea [70].

There is evidence in men, but not women, for a relationship between dietary sodium consumption and airway hyperresponsiveness. Burney [71], in an ecological study of asthma mortality rates in England and Wales found an association between regional variation in purchases of table salt and asthma mortality in adult men and children, but not in women. It was subsequently found in adult men that the higher their 24-h urinary sodium excretion (an indirect measure of salt consumption), the greater their airway responsiveness to inhaled histamine [72]. A subsequent intervention study showed that a decrease in salt intake was associated with a reduction in airway hyperresponsiveness in men but not women, consistent with the results of the ecological survey [73].

The relevance of these observations is unclear. Differences in salt intake have been suggested as a possible explanation for the difference in asthma prevalence between developing and developed countries. However, the lack of such a relationship in women remains unexplained and casts serious doubt on the validity of the hypothesis.

Respiratory tract infections

Viral respiratory tract infections, both colds (defined as uncomplicated upper respiratory tract infections [74]) and influenza A infections [75] are associated with a transient increase in non-specific airway responsiveness. The ability of viruses to cause a transient increase in airway hyperresponsiveness in both normal and asthmatic individuals is not, however, the same as a capacity to induce asthma, for which the evidence remains weak. The most convincing evidence for a causal relationship between virus respiratory tract infection and asthma comes from studies of children with respiratory syncytial virus (RSV) bronchiolitis: asthma has been reported to follow bronchiolitis in some 50% of cases. Rooney and Williams [76] found that 56% of 62 children who had had RSV bronchiolitis in infancy reviewed between the ages of 2 and 7 years, had had subsequent episodes of wheezing; 43% had suffered more than five episodes of wheezing during this period. First-degree relatives of infants who had had wheezy episodes had a higher incidence of asthma than those who had not.

Welliver *et al.* [77] demonstrated cell-bound IgE in exfoliated nasopharyngeal epithelial cells infected with RSV, which persisted longer in patients who developed asthma or bronchiolitis than in those with upper respiratory tract symptoms of pneumonia. In a subsequent report [78] they demonstrated RSV-specific IgE antibody in nasopharyngeal secretions in 60% of RSV-infected patients who developed wheezing, but in only one of 19 who did not. RSV IgE was implicated in the pathogenesis of the airway disease by the finding of histamine more often, and in higher concentrations, in the nasopharyngeal secretions of patients with wheezing and the observation that RSV IgE titres and histamine concentrations correlated with the degree of hypoxia. The close relationship of RSV IgE and histamine to the development of airway disease suggests that asthma may be the expression of an allergic IgE-mediated response to RSV in the airways and may initiate continuing asthma. However, the importance of these findings to asthma in general remains unclear: few children who develop asthma have had bronchiolitis in infancy.

References

1. Burrows B, Lebowitz M, Barbee RA. Respiratory disorders and allergy skin test reactions. *Ann Intern Med* 1976; **84:** 134.

2. Cockroft DW, Murdoch KY, Bershceid BA. Relationship between atopy and bronchial responsiveness to histamine: a random population. *Ann Allergy* 1984; **53:** 26–29.
3. Burrows B, Martinez FD, Halonen M, Barbee RA, Cline MG. Association of asthma with serum IgE skin reactivity to allergens. *N Engl J Med* 1989; **320:** 271–277.
4. Cookson WOCM, Hopkin JM. Dominant inheritance of atopic immunoglobulin-E responsiveness. *Lancet* 1988; **i:** 86–87.
5. Cookson WOCM, Sharp PA, Faux JA, Hopkin JM. Linkage between immunoglobulin E response underlying asthma and rhinitis and chromosome 11q. *Lancet* 1989; **i:** 1292–1294.
6. Marsh DG, Hsu SH, Roebber M *et al*. HLA DW2: A genetic marker for human immune response to short ragweed pollen allergen Ra5. *J Exp Med* 1982; **155:** 1439–1452.
7. Falliers CJ, Cardoso RR de A, Bane HN *et al.* Discordant allergic manifestations in monozygotic twins:genetic identity versus clinical physiologic and biochemical differences. *J Allergy* 1971; **47:** 207.
8. Schade H. Allergische Krankeiten in Human genetic. In: *Kurzes Handbuck.* (Becker PE ed). Stuttgart: Thieme, 1964; 551.
9. Lubs MLE. Allergy in 7000 twin pairs. *Acta Allerg* 1971; **26:** 249.
10. Townley R, Bewtra A, Wilson AF *et al*. Segregation analysis of bronchial response to methacholine inhalation challenge in families with and without asthma. *J Allergy Clin Immunol* 1986; **77:** 101–107.
11. Waite DA, Eyles EF, Tonkin SL, O'Donnell TV. Asthma prevalence in Tokelauan children in two environments. *Clin Allergy* 1980; **10:** 71–75.
12. van Niererk Ch, Weinberg EG, Shore SC, Heese HdeV, Schalioyk DJ. Prevalence of asthma; a comparative study of urban and rural Xhosa. *Clin Allergy* 1979; **9:** 319–324.
13. Morrison Smith J, Harding K, Cumming G. The changing prevalence of asthma in school children. *Clin Allergy* 1971; **1:** 57–61.
14. Mitchell EA. Increasing prevalence of asthma in children. *N Z Med J* 1983; **13:** 291–292.
15. Fleming DM, Crombie DL. Prevalence of asthma and hay fever in England and Wales. *BMJ* 1987; **294:** 279–283.
16. Burney PGJ, Chinn S, Rona RJ. Has the prevalence of asthma increased in children? Evidence from national study of health and growth 1973–86. *BMJ* 1990; **300:** 1306–1310.
17. Haahtela T, Linholm H, Bjorksten F, Koskenuvo K, Laitinen LA. Prevalence of asthma in Finnish young men. *BMJ* 1990; **301:** 266–268.
18. Aberg N. Asthma and allergic rhinitis in Swedish conscripts. *Clin Exp Allergy* 1989; **19:** 59–63.
19. Burr ML, Butland BK, King S, Vaughan-Williams E. Changes in asthma prevalence: two surveys 15 years apart. *Arch Dis Child* 1989; **64:** 1452–1456.
20. Ellul Micallef R, Ali-Ali S. The spectrum of asthma in Kuwait. *Clin Allergy* 1982; **11:** 675–678.
21. Woolcock AJ, Green W, Alpers MP. Asthma in a rural highland area of Papua New Guinea. *Am Rev Respir Dis* 1981; **123:** 565–567.
22. Woolcock AJ, Dowse GK, Temple K, Stanley H, Alpers MP, Turner K. The prevalence of asthma in the South Fore people of New Guinea: A method for field studies of bronchial reactivity. *Eur J Respir Dis* 1983; **64:** 571–581.
23. Anto JM, Sunyer J, Rodriguez-Roison R, Vazquez L. Community outbreak of asthma associated with inhalation of soy bean dust. *N Engl J Med* 1989; **320:** 1097–1102.
24. Anto JM, Sunyer J, Gunalt J, Aceves M, Reed CE. Outbreak of asthma associated with soybean dust. *N Engl J Med* 1989; **321:** 1128.
25. Sunjer J, Anto JM, Rodrigo MJ, Morell F. Case control study of serum immunoglobulin E antibodies reactive with soybean in epidemic asthma. *Lancet* 1989; **i:** 179–182.
26. Anto JM. Epidemiological studies of asthma epidemics in Barcelona. *Chest* 1990; **98:** 185s–190s.
27. Cockroft DW, Ruffin RE, Dolovitch J, Hargreave FE. Allergen induced increase in non-allergic bronchial reactivity. *Clin Allergy* 1977; **7:** 503
28. Boulet LP, Cartier A, Thomson NC, Roberts RS, Tech M, Dolovilch J, Hargreave F. Asthma and increases in non-allergic bronchial responsiveness from seasonal pollen exposure. *J Allergy Clin Immunol* 1983; **71:** 399–406.
29. Pollard SM, Chapman MD, Fiocco GP, Rose G, Platts Mills TAE. Epidemiology of acute asthma: IgE antibodies to common inhalant allergens as a risk factor for emergency room visits. *J Allergy Clin Immunol* 1989; **83:** 875–882.
30 Kerrebijn KJ. Endogenous factors in childhood CNSLD: methodological aspects in population studies. In: *Bronchitis III.* (Orie NGM, Van der Lende R eds) Netherlands: Royal Vangorcum Assem, 1970; 38–48.
31. Platts Mills TAE, Tovey ER, Mitchell EB, Moszoro H, Nock P, Wilkins SR. Reduction of bronchial reactivity during prolonged allergen avoidance. *Lancet* 1982; **ii:** 675-678.
32. Sporik R, Holgate ST, Platts Mills TAE, Cogswell JJ. Exposure to house dust mite allergen (Der pl) and the developmemt of asthma in childhood. *N Engl J Med* 1990; **323:** 502–507.

33. Meredith SK, Taylor UM, McDonald JC. Occupational respiratory disease in United Kingdom 1989; A report to the British Thoracic Society and the Society of Occupational Medicine by the SWORD project group. *Br J Ind Med* 1991; **48:** 292–298.
34. Newhouse ML, Tagg B, Pocott SJ, McEwan AC. An epidemiological study of workers producing enzyme washing powders. *Lancet* 1970; **i:** 689–693.
35. Greenberg M, Milne JF, Watt J. 1970. Survey of workers exposed to dust containing derivitives of *Bacillus subtilis*. *BMJ* 1970; **ii:** 629–633.
36. Weill H, Waddell LC, Ziskind M. A study of workers exposed to detergent enzymes. *J Am Med Assoc* 1971; **217:** 425–433.
37. Mitchell CA, Gandevia B. Respiratory symptoms and skin reactivity in workers exposed to proteolytic enzymes in the detergent industry. *Am Rev Respir* 1971; **104:** 1–12.
38. Juniper CP, How MJ, Goodwin BFJ, Kinshott AK. *Bacillus subtilis* enzymes: a seven year clinical epidemiological and immunological study of an industrial allergen. *J Soc Occup Med* 1977; **27:** 32.
39. Venables KM, Dally MB, Burge PS, Pickering CAC, Newman Taylor AJ. Occupational asthma in a steel coating plant. *Br J Ind Med* 1985; **42:** 517–524.
40. Howe W, Venables KM, Topping MD *et al.* Tetrachlorophthalic anhydride asthma: evidence for specific IgE antibody. *J Allergy Clin Immunol* 1983; **71:** 5–11.
41. Durham SR, Graneek BJ, Hawkins R, Newman Taylor AJ. The temporal relationship between increases in airway responsiveness to histamine and late asthmatic responses induced by occupational agents. *J Allergy Clin Immunol* 1987; **79:** 398–406.
42. Burge PS. Single and serial measurements of lung function in the diagnosis of occupational asthma. *Eur J Respir Dis* 1982; **63** (Suppl. 123):47–59.
43. Cartier A, Pineau L, Malo J-L. Monitoring of maximum expiratory peak flow rates and histamine inhalation tests in the investigation of occupational asthma. *Clin Allergy* 1984; **14:** 193–196.
44. Malo JC, Cartier A, Ghezzo H, Lafrance M, Cante M, Lehrer SB. Patterns of improvement in spirometry, bronchial hyperresponsiveness and specific IgE antibody levels after cessation of exposure in occupational asthma caused by snowcrab processing. *Am Rev Respir Dis* 1988 ; **138:** 807–812.
45. Venables KM, Topping MD, Nunn AJ, Howe W, Newman Taylor AJ. Immunologic and functional consequences of chemical (tetrachlorophthalic anhydride) induced asthma after four years of avoidance of exposure. *J Allergy Clin Immunol* 1987; **80;** 212–218.
47. Gerrard JW, Heiner DC, Ko CG, Muik J, Meyers A, Dosman J. Immunoglobulin levels in smokers and non-smokers. *Ann Allergy* 1980; **44:** 261–262.
48. Burrows B, Halonen M, Barbee RA, Lebowitz MD. The relationship of serum immunoglobulin E to cigarette smoking. *Am Rev Respir Dis* 1981; **124:** 523–525.
49. Taylor RG, Gross E, Holland F, Pride NB. Smoking allergy and the differential white cell count. *Thorax* 1985; **40:** 17–22.
50. Venables KM, Topping MD, Howe W, Newman Taylor AJ. Interaction of smoking and atopy in producing specific IgE antibody against a hapten protein conjugate. *BMJ* 1985; **290:** 201–204 .
51. Venables KM, Dally MB, Nunn AJ *et al.* Smoking and occupational allergy in a platinum refinery. *BMJ* 1989; **299:** 939–942.
52. Cartier A, Malo J-L, Forest F *et al.* Occupational asthma in snow crab processing workers. *J Allergy Clin Immunol* 1984; **74:** 261–269.
53. Biagini RE, Moorman WJ, Lewis TR, Bernstein IL. Ozone enhancement of platinum asthma in a primate model. *Am Rev Respir Dis* 1986; **134:** 719–725.
54. Riedel F, Kramer M, Scheibenbogen C, Rieger CHL. Effects of SO_2 exposure on allergic sensitation in the guinea pig. *J Allergy Clin Immunol* 1988; **82:** 527–534.
55. Burr ML, Miskelly FG, Butland BK, Merrete TG, Vaughan-Williams E. Environmental factors and symptoms in infants at high risk of allergy. *J Epidemiol Community Health* 1989; **43:** 125–132.
56. Magnusson CG. Maternal smoking influences cord serum IgE levels and increases the risk of subsequent infant allergy. *J Allergy Clin Immunol* 1986; **78:** 898–904.
57. Ownby DR, Johnson CD, Peterson EL. Maternal smoking does not influence cord serum IgE or IgD concentrations. *J Allergy Clin Immunol* 1991; **88:** 555–560.
58. Anderson HR. Respiratory abnormalities in Papua New Guinea children:the effects of locality and domestic wood smoke pollution. *Int J Epidemiol* 1978; **7:** 63–71.
59. Miyamoto T, Takafuji S, Suzuki S, Tadokoro K, Muranaka M. Allergy and changing environments – industrial/urban pollution. In: *Progress in Allergy and Clinical Immunology* (Pichler WJ, Stadler BM, Dakinden C *et al.* eds) Toronto: Hojrefe & Huber, 1988; 265–270.
60. Schachter EN, Witek TJ, Berk GJ, Hosein HR, Colic G, Caen W. Airway effects of low concentration of sulphur dioxide: Dose–response characteristics. *Arch Environ Hlth* 1984; **39:** 34–42.
61. Koenig JQ, Covert DS, Marshall SG, Belle G, Pierson WE. The effects of ozone and nitrogen dioxide on pulmonary function in healthy and asthmatic adolescents. *Am Rev Respir Dis* 1987; **136:** 1152–1157.

62. Koenig JW, Covert DS, Hanley QS, van Belle G, Pierson WE. Prior exposure to ozone potentiates subsequent response to sulphur dioxide in adolescent asthmatic subjects. *Am Rev Respir Dis* 1990; **141:** 377–380.
63. Molfino NA, Wright SC, Katz I *et al.* Effect of low concentrations of ozone on inhaled allergen responses in asthmatic subjects. *Lancet* 1991; **338:** 199–203.
64. Bates DV, Sizto R. Relationship between air pollution levels and hospital admissions in Southern Ontario. *Can J Publ Hlth* 1987; **74:** 117–122.
65. Bates DV, Sizto R. Air pollution and hospital admissions in Southern Ontario: The acid summer haze effect. *Environ Res* 1987; **43:** 317–331.
66. Bates DV, Sizto R. The Ontario air pollution study: Identification of the causative agent. *Environ Health Perspect* 1989; **79:** 69–72.
67. Bates DV, Baker-Anderson M, Sizto R. Asthma attack periodicity: A study of hospital emergency visits in Vancouver. *Environ Res* 1989; **50:** 1–21.
68. Magnusson K, Kjellman NIM. Development of atopic disease in babies whose mothers were on exclusion diets during pregnancy – a randomised study. *J Allergy Clin Immunol* 1987; **80:** 868–875.
69 Hattervig G, Kjellman B, Sigurst N, Bjorksten B, Kjellman NIM. Effect of maternal avoidance of eggs, cows milk and fish during lactation upon allergic manifestation in infants. *Clin Exp Allergy* 1989; **19:** 27–32.
70. Merrett TG, Burr ML, Butland BK, Merret J, Miskelly FG, Vaughan Williams E. Infant feeding and allergy: 12 month prospective study of 500 babies born into allergic families. *Ann Allergy* 1988; **61:** 13–20.
71. Burney P. A diet rich in sodium may potentiate asthma. *Chest* 1987; **91:** 1435–1485.
72. Burney P, Britton JR, Chinn S *et al.* Response to inhaled histamine and 24 hour sodium excretion. *BMJ* 1986; **292:** 1483–1486.
73. Burney P, Neild JE, Twort CHC *et al.* The effect of changing dietary sodium on the bronchial response to histamine. *Thorax* 1989; **44:** 36–41.
74. Empey DW, Laitinen LA, Jacobs L, Gold WM, Nadel JA. Mechanisms of bronchial hyper-reactivity in normal subjects after respiratory tract infection. *Am Rev Respir Dis* 1976; **113:** 131.
75. Little JW, Hall WJ, Douglas RJ Jr, Mudholkar GS, Speers DM, Patel K. Airway hyper-reactivity and peripheral airway dysfunction in influenza A infection. *Am Rev Respir Dis* 1978; **118:** 295.
76. Rooney JC, Williams HE. The relationship between proved bronchiolitis and subsequent wheezing. *J Paed* 1971; **79:** 744.
77. Welliver RC, Kaul TN, Ogra PL. The appearance of cell bound IgE in respiratory epithelium after respiratory-syncytial virus infection. *N Engl J Med* 1980; **303:** 1198–1202.
78. Welliver RC, Wong DT, Sun M, Middleton E, Vaughan RS, Ogra PL. The development of respiratory-syncytical-virus IgE release of histamine in naso-pharyngeal secretions after infection. *N Engl J Med* 1981; **305:** 841–846.

4

Asthma therapy in the future

P.J. Barnes

Introduction

There is evidence that morbidity and mortality from asthma are increasing, despite increases in the amount of treatment prescribed. This suggests that currently available therapy may be contributing to these statistics or that it is not being used optimally. Despite considerable efforts by the pharmaceutical industry no new types of drug have been introduced for asthma therapy over the last 20 years. It may be important to understand more about the mechanisms of asthma and also how the currently used drugs work before rational improvements in therapy can be expected. Advances in smooth muscle and receptor pharmacology have opened the way to the development of new classes of bronchodilator, and the further understanding of inflammatory mechanisms in asthma has encouraged exploration of new mediator antagonists, anti-inflammatory and immunomodulatory drugs. Advances in delivery systems are also important for inhaled drugs.

There are two main approaches to the development of new anti-asthma treatments – improvement in an existing class of effective drug, or development of novel compounds.

New bronchodilators

Bronchodilators are presumed to act by reversing contraction of airway smooth muscle, although some may have additional effects on mucosal oedema or inflammatory cells. The biochemical basis of airway smooth muscle relaxation has been studied extensively, yet few new classes of bronchodilator have had any clinical impact. The molecular basis of bronchodilation may involve an increase in intracellular cyclic 3' 5' adenosine monophosphate (cAMP) and a reduction in cytosolic calcium ion concentration. In addition, recent studies suggest that the rise in cAMP is linked to the opening of calcium-activated potassium channels in airway smooth muscle [1, 2]. All of these mechanisms may be amenable to pharmacological manipulation. Several new bronchodilators are under development (Figure 4.1).

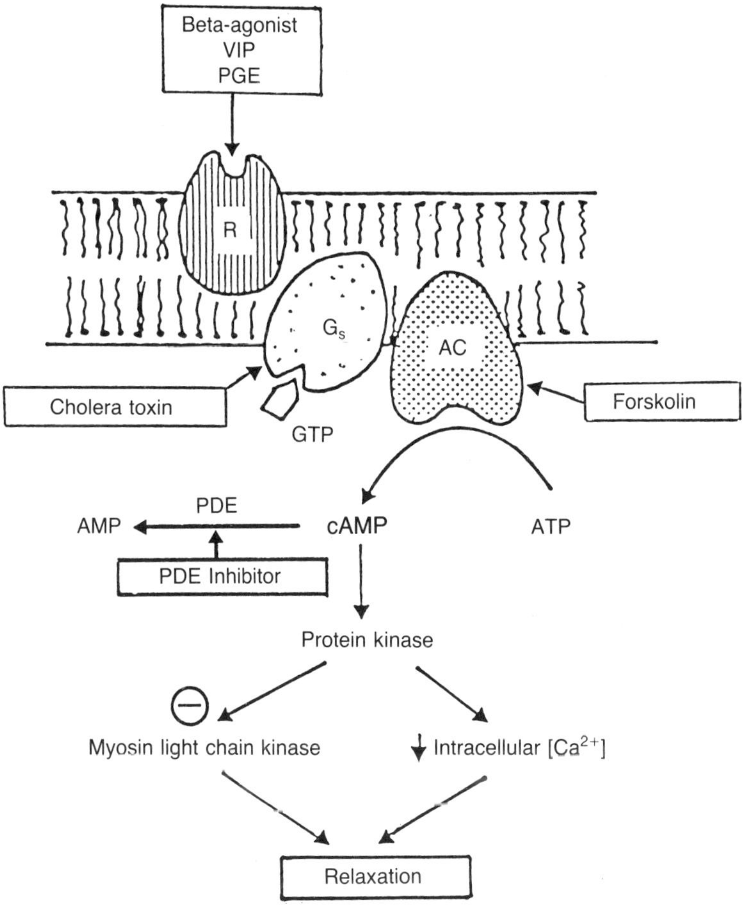

Figure 4.1 Mechanisms of bronchodilatation. Stimulation of surface receptors (R) (β_2-adrenergic, vasoactive intestinal peptide (VIP) or prostaglandin E (PGE) receptors) activates adenylyl cyclase (AC) via a G-protein (G_s), resulting in an increase in intracellular concentration of cAMP, which leads to relaxation of airway smooth muscle via activation of protein kinase A. cAMP is rapidly broken down by phosphodiesterases (PDE). There are several mechanisms of bronchodilatation based on an increase in cAMP concentration

β_2-Agonists

β_2-Agonists remain the most widely used and effective bronchodilators in clinical practice. They act as functional antagonists and reverse airway smooth muscle contraction irrespective of the spasmogen. They are equally effective on large and small airways, and may have effects on cells other than airway smooth muscle, such as mast cells, to prevent mediator release, on microvascular leak, on cholinergic neurotransmission and on release of epithelial factors. Many selective β_2-agonists are now available and there has been a search for β-agonists which have even greater selectivity for β_2-receptors. However, it is unlikely that any greater selectivity would be an advantage clinically, because when the drugs are given by inhalation a high degree of functional β_2-selectively is obtained. Furthermore, many of the side-effects of β-agonists (tremor, tachycardia, hypokalaemia) are mediated via β_2-receptors.

The most important recent advance has been the introduction of inhaled β_2-agonists with a long duration of action, such as salmeterol and formoterol, which cause bronchodilatation and protection against bronchoconstriction for over 12 h [3]. They are highly effective in preventing nocturnal asthma and in controlling 'brittle' asthma. Clinical trials show that both of these long-acting β_2-agonists are highly effective in controlling chronic asthma, have no significant side-effects and (perhaps surprisingly) tachyphylaxis (tolerance) does not develop [4]. It is difficult to imagine that any future drug could be more effective than a β_2-agonist as a bronchodilator, but doubts have recently been expressed about the role of inhaled β-agonists in the control of asthma. Regular use of inhaled β-agonists appears to give worse control of asthma than their use 'on demand' for symptom control [5]. It is probable that while these drugs may control the acute inflammatory response, they do not have an effect on the *chronic* inflammatory component of asthma [6].

Drugs which increase cAMP

Further understanding of the molecular mechanism of β-agonists has prompted a search for other drugs which might increase intracellular cAMP concentrations in airway smooth muscle (Table 4.1). Such drugs might also be effective in inhibiting the activation and secretion of inflammatory cells. Several airways smooth muscle receptors other than β-receptors may activate adenylyl cyclase via a stimulatory G-protein (G_s).

Vasoactive intestinal peptide (VIP)

This is a potent relaxant of human bronchi *in vitro* [7], yet it has no action in asthmatic subjects, when inhaled [8], probably because of problems with diffusion and

Table 4.1 New bronchodilators

Existing

- β_2 agonists: long-acting (salmeterol, formoterol)
- Methylxanthines: fewer side-effects (enprofylline)
- Anticholinergics: more selective (M_3 antagonists)

Novel

- VIP/VIP analogues
- Selective phosphodiesterase (type III, IV, V) inhibitors
- K^+ channel openers
- Nitrodilators (nitroprusside, ANP)

degradation by airway enzymes. When given by infusion the cardiovascular effects preclude a dose that causes bronchodilatation [9]. It is unlikely that a VIP analogue resistant to enzymatic degradation would offer any great advantage over the β_2-agonists already available.

Prostaglandins

Prostaglandin E (PGE) stimulates adenylyl cyclase and relaxes airways *in vitro*, but has not proved to be effective as a bronchodilator *in vivo*, and may even lead to constriction and coughing in asthmatics because it also stimulates afferent nerve endings in airways [10].

G-protein/adenylyl cyclase stimulation

Receptor-mediated stimulation of adenylyl cyclase involves activation of G_s, which may be stimulated irreversibly by cholera toxin. Less toxic compounds which stimulate G_s are under investigation. Forskolin directly activates the catalytic subunit of adenylyl cyclase, and increases cAMP in airway smooth muscle, but has not proved very effective as a bronchodilator *in vitro* [11], possibly because there is a compartmentalization of cAMP stimulated by certain receptors.

Selective phosphodiesterase inhibitors

By inhibiting the breakdown of cAMP by phosphodiesterase (PDE), it should be possible to increase intracellular concentrations and thereby relax airway smooth muscle and also potentiate the bronchodilator effect of β-agonists. Several isozyme families of PDE are now recognized and several selective inhibitors have recently been developed [12, 13]. The isoenzymes which are involved in relaxation of airway smooth muscle (types III and IV) make up less than 5% of the total enzyme activity [14]. Selective inhibitors of these isoenzymes, such as SK&F 94836 (which inhibits type III isoenzyme), may therefore be useful as bronchodilators. Evidence now suggests that type IV isoenzyme may be important in inflammatory cells such as mast cells, eosinophils and macrophages [13, 15], and that type IV isoenzyme inhibitors, such as rolipram and denbufylline, may be useful as anti-inflammatory drugs in asthma. Drugs that inhibit both type III and type IV enzymes, such as AH 21-132 and zardaverine [16, 17], may be both bronchodilatory and anti-inflammatory, and are therefore of particular interest for future development. The main problem with PDE inhibitors appears to be the profile of side-effects. Type III inhibitors are associated with cardiovascular side-effects, whereas the major problems with type IV inhibitors are nausea and vomiting.

Methylxanthines

Theophylline has remained an important treatment in asthma for over 50 years, yet its mode of action is still unknown. It now seems unlikely that bronchodilatation plays an important role in the anti-asthma effect of theophylline, and increasingly likely that some anti-inflammatory or immunomodulatory effect is important. Several molecular mechanisms have been proposed to explain the actions of theophylline, but perhaps the most likely is that it non-selectively inhibits PDE. There is little doubt that theophylline has a critical role in the management of more severe asthma and it is important that its mode of action in these patients is elucidated. The currently used 'therapeutic concentration' of plasma theophylline is derived from the belief that theophylline is a bronchodilator, but it is likely that the other anti-asthma effects of theophylline might be achieved at lower plasma concentrations, thereby avoiding the problems of toxicity and side-effects which currently limit the use of this drug.

The major problem with theophylline is the relatively high frequency of adverse effects, several of which are due to antagonism of adenosine receptors. The development of enprofylline (3-propylxanthine), which retains the bronchodilator and PDE inhibitory effect but is not an adenosine antagonist is therefore an advance. Enprofylline is an effective bronchodilator [18] and shares other anti-asthma properties of adenosine, but is not an adenosine antagonist at therapeutic concentrations [19]. Side-effects, such as diuresis, seizure and cardiac arrhythmias, are less common than with theophylline, although headache is a problem. Although enprofylline is not being developed because of toxicological problems, other related drugs are under investigation.

Drugs which increase cyclic GMP

Atrial natriuretic factor when given by intravenous infusion produces a significant bronchodilator response and protects against bronchoconstrictor challenges [20]. It is likely that the effects of ANF on airways are mediated by stimulation of *particulate* guanylyl cyclase and subsequent generation of cyclic GMP (cGMP) [21]. Nitro compounds such as isosorbide dinitrate, glyceryl trinitrate and sodium nitroprusside are thought to activate *soluble* guanylyl cyclase. A dose-dependent relaxant effect of various nitro compounds has been demonstrated on airway smooth muscle in a number of animal studies, and this effect appears to be mediated via stimulation of soluble guanylyl cyclase and subsequent generation of cGMP [21, 22]. Intravenous glyceryl trinitrate relaxes human tracheal smooth muscle in normal subjects undergoing cardiac surgery [23]. Sublingual glyceryl trinitrate and isosorbide dinitrate have been reported to have a bronchodilator effect in patients with asthma [24, 25]. Others have not confirmed the beneficial effects of nitrodilators, however [26]. These studies suggest that bronchodilators with an alternative intracellular mechanism of action to β2-agonists may be possible and that further investigation is warranted, particularly with inhaled formulations in order to avoid vasodilator side-effects.

Selective anticholinergics

It has recently been established that there are several distinct subtypes of muscarinic receptor with differing physiological roles in the airway [27]. Muscarinic receptors which inhibit the release of acetylcholine have been described in airway cholinergic nerves of animal and are classified as M_2 receptors, which are clearly different from the receptors on airway smooth muscle (M_3 receptors). Non-selective antagonists, such as ipratropium bromide, will inhibit prejunctional M_2 receptors and thus increase the amount of acetylcholine released as vagal stimulation, which may then overcome the postjunctional blockade of M_3 receptors, and may therefore not be as effective against reflex bronchoconstriction. Selective M_3-antagonists that block only postjunctional receptors on smooth muscle should be more effective, but have proved difficult to develop because the binding site for acetylcholine in the muscarinic receptor is very similar for each subtype of receptor [28].

Calcium antagonists

Contraction of airway smooth muscle and release of inflammatory mediators results from an increase in intracellular Ca^{2+} concentration and subsequent activation of calmodulin. Several important advances have been made in understanding the regulation of intracellular Ca^{2+} and many new types of drug are under development. Drugs which block calcium entry through voltage-dependent calcium channels, such as nifedipine, verapamil and diltiazem, have not proved effective in asthma. This suggests that Ca^{2+} entry via these channels is not important in human airway smooth muscle contraction. Calcium entry via receptor-operated channels may be more important in airway smooth muscle, and drugs which act on these channels are currently under development.

Release of Ca^{2+} from intracellular stores is probably the most important source of calcium for contraction of airway smooth muscle. Drugs that inhibit calcium release, such as TMB-8, may have effects on airway smooth muscle, but they lack selectivity and will probably be too toxic for clinical use.

Most spasmogens contract airway smooth muscle by stimulating phosphoinositide hydrolysis [29]. Drugs which inhibit the turnover or effects of phosphoinositide may, therefore, be of potential use in asthma. Inositol (1,4,5)trisphosphate (IP_3) generated by phosphoinositide hydrolysis, causes release of intracellular calcium by binding to specific sites on endoplasmic reticulum. Heparin is a potent competitive inhibitor of IP_3 binding in airway smooth muscle [30], but is not of therapeutic use because it docs not penetrate cells. Analogues of IP_3 are currently under development.

Breakdown of phosphoinositide also leads to the function of diacylglycerol, which activates protein kinase C. This enzyme regulates many cellular events, including slow contractile responses. Antagonists of protein kinase C, such as staurosporine, lack specificity, but more selective protein kinase C inhibitors are under development. The recognition of several isoenzymes of protein kinase C may make it possible to develop blockers selective to certain cell types or functions in the future [31].

Potassium channel activators

Potassium channels play an important role in the recovery of excitable cells after activation, and in maintaining cell stability. Opening of these channels results in relaxation of smooth muscle and inhibition of secretion. Many different types of potassium channel have been recognized electrophysiologically, with the discovery of several selective toxins and drugs. Drugs that selectively activate such a channel in smooth muscle, such as BRL3491 (cromakalim), have been developed for the treatment of hypertension. These drugs inhibit spontaneous and induced tone in airway smooth muscle *in vitro* and might, therefore, have a role in *normalizing* 'hyperreactive' airway smooth muscle. Potassium channel activators are currently under investigation as potential anti-asthma compounds [32]. The active enantiomer of cromakalim, BRL 38227 (lemakalim), is a relatively effective relaxant of human bronchi *in vitro* and appears equally active against several spasmogens [33]. *In vivo* it has no bronchodilator or protective effect against bronchoconstrictor challenge at maximally tolerated oral doses [34], but cromakalim has been shown to have a small protective effect against the fall in lung function at night in asthmatic patients [35]. Side-effects include headache, flushing and postural hypotension due to vasodilatation. It will therefore be necessary to develop these drugs for inhalational use, although it may be possible to develop activators more selective for airway than vascular smooth muscle, in view of the diversity of potassium channels.

The future success of these compounds in the treatment of asthma will probably depend on whether they have any additional effects not shared with β-agonists. Potassium channel activators inhibit the release of neuropeptides from sensory nerves and modulate neurotransmission in the airways [36], but whether they have effects on inflammatory cells is not certain. Many different types of channel have now been characterized; cromakalim and related drugs appear to open a low-affinity ATP-dependent channel. Relaxation of airway smooth muscle in response to β-agonists and theophylline appears to involve another type of channel, a calcium-activated potassium channel which is selectively blocked by charybdotoxin [1, 2]. Development of activators of this channel may therefore be an important area for future study.

Anti-inflammatory drugs

There are several new approaches to controlling inflammation in asthmatic airways (Table 4.2).

Corticosteroids

Corticosteroids are the most efficacious treatment currently available for the long-term management of asthma. Steroids of high topical potency, such as budesonide and beclomethasone, are highly effective when given by inhalation. Future developments will depend upon the development of inhaled steroids of even higher topical potency or which are metabolized locally ('hit and run' steroids), so that the local dose of steroids in the airways will be increased without the systemic effects which currently limit dose [37]. Perhaps steroids that are 'targeted' to key inflammatory cells such as macrophages would also be useful, and the use of liposomes to deliver steroids to specific sites may be considered.

Table 4.2 Anti-inflammatory drugs

Existing drugs

- Corticosteroids: increased topical effect (budesonide, fluticasone)
- Cromoglycate: increased potency/effect (nedocromil, frusemide)

Novel drugs

- Mediator antagonists (LTD_4, 5-lipoxygenase, PAF antagonists)
- Phospholipase A_2/C/D inhibitors
- Neurogenic inflammation inhibitors (μ opioids, SP antagonists)
- Immunomodulators (cyclosporin A, FK 506, rapamycin)
- Cytokine inhibitors (IL-5 inhibitor)
- IgE suppressors (IL-4 inhibitor)

Because steroids are so effective in the control of asthma, an important goal of research is to identify the particular cellular and molecular mechanisms which are of critical importance in asthmatic inflammation. This may lead to non-steroidal drugs which mimic the beneficial effects, without the side-effects which are due to the other actions of steroids. The molecular basis of steroid action involves interaction with a cytosolic glucocorticosteroid receptor, which then interacts with specific nucleotide sequences on the upstream regulatory elements of certain target genes either to increase or decrease the rate of transcription [38]. It might be possible in the future to mimic certain aspects of steroid action by developing agents which selectively influence the transcription of the same genes.

Lipocortin

Steroids stimulate the production of a protein, lipocortin, which inhibits phospholipase A_2 [39], the enzyme that leads to the generation of arachidonic acid and platelet-activating factor (PAF). Recombinant human lipocortin is now available, but there could be problems in its delivery, and it may be degraded at inflammatory sites. The presumed advantage of lipocortin might be reduction in glucocorticoid side-effects, but there are doubts as to whether many of the effects of steroids are mediated via PLA_2 inhibition.

Mediator antagonists

Many different inflammatory mediators have been implicated in asthma, and several specific receptor antagonists and synthesis inhibitors have been developed that will prove invaluable in working out the contribution of each mediator. Because many mediators probably contribute to the pathological features of asthma, it seems unlikely that a single antagonist will have a major clinical effect, compared with non-specific agents such as β-agonists and corticosteroids. However, until such drugs have been evaluated in careful clinical studies, it is not possible to predict their value.

Lipid mediators may play an important role in asthmatic inflammation. Several potent leukotriene, PAF and thromboxane antagonists have been developed and are currently undergoing clinical trials. Initial results appear to suggest that potent leukotriene antagonists, such as MK-571 and ICI 204,219, have a significant protective effect against some constrictor challenges, such as exercise and allergen [40, 41], and long-term clinical trials are now under way, with preliminary encouraging results. Although PAF has several properties which suggest that it may play an important role in asthma [42], recent studies with potent PAF antagonists show no effect on allergen challenge [43, 44]. It seems rather unlikely that antagonizing a single mediator will ever be as useful as less specific therapies, but such therapies may have the advantage of fewer side-effects and oral administration. Certain types of asthmatic patient may respond much better to these more specific therapies.

Enzyme inhibitors

An alternative to antagonists of mediator receptors are drugs which inhibit the enzymes involved in mediator synthesis. Because PLA_2 appears to be of critical importance in the generation of all lipid mediators, it is a suitable target for inhibitory drugs. Drugs, other than steroids, that inhibit PLA_2 (such as mepacrine) might be expected to share the beneficial effects of steroids, but mepacrine is weak acting and non-specific. Perhaps more potent and selective PLA_2 inhibitors, such as manoalide (derived from a sponge), may be useful leads in developing such inhibitors in the future [45]. Inhibition of phospholipase C, which is the enzyme leading to breakdown of phosphoinositide, could also be useful, as discussed above.

Cyclo-oxygenase inhibitors, which inhibit the formation of prostaglandins and thromboxane, are of no obvious therapeutic value in asthma, and in a small group of asthmatics with aspirin-sensitive asthma they may cause a deterioration in asthma .

5-Lipoxygenase is the critical enzyme involved in the generation of leukotrienes. Several drugs have been developed which inhibit this enzyme, although most of these compounds are very weak. Thus zileuton, the most effective of these drugs available for clinical use, has only a trivial inhibitory effect on allergen induced responses and leukotriene production [46]. Zileuton, as most other 5-lipoxygenase inhibitors, appears to work as a redox inhibitor of the enzyme, but more recently a novel inhibitor MK-886 has been developed, which appears to bind to a 5-lipoxygenase activating protein in the cell membrane, to which cytosolic 5-lipoxygenase must bind in order to be active [47]. There is a theoretical advantage to using 5-lipoxygenase inhibitors over leukotriene antagonists because the formation of LTB_4 and other 5-lipoxygenase products, as well as sulphidopeptide leukotrienes, will be inhibited.

Inhibitors of neurogenic inflammation

Neuropeptides, which may be released from sensory nerves in airways in asthma via an axon reflex, might amplify the inflammatory response [48]. There are several approaches to inhibiting these local reflexes [49] (Figure 4.2). Antagonists of sensory neuropeptides, such as substance P, neurokinin A and calcitonin gene-related

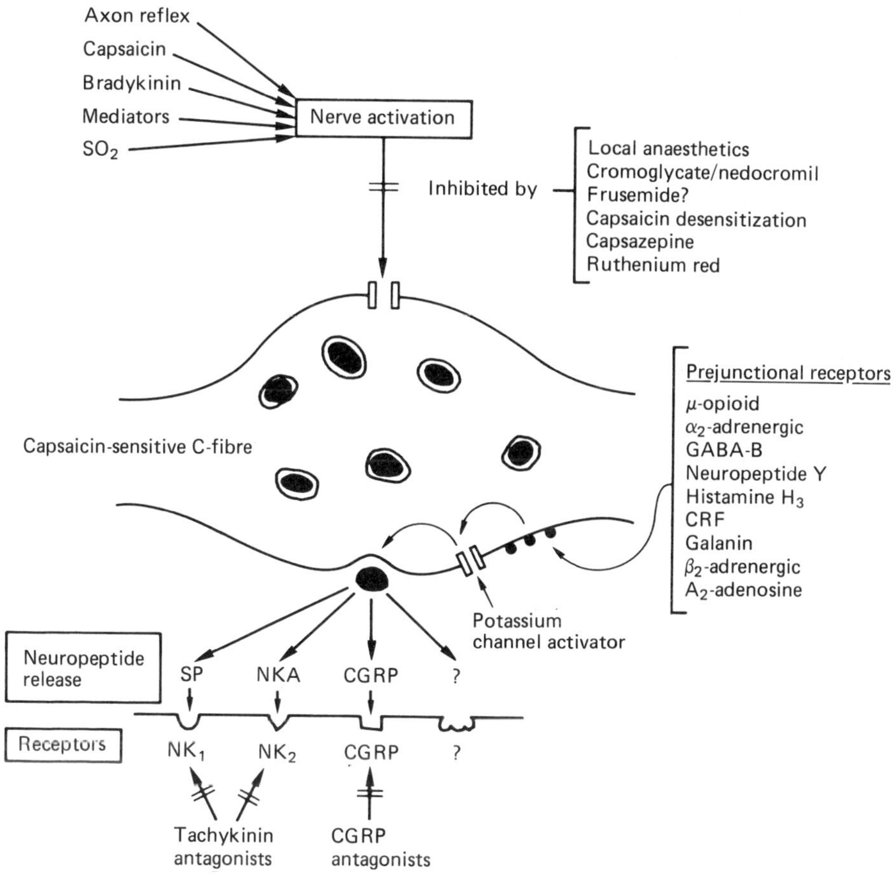

Figure 4.2 Modulation of neurogenic inflammation. Neurogenic inflammation may be blocked by antagonizing neuropeptide receptors, by inhibiting release of neuropeptides via prejunctional receptors, or by inhibiting the activation of sensory nerves

peptide, are currently under development. Most of the inflammatory effects of tachykinins are mediated by NK_1-receptors and several selective antagonists have been developed. A potent non-peptide NK_1-antagonist, CP-96,345, has recently been described, and may prove to be a very useful lead compound which avoids all the problems associated with the development of peptide antagonists [50]. This antagonist is extremely effective in blocking the inflammatory effects of tachykinins released endogenously by nerve stimulation [51].

Another approach is to inhibit the *release* of these peptides from C-fibres rather than to block their effects, because several peptides are likely to be released from sensory nerves. Opioids markedly inhibit sensory neuropeptide release and have been shown to block neurogenic plasma exudation, mucus secretion and bronchoconstriction in guinea pigs and neurogenic mucus secretion in human airways [8]. Opioids which act peripherally, such as the opioid peptide BW443C, may be effective in reducing neurogenic inflammation in asthma (and also the associated sensory symptoms such as cough) [52]. Inhaled BW443C has no effect on resting lung function or on bronchoconstriction induced by metabisulphite [53], although it is likely to be rapidly degraded by epithelial enzymes. More stable peripherally active opioid agonists are now under development. Several other agonists act on prejunctional receptors on sensory nerves in airways to inhibit neuropeptide release; these include α_2-agonists, γ-amino butyric acid, and histamine H_3 agonists, which all appear to open a common potassium channel that is blocked by charybdotoxin [8].

A third possibility is to inhibit activation of sensory nerves. This may be achieved by drugs such as sodium cromoglycate and nedocromil sodium, which appear to stabilize unmyelinated nerves in airways [54]. Another drug with a similar profile of activity is the loop diuretic frusemide.

A more radical solution is to deplete sensory nerves of neuropeptides using capsaicin. This approach has been successful in vasomotor rhinitis, and local application of capsaicin markedly reduces symptoms of rhinitis for several months [55].

Frusemide

Inhaled frusemide protects against 'indirect' bronchoconstrictor challenges such as exercise, fog, allergen, sodium metabisulphite and adenosine, but has no effect against direct bronchoconstrictor challenges such as histamine, methacholine and $PGF_{2\alpha}$ [56]. These effects mimic those of sodium cromoglycate but inhaled frusemide also inhibits certain types of induced cough [57]. The mechanism of action of frusemide in asthma is not certain, but it is ineffective sytemically, suggesting that it acts at the airway surface. Frusemide works as a diuretic by inhibiting the $Na^+/K^+/Cl^-$ cotransporter in renal tubular cells, but the more potent inhibitor bumetanide is ineffective in the same challenges [58]. Some effects of frusemide are mediated by the release of PGE_2, but cyclo-oxygenase inhibition does not abolish the anti-asthma effect. The most likely possibility is that frusemide blocks a certain type of Cl^- channel that is necessary for the activation of inflammatory cells and sensory nerves. Indeed, frusemide is effective in blocking eosinophil activation and airway sensory nerves, and its actions are mimicked by Cl^-- channel-blocking drugs [59]. Frusemide itself causes diuresis when inhaled in high concentrations, but it is possible that derivatives with lower diuretic potency or selective Cl^- channel blockers may be developed for use in asthma in the future.

Immunomodulators

T lymphocytes may play a critical role in initiating and maintaining the inflammatory process in asthma via the release of cytokines. Methotrexate has a steroid-sparing effect in asthma, probably acting as a non-specific immunosuppressive or anti-inflammatory agent [60, 61]. The side-effects of methotrexate (particularly nausea and blood dyscrasias) preclude its use in all but the most severe asthmatic patients who have problems with oral steroids.

More specific immunomodulators, such as cyclosporin A, which have an inhibitory effect on T lymphocyte function, might be more useful in controlling asthma, and there is some evidence that low-dose cyclosporin A improves lung function in steroid-dependent asthmatics [62]. The nephrotoxicity of cyclosporin A would limit its widespread use but derivatives with lower nephrotoxicity are being developed and the possibility of using inhaled cyclosporin is being explored. Other immunomodulators such as FK506 and rapamycin appear to be more potent and less toxic.

Cytokine inhibitors

There is increasing evidence that cytokines may participate in the inflammatory response in asthma. Interleukin (IL)-1, IL-8 tumour necrosis factor and GM-CSF from macrophages, and IL-3, IL-4 and IL-5 from CD4+ T lymphocytes may all be involved in the chronic inflammation in asthmatic airways, together with additional cytokines (GM-CSF, IL-6, IL-8) which may be released from epithelial cells of the airways. Drugs that interfere with the production or action of these cytokines may therefore prove to be of benefit in asthma. Indeed corticosteroids may be effective in asthma by suppressing cytokine synthesis in inflammatory cells [63]. It may prove difficult to develop specific receptor antagonists for cytokines, because they are large peptides and have a very high affinity for their receptors. Strategies such as antisense nucleotides, which would inactivate the specific mRNA encoded by cytokine genes, may be a more optimistic approach [64]. A naturally occurring antagonist of IL-1 has been isolated, and similar antagonists of other cytokines may be discovered, which could lead to the development of future antagonists. Specific antibodies to various cytokines have been developed, but while these may be suitable for revealing the roles of various cytokines [65], they would not be suitable for long-term administration.

Cell adhesion blockers

It is now recognized that the infiltration of inflammatory cells into tissues is dependent on adhesion of blood-borne inflammatory cells to endothelial cells prior to migration to the inflammatory site [66]. This depends upon specific glycoprotein adhesion molecules (integrins) on leucocytes, lymphocytes and on endothelial cells, which may be upregulated, or expressed on the cell surface in response to various stimuli such as cytokines or mediators such as PAF or leukotrienes. Monoclonal antibodies that inhibit these adhesion molecules therefore may prevent inflammatory cell infiltration. Thus, a monoclonal antibody to ICAM-1 on endothelial cells prevents the eosinophil infiltration into airways and the increase in bronchial reactivity after allergen exposure in sensitized primates [67]. Synthetic peptides containing the sequence critical for adhesion may have therapeutic potential. Some integrins bind to the tripeptide sequence Arg–Gly–Asp, and may therefore inhibit leucocyte adhesion. Another possibility is to inhibit the expression of adhesion molecules on the cell surface, for example 3-deazoadenosine inhibits cytokine-mediated induction of ICAM-1 [68].

IgE suppression

Release of mediators in asthma may be IgE-dependent, and therefore an alternative approach may be to inhibit the synthesis of IgE. Suppressor factors which inhibit IgE synthesis and which are related in structure to the IgE receptor have been described, but have proved disappointing *in vivo*. IgE synthesis by B lymphocytes is dependent on IL-4, so that IL-4 synthesis inhibitors or receptor antagonists would be useful in allergy suppression [69].

Conclusions

Many different therapeutic approaches to the treatment of asthma may be possible, yet few new drugs have been developed. By far the most effective bronchodilator drugs are the β_2-agonists, which lead to rapid symptomatic relief. Now that inhaled β_2-agonists with a long duration of action have been developed it is difficult to imagine that more effective bronchodilators could be discovered. Similarly, inhaled corticosteroids are extremely effective as long-term treatment in asthma and suppress the underlying inflammatory process. It follows that a combination of inhaled steroids and β-agonists is required and combined inhalers would seem to be a sensible development, since they will improve the compliance of inhaled steroids (which is poor because of the lack of immediate bronchodilator effect). The ideal drug for asthma treatment would probably be a tablet that can be administered once daily to improve compliance: it should have no side-effects, which means that it should be specific for the abnormality of asthma (or allergy).

Future developments in asthma therapy should be directed towards the inflammatory mechanisms and perhaps more specific therapy may one day be developed. The possibility of developing a 'cure' for asthma seems remote, but when more is known about the genetic abnormalities of asthma such a therapy may be possible. Advances in molecular biology may aid the development of drugs that can specifically switch off relevant genes, but more must be discovered about the basic mechanisms of asthma before such advances are possible.

References

1. Jones TR, Charette L, Garcia ML, Kaczorowski GJ. Selective inhibition of relaxation of guinea-pig trachea by charybdotoxin, a potent Ca^{++}-activated K^+ channel inhibitor. *J Pharmacol Exp Ther* 1990; **225:** 697–706.
2. Miura M, Belvisi MG, Stretton CD, Yacoub MH, Barnes PJ. Role of potassium channels in bronchodilator responses in human airways. *Am Rev Respir Dis* 1992; **146:** 132–136.
3. Lofdahl CG, Chung KF. Long-acting β_2-adrenoceptor agonists: a new perspective in the treatment of asthma. *Eur Respir J* 1991; **4:** 218–226.
4. Ullman A, Hedner J, Svedmyr N. Inhaled salmeterol and salbutamol in asthmatic patients. An evaluation of asthma symptoms and the possible development of tachyphylaxis. *Am Rev Respir Dis* 1990; **142:** 571–575.
5. Sears MR, Taylor DR, Print CG *et al.* Regular inhaled beta-agonist treatment in bronchial asthma. *Lancet* 1990; **336:** 1391–1396.
6. Barnes PJ, Chung KF. Questions about inhaled β_2-agonists in asthma. *Trends Pharmacol Sci* 1992; **13:** 20–23.
7. Palmer JBD, Cuss FMC, Barnes PJ. VIP and PHM and their role in nonadrenergic inhibitory responses in isolated human airways. *J Appl Physiol* 1986; **61:** 1322–1328.

8. Barnes PJ, Dixon CMS. The effect of inhaled vasoactive intestinal peptide on bronchial reactivity to histamine in man. *Am Rev Respir Dis* 1984; **130:** 162–166.
9. Palmer JBD, Cuss FMC, Warren JB, Barnes PJ. The effect of infused vasoactive intestinal peptide on airway function in normal subjects. *Thorax* 1986; **41:** 663–666.
10. Walters EH, Davies BH. Dual effect of prostaglandin E_2 on normal airways smooth muscle *in vivo*. *Thorax* 1982; **37:** 918–922.
11. Waldeck B, Widmark E. Comparison of the effects of forskolin and isoprenaline on tracheal, cardiac and skeletal muscles from guinea-pig. *Eur J Pharmacol* 1985; **112:** 349–353.
12. Beavo JA, Reifsnyder DH. Primary sequence of cyclic nucleotide phosphodiesterase isoenzymes and the design of selective inhibitors. *Trends Pharmacol Sci* 1990; **11:** 150–155.
13. Nicholson CD, Challiss RAJ, Shahid M. Differential modulation of tissue function and therapeutic potential of selective inhibitors of cyclic nucleotide phosphodiesterase isoenzymes. *Trends Pharmacol Sci* 1991; **12:** 19–27.
14. Torphy TJ, Undem RJ. Phosphodiesterase inhibitors: new opportunities for the treatment of asthma. *Thorax* 1991; **46:** 499–503.
15. Dent G, Giembycz MA, Rabe KF, Barnes PJ. Inhibition of eosinophil cyclic nucleotide PDF activity and opsonized zymosan-stimulated respiratory burst by 'type IV' PDE inhibitors. *Br J Pharmacol* 1991; **103:** 1339–1346.
16. Giembycz MA, Barnes PJ. Selective inhibition of a high affinity type IV cAMP phosphodiesterase in bovine trachealis by AH 21-132. *Biochem Pharmacol* 1991; **42:** 663–677.
17. Dent G, Evans PM, Chung KF, Barnes PJ. Zardaverine inhibits respiratory burst activity in human eosinophils. *Am Rev Respir Dis* 1990; **141:** A392.
18. Chapman KP, Boucher S, Hyland RH *et al.* A comparison of enprofylline and theophylline in the maintenance therapy of chronic reversible obstructive airway disease. *J Allergy Clin Immunol* 1990; **85:** 514–521.
19. Persson CGA. Development of safer xanthine drugs for the treatment of obstructive airways disease. *J Allergy Clin Immunol* 1986; **78:** 817–824.
20. Hulks G, Jardine AG, Connell JMC, Thomson NC. Bronchodilator effect of atrial natriuretic peptide in asthma. *BMJ* 1989; **292:** 1081–1082.
21. Ishii K, Murad F. ANP relaxes bovine tracheal smooth muscle and increase cGMP. *Am J Physiol* 1989; **256:** C495–500.
22. Gruetter CA, Childers CC, Bosserman MK, Lemke SM, Ball JG, Valentovic MA. Comparison of relaxation induced by glyceryl trinitrate, isosorbide dinitrate and sodium nitroprusside in bovine airways. *Am Rev Respir Dis* 1989; **139:** 1192–1197.
23. Byrick RJ, Hobbs EG, Martineau R, Noble WH. Nitroglycerin relaxes large airways. *Anesth Analg* 1983; **62:** 421–425.
24. Hirschleiter L, Arora Y. Nitrates in the treatment of bronchial asthma. *Br J Dis Chest* 1961; **39:** 275–283.
25. Okayama M, Sasaki H, Takishima T. Bronchodilator effect of sublingual isosorbide dinitrate in asthma. *Eur J Clin Pharmacol* 1984; **26:** 151–155.
26. Miller WC, Shultz TF. Failure of nitroglycerin as a bronchodilator. *Am Rev Respir Dis* 1979; 120: 471–472.
27. Barnes PJ. Muscarinic receptors in airways: recent developments. *J Appl Physiol* 1990; **68:** 1777–1785.
28. Kurtenbach E, Curtis CAM, Pedder EK, Aiken A, Harris ACM, Hulme EC. Muscarinic acetylcholine receptors. *J Biol Chem* 1990; **265:** 13702–13708.
29. Hall I, Chilvers ER. Inositol phosphates and airway smooth muscle. *Pulmon Pharmacol* 1989; **2:** 113–120.
30. Chilvers ER, Challiss RAJ, Willcocks AL, Potter BUL, Barnes PJ, Nahorski SR. Characterisation of stereospecific binding sites for inositol 1,4,5-trisphosphate in airway smooth muscle. *Br J Pharmacol* 1990; **99:** 297–302.
31. Nishizuka Y. The molecular heterogeneity of protein kinase C and its implications for cellular regulation. *Nature* 1988; **334:** 661–665.
32. Black JL, Barnes PJ. Potassium channels and airway function: new therapeutic approaches. *Thorax* 1990; **45:** 213–218.
33. Black JL, Armour CL, Johnson PRA, Alouan LA, Barnes PJ. The action of a potassium channel activator BRL 38227 (lemakalim) on human airway smooth muscle. *Am Rev Respir Dis* 1990; **142:** 1384–1389.
34. Kidney JC, Wordsell YM, Lavender EA, Chung KF, Barnes PJ. The effect of an ATP-dependent potassium channel activator BRL 38227 in asthmatics. *Am Rev Respir Dis* 1991; **142:** A423.
35. Williams AJ, Lee TH, Cochrane GM *et al.* Attenuation of nocturnal asthma by cromakalim. *Lancet* 1990; **336:** 334–336.
36. Ichinose M, Barnes PJ. A potassium channel activator modulates both noncholinergic and cholinergic neurotransmission in guinea pig airways. *J Pharmacol Exp Ther* 1990; **252:** 1207–1212.

37. Brattsand R. Glucocorticosteroids for inhalation. In: Barnes PJ, ed. *New Drugs for Asthma*. London: IBC Technical Services Ltd, 1989:117–130.
38. Beato M. Gene regulation by steroid hormones. *Cell* 1989; **56:** 335–344.
39. Flower RJ. Lipocortin and the mechanism of action of the glucocorticoids. *Br J Pharmacol* 1988; **94:** 987–1015.
40. Manning PJ, Watson RM, Margolskee DJ., Williams VC, Schwartz JI, O'Byrne PM. Inhibition of exercise-induced bronchoconstriction by MK-571, a potent leukotriene D_4-receptor antagonist. *N Engl J Med* 1990; **323:** 1736–1739.
41. Taylor IK, O'Shaughnessy KM, Fuller RW, Dollery CT. Effect of cysteinyl-leukotriene receptor antagonist ICI 204,219 on allergen-induced bronchoconstriction and airway hyperreactivity in atopic subjects. *Lancet* 1991; **337:** 690–694.
42. Barnes PJ, Chung KF, Page CP. Platelet-activating factor as a mediator of allergic disease. *J Allergy Clin Immunol* 1988; **81:** 919–934.
43. Bel EH, de Smet M, Rossing T, Timmers MC, Dijkman JH, Sterk PJ. The effect of a specific oral PAF-antagonist MK-287 on antigen-induced early and late asthmatic reactions in man. *Am Rev Respir Dis* 1991; **143:** A811.
44. Wilkens M, Wilkens JH, Busse S *et al.* Effects of an inhaled PAF antagonist (WEB 2086BS) on allergen-induced early and late asthmatic responses and increased bronchial responsiveness to methacholine. *Am Rev Respir Dis* 1991; **143:** A812.
45. Lombardo D, Dennis EA. Cobra venom phospholipase A_2 inhibition by manoalide: a novel type of phospholipase inhibitor. *J Biol Chem* 1985; **260:** 7234–7240.
46. Hui KP, Taylor IK, Taylor GW *et al.* Effect of a 5-lipoxygenase inhibitor on leukotriene generation and airway response after allergen challenge in asthmatic patients. *Thorax* 1991; **46:** 184–189.
47. Miller DK, Gillard JW, Vickers PJ. Identification and isolation of a membrane protein necessary for leukotriene production. *Nature* 1990; **343:** 278–281.
48. Barnes PJ, Baraniuk J, Belvisi MG. Neuropeptides in the respiratory tract. *Am Rev Respir Dis* 1991; **144:** 1187–1198.
49. Barnes PJ, Belvisi MG, Rogers DF. Modulation of neurogenic inflammation: novel approaches to inflammatory diseases. *Trends Pharmacol Sci* 1990; **11:** 185–189.
50. Snider RM, Constantine JW, Lowe JA *et al.* A potent nonpeptide antagonist of the substance P (NK_1) receptor. *Science* 1991; **251:** 435–437.
51. Lei Y-H, Barnes PJ, Rogers DF. Inhibition of neurogenic plasma exudation in guinea pig airways by CP-96,345, a new non-peptide NK_1-receptor antagonist. *Br J Pharmacol* 1992; **105:** 261–262..
52. Posner J, Dear K, Jeal S *et al.* A preliminary study of the pharmacodynamics and pharmacokinetics of a novel enkephalin analogue [Tyr-D.Arg-Gly-Phe(4NO_2).Pro.NH_2] (BW 443C) in healthy volunteers. *Eur J Clin Pharmacol* 1988; **34:** 67–71.
53. O'Connor BJ, Chen-Wordsell M, Barnes PJ, Chung KF. Effect of an inhaled opioid peptide on airway responses to sodium metabisulphite in asthma. *Br J Clin Pharmacol* 1993; in press.
54. Jackson DM, Norris AA, Eady RP. Nedocromil sodium and sensory nerves in the dog lung. *Pulmon Pharmacol* 1989; **2:** 179–184.
55. Lacroix J-S, Buvelot JM, Polla BS, Lurdberg JM. Improvement of symptoms of non-allergic chronic rhinitis by local treatment with capsaicin. *Clin Exp Allergy* 1991; **21:** 595–600.
56. Chung KF, Barnes PJ. Loop diuretics and asthma. *Pulmon Pharmacol* 1992; **5:** 1–7.
57. Ventresca GP, Nichol GM, Barnes PJ, Chung KF. Inhaled furosemide inhibits cough induced by low chloride content solutions but not by capsaicin. *Am Rev Respir Dis* 1990; **142:** 143–146.
58. O'Connor BJ, Chung KF, Chen-Wordsell YM, Fuller RW, Barnes PJ. Effect of inhaled furosemide and bumetamide on adenosine 5'-monophosphate and sodium metabisulphite-induced bronchoconstriction. *Am Rev Respir Dis* 1991; **143:** 1329–1333.
59. Perkins RS, Dent G, Chung KF, Barnes PJ. Effects of anion transport inhibitors and chloride ions on eosinophil respiratory burst activity. *Am Rev Respir Dis* 1991; **143:** A331.
60. Mullarkey MF, Lammert JK, Blumenstein BA. Long-term methotrexate treatment in corticosteroid-dependent asthma. *Ann Intern Med* 1990; **112:** 577–581.
61. Shiner RJ, Nunn AJ, Chung KF, Geddes DM. Randomized, double-blind, placebo-controlled trial of methotrexate in steroid-dependent asthma. *Lancet* 1990; **336:** 137–140.
62. Alexander A, Barnes NC, Kay AB. Cyclosporin A in chronic severe asthma: a double-blind placebo-controlled trial. *Am Rev Respir Dis* 1991; **143:** A633.
63. Guyre PM, Girard MT, Morganelli PM, Manginiello PD. Glucocorticoid effects on the production and action of immune cytokines. *J Steroid Biochem* 1988; **30:** 89–93.
64. Colman A. Antisense strategies in cell and developmental biology. *J Cell Sci* 1990; **97:** 399–409 .
65. Coffman RL, Seymour BWP, Hudak S, Jackson J, Rennick D. Antibody to interleukin-5 inhibits helminth-induced eosinophilia in mice. *Science* 1989; **245:** 308–310.

66. Albelda SM. Endothelial and epithelial cell adhesion molecules. *Am J Respir Cell Mol Biol* 1991; **4:** 195–203.
67. Wegner CD, Gundel L, Reilly P, Haynes N, Letts LG, Rothlein R. Intracellular adhesion molecule-1 (ICAM-1) in the pathogenesis of asthma. *Science* 1990; **247:** 456–459.
68. Jurgensen CH, Huber BC, Zimmermann TP, Wolberg G. 3-Denzoadenosine inhibits leukocyte adhesion and ICAM-I biosynthesis in TNF-stimulated human endothelial cells. *J Immunol* 1990; **144:** 653–661.
69. Ricci M, Rossi O. Dysregulation of IgE responses and airway allergic inflammation in atopic individuals. *Clin Allergy* 1990; **20:** 601–609.

5

Mechanisms and treatment of coughing

R.W. Fuller

Introduction

Coughing is the most common respiratory symptom and perhaps the most difficult to treat. It will be reported by most patients with a respiratory disease and in a proportion of people who are otherwise healthy. The incidence within a population differs, depending upon many factors such as smoking habits, pollution and the incidence of causative diseases such as asthma. The surveys report incidence between 5 and 40% [1]. However, in view of the occurrence of coughing during viral upper respiratory tract infection, it will be a rare person who never experiences cough.

Part of the difficulty of treating cough has been the relative paucity of research into its mechanisms in humans and hence few novel approaches have been taken until recently. This has been confounded by confusion over the role of asthma in the genesis of cough as emphasis has been placed on the importance of cough as a presenting symptom of asthma [2], however, this leads to a belief that the two conditions are intimately related, which is not the case. The second confounding problem was the belief that reduction of cough would lead to deleterious effects in the patient due to retention of secretion as all cough was viewed as a part of mucociliary clearance. This is not the full story as a large proportion of patients have non-productive cough and suppression in these patients would bring welcome relief.

This chapter will review the known mechanisms and pharmacology of cough in humans and outline a plan for the management of patients with cough.

The physiology of the normal cough reflex

Afferent input

The majority of cough sensory nerves are found in the walls of the larynx, trachea and large intrathoracic airways. There are few, if any, in peripheral airways, nasopharynx or mouth [3]. Cough has, however, been reported due to stimulation of the external auditory meatus. Animal physiology has revealed three sensory nerve types which can influence the cough reflex. These are the non-myelinated c fibres [4], the myelinated irritant fibres [5], and the myelinated stretch fibres [6]. In animals, depending upon the species, either the c or irritant fibres predominate as the main tussive fibre. In particular, the dog shows no response to c-fibre stimulation [7], whereas the guinea-pig has a predominantly c-fibre sensitive cough [8]. Stretch fibres appear to have no direct effect on the cough reflex but do have a modulatory role [1].

In humans it is not known which fibres are involved. Capsaicin, the classic c-fibre stimulant, causes coughing, but whether this is due solely to c-fibre stimulation is uncertain [9]. It is, however, inconceivable that c-fibre stimulation has no effect on the human cough reflex. Other stimuli which induce coughing, such as citric acid [10] and the more recently examined low chloride [11], differ in some respects in their human physiology and pharmacology (see Table 5.1). The characteristic loss of response to low chloride has led some to ascribe the cough to irritant-fibre stimulation as these show rapid adaptation in animal studies [12]. There are other, less fundamental, explanations, and it should be remembered that irritant fibres, although adapting during stimulation, will respond again to challenge shortly afterwards which is not the case with human challenge with low chloride. Other intriguing differences, including the sex difference in the sensitivity to low-chloride cough and the differences in the challenges and sensitivities to prostaglandins, may all reflect differences in the mechanisms of the challenge. However, whether these are due to differences in the fibre type involved in the response is as yet unknown. The knowledge of which fibre is the main fibre involved in the human cough reflex is important as these fibres cannot be targeted in the development of novel locally acting therapies until the fibre type is identified.

Table 5.1 Comparison of capsaicin and low chloride-induced cough in humans

	Sex prevalence	*Tachy-phylaxis*	*Abnormal non-productive cough*	*Inhaled β_2-agonists*	*Inhaled diuretics*	*PGE_2 potentiation*	*$PGF_{2\alpha}$ potentiation*
Capsaicin	M=F	±	+++	0	0	+	+
Low choride	F>M	++	+	↓	↓	0	++

± = equivocal; + = increase; ↓ = decrease; 0 = no change

Central relay

In the mid-brain close to the medulla oblongata, at least in the cat [12], the sensory fibres relay with the efferent fibres which serve the larynx and respiratory muscle [13]. This relay allows input from the cortex, as cough can be suppressed and activated voluntarily. In animals it is known that both 5HT acting at $5HT1_a$ receptors [14] and benzodiazepines [15] suppress cough, but the facilitatory transmitters are not yet known. It is yet to be shown whether 5HT is involved in humans, although studies with monoamine oxidase inhibitors [16] and a $5HT_3$ agonist [17] fail to show any effect on the cough reflex, suggesting that 5HT does not have a tonic influence. Opiates do suppress coughing [18] by a naloxone-sensitive mechanism which is probably not solely due to sedation, as sedative doses of clonidine failed to reduce coughing [19].

Efferent limb

Coughing has four phases arising from coordinated efferent input to the glottis, chest wall and diaphragm as well as airway smooth muscle [13]. It begins with an inspiration. This is followed by glottic closure and activation of the respiratory muscles with a large increase in intrathoracic pressure. The glottis then opens rapidly, air is expelled and there is contraction of airway smooth muscle to aid turbulence and clearance of airway particles. This expiration is followed by a relaxation of the airways and respiratory muscle.

Cough mechanisms

In the presence of a normal cough reflex

Cough clearance is part of the mucociliary clearance system, being the ultimate fate of mucus as it ascends the ciliary elevator from the more peripheral airways to the central airways which possess the majority of cough fibres [3]. It is probable that mechanical stimulation of the fibres by the presence of mucus will stimulate the cough reflex, although the stimulus could follow the generation of tussive mediators from cells within the mucus, or some other environmental change which triggers the nerve.

This mechanism will account for coughing following foreign body inhalation and in diseases associated with increased mucus secretion, such as chronic bronchitis and bronchiectasis. This mechanism may also occur in some coughing associated with acute respiratory infection and postnasal drip.

Little is known of how manipulation of the quantity and quality of mucus alters the processes and therefore how it could be useful for altering coughing associated with these conditions. However, drugs which reduce the volume of mucus will reduce the symptoms and perhaps those which aid its clearance by the airflow during coughing may also reduce the total amount of stimulation. Any increase in mucus secretion caused by expectorants may increase, not decrease, coughing.

Asthma

Coughing is a predominant symptom of asthma and emphasis has been placed upon isolated coughing, especially at night, as a presenting symptom of asthma [2]. In view of this, the diagnosis of asthma should be excluded in patients with unexpected coughing. There are three possible mechanisms for coughing in asthma. Bronchoconstriction itself induces coughing, either by altering input from the stretch fibres, or directly activating the pro-tussive nerves. The degree of bronchoconstriction required to cause a cough is large, as a 20% fall in FEV_1 caused by histamine or methacholine inhalation will rarely cause coughing but greater changes do induce cough in both normal and asthmatic subjects. Secondly, tussive mediators, such as prostaglandins [20] and bradykinin [21], may be released; these will be directly tussive and perhaps their release in the late phase of antigen response is the cause of coughing in the absence of profound bronchoconstriction. The third possibility is that there is an abnormal cough response in asthma analogous to the abnormal bronchoconstrictor response. This can indeed be demonstrated in some (but not all) asthmatics and in our experience is associated with the symptom of cough in these patients [22]. Mild asthmatics with no current cough do not usually show an abnormal response, so the abnormality is not an inevitable consequence of asthma and is not due solely to the airway hyperreactivity of asthma.

All these mechanisms will have a role, depending upon the state of the asthmatic process. It is likely that all three will respond to adequate treatment with anti-inflammatory therapy such as glucocorticosteroids.

The abnormal cough reflex

The sensitivity of such an important protective reflex as coughing is finely balanced and the sensitivity within the normal population varies over only a small range [23]. This balance allows the reflex to be sensitive enough to protect the airways fully but not so sensitive that it will be triggered during the normal environmental changes associated with breathing. Therefore, it is not surprising that any change in sensitivity will be associated with morbidity. We have observed reduced sensitivity in patients with cerebrovascular accident who could still cough voluntarily and others have observed the same in postoperative patients [24]. Both groups are susceptible to chest infection, perhaps because of the loss of this protective reflex.

Increased sensitivity has been reported in asthma and in association with viral infection [25]. We have also shown that this is the case in patients with cough associated with angiotensin-converting enzyme inhibitor therapy [23] and various diseases associated with non-productive cough [22].

The mechanism for the increase may vary with the disease state: that associated with angiotensin-converting enzyme inhibitor therapy is likely to be due to increased prostaglandin production [26], whereas this is not the case with other causes. Others have reported inflammatory changes in the airways associated with abnormal cough, but the cough reflex has not been tested [27]. The abnormality is likely to follow airway inflammation in most cases as most persistent unproductive coughs follow viral infection. Other possible explanations, such as an abnormality of the central relay and a change in the nature of the sensory nerves involved, need to be explored.

Clearly, the observation of an abnormal increase in the sensitivity of the cough reflex in association with coughing is important, as it alters the management of patients and may alter the philosophy of therapy; it is also less damaging to reduce an abnormally increased reflex than to reduce the sensitivity of a normal reflex.

Pharmacology of the cough reflex

The known pharmacology of the normal human cough reflex is shown in Table 5.2. Opiates in high doses given systemically [18] and local anaesthetics [28] given topically not surprisingly reduce the sensitivity of the reflex in normal volunteers.

Table 5.2 Pharmacology of the normal human cough reflex challenged by capsaicin

Treatment	*Effect on cough*
Systemic opiates	Great reduction
Local opiates	None
Inhaled β_2 agonists	None
Inhaled anticholinergic drugs	None
Inhaled diuretics	None
Sodium cromoglycate	None
Nedocromil sodium	None
Monoamine oxidase A + B inhibitors	None
Clonidine	None
Granisetron	None
Local anaesthetics	Reduction
Demulcents	Reduction
Terfenadine	None

However, topically applied [18] and topically acting [29] opiates are, disappointingly, without effect on the normal cough reflex. Some agents, such as diuretics [30] and bronchodilators [31, 32], appear to give different results depending upon the tussive challenge used. Both classes have no effect on capsaicin-induced cough but reduce that due to low chloride solution. Novel attempts to modify the response using $5HT_3$-receptor agonists [17], monoamine oxidase inhibitors [16] and α_2-agonists were without effect [9]. Also, unexpected from the available animal data, was the lack of action of either sodium cromoglycate [9] or nedocromil sodium [33] on induced cough.

Few studies have been performed in patients with proven abnormal cough reflex. However, some details can be inferred from studies of drugs in patients in whom the cough reflex is likely to be abnormal: 1 week of therapy with a non-steroidal anti-inflammatory agent, sulindac, had no effect on patients with an abnormal cough reflex [26]; nor did nedocromil sodium given for 1 month. Studies with opiates do not suggest any greater sensitivity in patients with cough [34, 35]. Bronchodilators have been shown to be effective in asthmatics [36] but not in normals when challenged with citric acid, which suggests a difference between the normal and asthmatic reflex, at least in this group. Treatment with inhaled steroids in patients with chronic cough but no asthma was also ineffective [37].

Treatment of coughing

This lies chiefly with the identification of an underlying cause, as non-specific therapy remains disappointing. The investigation of a cough following simple routine history and examination is fairly straightforward: chest radiology and simple lung function (spirometry, gas transfer) should give pointers to most pulmonary causes. Inhaled foreign bodies may be difficult to detect in the absence of a clear history if the chest radiograph is normal and if a foreign body or central airway tumour is suspected then the patient requires computed tomography (CT) scanning or bronchoscopy to exclude the diagnosis. The pick-up of these diagnoses on 'blind' bronchoscopy in otherwise uncomplicated cough is too small to justify the procedure and careful follow-up is advisable.

The difficult patients to treat are inevitably those with non-productive cough; these patients require bronchoconstrictor challenge to rule out asthma; ear, nose and throat examination and upper gastrointestinal investigation may also be helpful. The treatment of occult asthma post-nasal drip and oesophageal reflux will often lead to resolution of the cough [38], but the treatment of post-nasal drip can itself be as difficult as treating idiopathic cough. The author uses high-dose topical glucocorticosteroids and anticholinergic therapy with oral non-sedative antihistamines, but control is not always successful even then. Even with no pointers 'blind' therapy of oesophageal reflux and post-nasal drip (but not asthma) is worthwhile, as these diagnoses can be difficult to rule out with certainty.

In the absence of an obvious cause, the therapy will be disappointing. High-dose opiates will be effective but toxic and a local anaesthetic too short-acting to be of much help. However, both may be used if justified. Over-the-counter preparations contain too low a dose of opiates to have clinically relevant antitussive actions but they do act as demulcents which have a real effect on the cough response. This demulcent action is invaluable if the cough is short-lived and in most cases will stop coughing temporarily.

Conclusions

The most common symptom of asthma still holds a number of challenges, for not only is the mechanism poorly explained in humans, but also there is little that has contributed to its therapy since the discovery of opiates and cocaine in ancient times. In view of the prevalence and morbidity of coughing, there is plenty of scope for its further investigation.

References

1. Fuller RW, Jackson DM. Physiology and treatment of cough. *Thorax* 1990; **45:** 425–430.
2. Corrao WM, Braman SS, Irwin RS. Chronic cough as the sole presenting manifestation of bronchial asthma. *N Engl J Med* 1979; **330:** 633–637.
3. Korpas J, Tomori Z. *Cough and Other Respiratory Reflexes*. Basel: Karger, 1979.
4. Coleridge HM, Coleridge JCG. Reflexes evoked from tracheobronchial tree and lungs. In: *Handbook of Physiology: The Respiratory System Control of Breathing*. Bethesda MD: American Physiological Society, 1986; 585–630.
5. Fillenz M, Widdicombe JG. Receptors of the lungs and airways. In: *Handbook of Sensory Physiology*. (Neil E, ed.) Berlin: Springer, 1972; 81–112.
6. Widdicombe JG. Respiratory reflexes from the trachea and bronchi of the cat. *J Physiol (Lond.)* 1954; **123:** 55–70.
7. Karlsson JA, Forsberg K, Sant'Ambrogio G, Palecek F, Mathew OP, Sant'Ambrogio FB. Respiratory and cardiovascular effects of bradykinin, PGE_2 and $PGF_{2\alpha}$ administered into the airways of dogs. *Eur Respir J* 1989; **2** (Suppl. 5): 390s.
8. Forsberg K. Karlsson J-A. Cough induced by stimulation of capsaicin-sensitive sensory neurons in conscious guinea-pigs. *Acta Physiol Scand* 1986, **128:** 319–320.
9. Collier JG, Fuller RW. Capsaicin inhalation in man and the effects of sodium cromoglycate. *Br J Pharmacol* 1984; **81:** 113–117.

10. Packman EW, London SJ. The utility of artificially induced cough as a clinical model for evaluating the antitussive effects of aromatics delivered by inunction. *Eur J Respir Dis* 1980; **110:** 101–109.
11. Higenbottam T. Cough induced by changes of ionic composition of airway surface liquid. *Bull Eur Physiopathol Respir* 1984; **20:** 553–562.
12. Fuller RW. Cough. In: *The Lung, vol.* 2. (Crystal RG, West JB, eds) New York: Raven Press, 1991; 1861–1867.
13. Leith DE, Butler JP, Sneddon SL, Brain JD. Cough. In: *Handbook of Physiology: The Respiratory System Control of Breathing*. Bethesda, MD: American Physiological Society 1986; 315–336.
14. Kamei J, Hosokawa T, Yanaura S, Hukuhara T. Involvement of central serotonergic mechanisms in the cough reflex. *Jpn J Pharmacol* 1986; **42:** 531–538.
15. Chou DT, Wang SC. Studies on the localization of central cough mechanism; site of action of antitussive drugs. *J Pharmacol Exp Ther* 1975; **194:** 499–505.
16. Choudry NB, Harland D, Studham J, Fuller RW. Effect of monoamine oxidase inhibition of capsaicin induced cough and increase in respiratory resistance. *Am Rev Respir Dis* 1991; **143:** A360.
17. Choudry NB, McEwan JR, Lavender EA, Williams AJ, Fuller RW. Hurnan responses to inhaled capsaicin are not inhibited by granisetron. *Br J Clin Pharmacol* 1991; **31:** 337–339.
18. Fuller RW, Karlsson J-A, Choudry NB, Pride NB. Effect of inhaled and systemic opiates on responses to inhaled capsaicin in humans. *J Appl Physiol* 1988; **65:** 1125–1130.
19. O'Connell F, Henderson J, Thomas V, Fuller RW. Effect of clonidine on capsaicin induced cough and reflex bronchoconstriction. *Eur Respir J* 1991; **4:** 341.
20. Costello JF, Dunlop LS, Gardiner PJ. Characteristics of prostaglandin induced cough in man. *Br J Pharmacol* 1985; **20:** 355–359.
21. Choudry NB, Fuller RW, Pride NB. Sensitivity of the human cough reflex: Effect of inflammatory mediators prostaglandin E_2, bradykinin, and histamine. *Am Rev Respir Dis* 1989; **140:** 137–141.
22. Fuller RW, Choudry NB. Sensitivity of the cough reflex in patients with chronic cough. *Eur Respir J* 1992; **5:** 296–301.
23. Fuller RW, Choudry NB. Increased cough reflex associated with angiotensin converting enzyme inhibitor cough. *BMJ* 1987; **295:** 1025–1026.
24. Dilworth JP, Pounsford JC. Cough following general anaesthesia and abdominal surgery. *Respir Med* 1991; **85** (Suppl A): 13–16.
25. Empey DW, Laitinen LA, Jacobs L, Gold WM, Nadel JA. Mechanisms of bronchial hyperreactivity in normal subjects after upper respiratory tract infection. *Am Rev Respir Dis* 1976; **113:** 131–139.
26. McEwan JR, Choudry NB, Fuller RW. The effect of sulindac on the abnormal cough reflex associated with dry cough. *J Pharmacol Exp Ther* 1990; **255:** 161–164.
27. Gibson PG, Dolovich J, Denburg J, Ramsdale EH, Hargreave FE. Chronic cough: eosinophilic bronchitis without asthma. *Lancet* 1989; **ii:** 1346–1348.
28. Choudry NB, Fuller RW, Anderson N, Karlsson J-A. Separation of cough and reflex bronchoconstriction by inhaled local anaesthetics. *Eur Respir J* 1990; **3:** 579–583.
29. Choudry NB, Gray SJ, Posner J, Fuller RW. The effect of 443C81, a μ opioid receptor agonist, on the response to inhaled capsaicin in healthy volunteers. *Br J Clin Pharmacol* 1991; **32:** 633–636.
30. Choudry NB, Fuller RW, Karlsson J-A. Effect of inhaled frusemide and hydrochlorthiazide on capsaicin-induced cough and increase in airways resistance in man. *J Physiol (Lond.)* 1990; **422:** 33P.
31. Lowry R, Higenbottam T, Johnson T, Godden D. Inhibition of artificially induced cough in man by bronchodilators. *Br J Clin Pharmacol* 1987; **24:** 503–510.
32. Smith CA, Adamson DL, Choudry NB, Fuller RW. The effect of altering airway tone on the sensitivity of the cough reflex in normal volunteers. *Eur Respir J* 1991; **4:** 1076–1079.
33. Hansson L, Choudry NB, Fuller RW, Pride NB. Effect of nedocromil sodium on the airway response to inhaled capsaicin in normal subjects. *Thorax* 1988; **43:** 935–936.
34. Eddy NB, Friebel H, Hahn K-J, Halbach H. Codeine and its alternatives for pain and cough relief. 3. The antitussive action of codeine – mechanism, methodology and evaluation. *Bull World Health Organ* 1969; **40:** 425–454.
35. Eddy NB, Friebel H, Hahn K-J, Halbach H. Codeine and its alternates for pain and cough relief. 4. Potential alternates for cough relief. *Bull World Health Organ* 1969; **40:** 639–719.
36. Pounsford JC, Birch MJ, Saunders KB. Effect of bronchodilators on the cough response to inhaled citric acid in normal and asthmatic subjects. *Thorax* 1985; **40:** 662–667.
37. Evald T, Munch EP, Kok-Jensen A. Chronic non-asthmatic cough is not affected by inhaled beclomethasone dipropionate. *Allergy* 1989; **44:** 510–514.
38. Irwin RS, Corrao WM, Pratter MR. Chronic persistent cough in the adult: the spectrum and frequency of causes and successful outcome of specific therapy. *Am Rev Respir Dis* 1981; **123:** 413–417.

6

Respiratory tract infections

R. Wilson and P. Cole

Introduction

Respiratory tract infection is common despite the protection provided by a sophisticated system of inter-related lung defences. Human evolution has involved developing the lungs from foregut tissues, and therefore the local defences of this new portal of entry have been adapted from those formerly protecting foregut in more primitive forms of life, and are not custom-built for this purpose in humans. For example, the site of the respiratory tract lies in vulnerable juxtaposition to the oropharynx and gullet. Furthermore, because of its function of gas exchange the lung is constantly exposed to noxious substances and potential infective agents from the environment.

Infection may occur because of the malfunction of a defence mechanism, which may be inherited or acquired, or because of the virulence of the microorganism. Chronic or recurrent infection of the airways is commonly caused by the former, and acute pneumonia by the latter, but this is not always the case. The pathogenesis of these two conditions is often quite different, which has implications on investigation and management of patients. In this chapter the respiratory tract defences will be reviewed, particularly with respect to infection, and the pathogenesis and management of acute pneumonia will be contrasted with chronic infections of the airways.

Respiratory tract defences

The respiratory tract possesses a complex array of defence mechanisms, some of which are local and 'first-line', while others are only called upon if the 'first-line' defences are breached [1–3]. Their normal function ensures that the lung is sterile from the first bronchial division to the alveoli. Nasal breathing creates a primary filter of inhaled particles. The vestibule of the nose is lined by skin with sebaceous glands and coarse hairs. Large particles are removed by these hairs, while the pattern of air flow through the baffle system of the nasal turbinates tends to deposit particles on the sticky mucus layer which lines the airways. The nose and paranasal sinuses are highly vascular and provided with abundant mucous glands and goblet cells. Thus inhaled air is warmed and humidified, and mucus acts as a lubricant, dilutes toxic substances, and most importantly traps inhaled particles. The origin and content of periciliary fluid is less well defined. However, there is a major contribution from active water and solute transport across respiratory epithelium [4, 5]. Mucus has physical properties which influence its transport including viscosity, elasticity, surface tension and stickiness; a high elastic recoil and low viscosity represent the best rheological combination for transport by cilia [6].

Mucociliary clearance

The mucociliary system provides a primary defence mechanism of the upper and lower respiratory tracts. Ciliated columnar epithelium lines the nasal passages, paranasal sinuses, middle ear and eustachian tube, and the lower respiratory tract from the trachea to the respiratory bronchioles. The surface of each ciliated columnar cell contains approximately 200 cilia of uniform length and diameter [4, 7, 8]. The cilia beat in a two-layered system of fluid, consisting of a watery periciliary fluid phase, which lies below the layer of mucus. The distance of the mucus layer from the cell surface is approximately the perpendicular height of a vertical cilium. Inhaled particles adhere to the mucus layer and are moved towards the back of the throat by the coordinated movement of cilia; each individual cilium beating in concert with its neighbours at about 14 times per second, producing metacronal waves of ciliary beating. Mucus is transported at about 5 mm per minute in the trachea, 2.5 mm per minute in the main bronchi and more slowly distally in the bronchial tree. About 10 ml of mucus per day is transported from the respiratory tract in health, but this may increase to 200–300 ml in certain disease states [2].

Mucus can be transported by other mechanisms besides ciliary beating. Coughing for example, provides a sudden, high air flow which expels mucus collected in the proximal airways. In the peripheral small airways, relatively low air flow rates occur during coughing, but the high intrathoracic pressures produced may compress small airways, resulting in a 'milking' action of mucus towards the large airways for subsequent expulsion. 'Two-phase air flow', the difference between inspiratory and expiratory air flow, may also make an important contribution to the movement of mucus.

Mucociliary clearance may be impaired when a primary defect occurs in one of its component parts, or secondary to a disease process. Primary ciliary dyskinesia (Kartagener's syndrome), cystic fibrosis and Young's syndrome are examples of the former; examples of the latter include the rheological properties of mucus which may change during disease, for example becoming less elastic during viral infections [9] or more viscous during bacterial infections [10]. An increase in the depth of the mucus layer may also cause inefficient ciliary transport due to uncoupling within it, so that the inner part is moved by the beating cilia while the outer part on which the particles stick remains stationary [4]. Changes in the depth of the periciliary fluid layer may have adverse effects on mucus transport, a layer which is too deep causes disconnection of the tips of the cilia from the overlying mucus, while one which is too shallow would cause entanglement of the cilia. In addition, loss of ciliated epithelium can occur during viral [11, 12] and bacterial [8, 13] infection, causing stasis of the overlying mucus. Finally, ciliary beating itself may either slow or become disorganized due to products of the bacteria themselves or the host's inflammatory reaction [8, 14]. Altered mucus rheology will also influence the effectiveness of cough, and bronchoconstriction leads to lower air flow rates and therefore less mucus clearance by two-phase flow [2].

Local defences

Mucus contains two antibacterial substances produced by the serous cells. Lysozyme is an enzyme which attacks the cell walls of Gram-positive bacteria, while lactoferrin binds iron, an important growth factor for many bacterial species. *Streptococcus pneumoniae* grown in the presence of human respiratory tissue in organ culture, developed changes very similar to bacteria treated with lysozyme *in vitro* [15, 16], suggesting that there are sufficient concentrations of this enzyme in organ culture secretions to influence bacterial morphology.

There are many proteins in lung secretions. Some of these are produced locally, while others diffuse into lung secretions from the circulation. Some proteins, such as protease inhibitors, complement components and immunoglobulin are produced locally to give a baseline defence to the lung, but are supplemented from the circulation during episodes of lung inflammation.

Immunological defences

The lymphoid cells of the respiratory tract are distributed singularly throughout the bronchial tree, and in addition there are well-defined follicles and aggregates of organized lymphoid tissue. It is thought that about half of IgA in the lung is produced locally [17]. In the large airways IgA-containing plasma cells predominate, whereas IgG-containing cells are more common in the peripheral airways. Most plasma IgA is monomeric, while IgA in lung secretions is a dimer consisting of two monomeric IgA molecules joined together by another protein called J protein. Secretory component is a protein inserted into the membrane on the basal lateral surface of some mucosal epithelial cells which binds dimeric IgA, and the complex is internalized by endocytosis and transported across the cell in vesicles. The complex is then released at the luminal surface as complete secretory IgA [3]. Two polymorphic variants of IgA are found in lung secretions, termed IgA1 and IgA2. In plasma 80–90% is IgA1, while in lung secretions it is about 70% [3, 17]. The IgG subclass distribution also differs between lung and plasma [17].

The role of IgA is not fully understood. It may prevent binding of bacteria and viruses to the epithelial surface. Secretory IgA can enhance macrophage phagocytosis [18], while secretory IgA and IgG act synergistically in stimulating antibody-dependent, cell-mediated cytotoxicity [19]. However, secretory IgA has in general been thought of as a poor opsonin compared with IgG, and it has been proposed that IgA could therefore block preferred opsonization by IgG [20]. The importance of IgA has been called into question by the observation that many subjects with selective IgA deficiency have few respiratory problems [21]. However, these results are from plasma levels and may not reflect levels in secretions [22]. It has also been observed that in the presence of IgA deficiency there may be an increase in IgG- and IgM-bearing cells in the mucosa to compensate [23]. Clinically, it is important to recognize the association of IgA deficiency with IgG subclass deficiency, although total IgG may lie within the normal range [24].

Bacteria that cause lower respiratory tract infections interact with the host's defences in complex and often poorly understood ways . For example, an interesting but poorly understood characteristic of some bacterial species pathogenic in the lower respiratory tract, including non-typable *Haemophilus influenzae,* is their ability to secrete IgA1 proteases. These enzymes selectively cleave IgA1 [25]. Cleavage of IgA1 occurs at the hinge region of the heavy chain of the immunoglobulin molecules. The amino acids involved in the two cleavage specificities lie within a repeating octapeptide. This octapeptide is deleted from IgA2, hence the specificity for IgA1. The importance of IgA1 proteases to pathogenicity is suggested by the observation that closely related non-pathogenic organisms do not secrete them [25]. Nevertheless, the role of IgA1 proteases in pathogenicity remains a mystery, as IgA1 comprises only a proportion of the IgA in secretions. One possibility is that by disabling IgA bacteria could protect themselves with non-functioning antibody which would block opsonization by effective antibody [26]. An alternative hypothesis has recently been proposed [27]: IgA1 protease enzyme is expressed on the surface of bacteria and could act as a novel adhesin for bacteria to IgA in mucus. This might be advantageous to the microorganism during colonization of the respiratory mucosa (see Chronic Bronchial Infection, page 110). The structural gene for *H. influenzae* IgA1 protease enzyme has been cloned and a frame-shift mutation has been introduced to permit the construction of isogenic variants that are IgA1 protease secreting or protease negative [28]. Such isogenic strains were studied in an organ culture of human adenoidal tissue obtained from children undergoing adenoidectomy [29]. However, in this study no effect of IgA1 protease on ciliary motility, invasiveness of epithelial cells, or levels of IgA1 could be demonstrated. The authors concluded that either IgA1 protease plays an insignificant role in these interactions between *H. influenzae* and epithelial cells, or the model is an inadequate biological system in which to show their effects.

The importance of IgG transudation into the lung during episodes of inflammation is emphasized by animal experiments in which bacterial proliferation in the lung was prevented by simultaneous administration of specific antibacterial IgG systemically [30]. However, large quantities of antibody in bronchial secretions may not necessarily be to the host's advantage, for example IgG2 subclass is a less good opsonin and yet predominates in the secretions of patients with cystic fibrosis [31].

The epithelium of the airways consists of ciliated, brush, goblet, serous and basal cells. In addition to producing the surface fluids which bathe the epithelium, these cells form an intact barrier against invasion. Tight junctions prevent passage of infective agents between cells, and injuries are followed by cell division to maintain integrity. Ciliary movement, as well as propelling mucus, may physically prevent bacteria from binding to and colonizing the epithelial surface. In bronchial epithelium and lamina propria a complicated series of cells mediate the host's specific mucosal immune response. This consists of humoral antibody responses and cell-mediated immune responses. Both types of response require presentation of the antigen to relevant cells of the lymphocyte series which then mediate an appropriate response.

A small pre-existing population of B lymphocytes, already committed to a particular antigen by possession of complementary surface immunoglobulin, is stimulated into division and secretion of specific antibody – the primary response. If successful this eliminates the antigen but leaves the mucosa primed with B memory cells for an even more effective secondary response should the antigen return. Helper T cells are required to enable B cells to be fully triggered. B cell types proliferate clonally and differentiate into mature functional cells. Mediators such as IL-1 from antigen-presenting cells and IL-2 from T cells themselves stimulate this proliferation. Crucial to these responses is presentation of the antigen to T and B cells by mature macrophages and specialized antigen-presenting cells. Successful presentation also requires the antigen to be presented with Ia molecules, which are T-cell regulators produced by the major histocompatibility complex gene locus present on the cell surfaces. Regulation of antibody response occurs by removal of antigen, by suppressor T cells, and by immunoglobulin feedback inhibition. T-cell cytotoxicity and macrophage killing also require T-cell help and antigen presentation. For example, for efficient killing of ingested bacteria, macrophages require activation by T cells that recognize altered Ia major histocompatibility antigens on their surface.

A number of studies have examined T-cell involvement in normal and inflamed epithelium. Bronchial biopsy samples were obtained from normal non-smoking subjects, smokers without clinical signs of chronic bronchitis, and patients who are smokers with chronic bronchitis and mild air flow limitation [32]. These samples were studied with a panel of monoclonal antibodies directed against cell-surface antigens to differentiate lymphocyte populations. Virtually no B cells were found in central airway epithelium from subjects of any group. Conversely, consistent infiltration of epithelial layers with T lymphocytes was observed in all subjects with a constant predominance of CD8/CD4+ cells. Mean lymphocyte numbers of both subsets were found to be increased in subjects with chronic bronchitis compared with the other two groups. Cigarette smoking alone was not found to influence the scores of intraepithelial T lymphocytes, and infective exacerbations that occur in chronic bronchitis might provide an explanation of this difference.

Cellular defences

The alveolar macrophage is the major phagocyte in the healthy bronchial tree in terms of cell numbers. It forms greater than 95% of total cells recovered by bronchoalveolar lung lavage from healthy subjects [33]. The population of alveolar macrophages in the lung is heterogeneous in that various combinations of surface membrane antigens can be detected with monoclonal antisera, and apparently similar cells have divergent properties *in vitro* after stimulation [34]. The cell fulfils many functions and is probably responsible for initiating and maintaining the secondary immune and inflammatory response when local defences have been breached. The functions of the macrophage include phagocytosis of a large range of matter, including microorganisms which may be killed by the production of superoxides and proteases. Phagocytosis is enhanced by opsonization and the presence of surface receptors to the Fc portion of immunoglobulins and to complement components on the macrophage surface. If this phagocytic capacity of the macrophages is overwhelmed and bacteria proliferate in the lung the macrophage is involved in the production of secondary chemotaxins and secondary phagocyte recruitment is engendered.

The macrophage is known to secrete in excess of 100 products with diverse functions [34]. The processes involved in determining the end products are largely unknown and complicated, and the same cell may, under different circumstances, produce factors with diametrically opposite functions, such as chemotaxins and inactivators of chemotaxins [3]. The cell is intimately involved with antigen presentation and by interleukin release activates lung lymphocytes. The macrophage is also involved in tissue remodelling during episodes of acute and chronic inflammation. It may release several proteases which can digest connective tissue, and conversely it can instigate repair by release of fibronectin [3]. The release of growth factors by the macrophage may stimulate fibroblasts into collagen synthesis. Finally the macrophage may have another protective function, as it can ingest and neutralize neutrophil elastase via specific cell receptors on its surface [35].

The presence of bacteria in the airways stimulates an influx of neutrophils from the circulation. It is thought that this may occur in response to receptors expressed on endothelial cells [3]. Neutrophils are attracted by chemotactic factors released by macrophages, complement components such as C5a and directly by chemotactic bacterial products [36]. They ingest bacteria and kill them using a variety of oxidative and non-oxidative antimicrobial systems.

During engulfment of bacteria by neutrophils, a small quantity of proteinase enzyme (e.g. neutrophil elastase) 'spills' from each cell. In the normal airway, the balance between enzyme inhibitor capacity in the surface fluids (e.g. α_1-antiproteinase) and potentially damaging proteinase enzymes favours the inhibitors and there is no potentially damaging free enzyme activity. However during infections the release of proteinase enzymes may overwhelm the ability of the antiproteinases to inhibit them, leading to free proteinase enzyme in epithelial fluids. This free enzyme, along with similarly 'spilled' toxic oxygen radicals, may damage the respiratory mucosa [37]. Another protective function of the alveolar macrophage may be the engulfment of dying neutrophils before they can release potentially damaging products [38].

The importance of the neutrophil and its ability to kill bacteria by superoxide radical production is emphasized by two congenital disorders which predispose to respiratory infections. First, the Chediak–Higashi syndrome is a disorder of microtubular function, and neutrophils show a reduced chemotactic response and delayed degranulation [39]. This leads to repeated pyogenic infections. Secondly, in chronic granulomatous disease there is a failure of protein phosphorylation which leads to inability to generate hydrogen peroxide and hydroxyl radicals. This leads to pyogenic and fungal infections [40].

Acute respiratory infection: pneumococcal pneumonia

Streptococcus pneumoniae accounts for the majority of cases of community-acquired pneumonia [41, 42]. In a prospective study of the causes of community-acquired pneumonia in Nottingham, which used countercurrent immunoelectrophoresis to identify pneumococcal antigen and serological evidence of other infective agents in paired samples of serum, a pathogen was implicated in 97% of 127 cases. *S. pneumoniae* accounted for 76%, *H. influenzae* 3% and *Staphylococcus aureus* 2.4% of cases [42]. The mortality and morbidity rates from pneumococcal infections remain significant, particularly in patients with well-documented negative prognostic features [43, 44], despite the use of potent antimicrobial agents and the introduction of intensive care facilities [45, 46]. In a review of 50 patients with severe community-acquired pneumonia admitted to the intensive care unit of a district general hospital, 16 cases were due to *S. pneumoniae* [47]. Assisted ventilation was required in 44 of the 50 patients, of whom 25 died, including 12 (75%) with pneumococcal pneumonia. In a recent British Thoracic Society study of severe community-acquired pneumonia, 59 patients were studied in whom a microbial aetiology was identified in 35. *S. pneumoniae* was the major pathogen (11 patients) and the overall mortality was 49% [48]. An increased mortality is seen with advanced age and in the presence of pre-existing illness [45, 49]. In a large retrospective study of 455 patients with bacteraemic pneumococcal disease, 30% of those with pre-existing illness died, but only 7% of those with no pre-existing illness [45]. In the same study [45] the frequency of the first eight capsular serotypes of *S. pneumoniae* was increased, which accounted for two-thirds of the cases of pneumococcal disease with bacteraemia. There was also increased fatality associated with type III pneumococcus, an observation which has been made in a number of studies, although this was partly accounted for by the greater age of patients infected with this type of organism. The variable pathogenicity of individual pneumococcal serotypes is incompletely understood, but may be related in part to the degree of resistance to phagocytosis afforded by the types of specific capsular polysaccharide, and in part to variability in their ability to stimulate an alveolar exudation of fluid in which the bacteria multiply and spread [44].

Complications of pneumococcal pneumonia can result from spread to adjacent structures giving rise to empyema or pericarditis, or from an accompanied bacteraemia, for example leading to septic arthritis (which is more often seen in children than in adults), acute bacterial endocarditis or meningitis. Classical pneumococcal pneumonia produces diffuse involvement of most of a lobe but more than one lobe may be involved in 10–25% of cases, although spread of consolidation throughout an entire lung is unusual, occurring in less than 1% of patients [44]. Mortality is greater in those patients in whom more than one lobe is involved [44, 49].

Colonization of the respiratory mucosa

S. pneumoniae colonizes the nasopharynx of up to 70% of healthy adults [50]. Several studies have suggested that the pneumococcus may adhere to dispersed buccal and nasopharyngeal epithelial cells [51–55] but relatively little is known about the interactions of the organism with the intact respiratory mucosa. It is likely that such interactions are important in the pathogenesis of *S. pneumoniae* infections because it has been proposed that adherence of microorganisms to epithelial surfaces may be an important determinant of colonization, at least in the case of some bacteria [56, 57]. Pneumococcal adherence to isolated buccal and nasopharyngeal cells has identified a putative adhesin with both heat-labile and heat-stable components [52], and a putative epithelial cell receptor in the GalNAcβ1–4Gal sequences of glycosphingolipids found abundantly in the respiratory tract [54, 58]. However, despite these findings, good adherence of the pneumococcus to epithelial cells is difficult to demonstrate, and it has been suggested that its polysaccharide capsule may interfere with the adherence process [55, 56], although strains from patients with frequent otitis media and from carriers have shown a higher adhesive capacity [51].

Pneumonia is predisposed to by conditions reducing host defence, particularly suppression of the cough reflex, impairment of mucociliary clearance, conditions leading to reduced phagocytic activity of alveolar macrophages and neutrophils, and impaired immunoglobulin production [44]. Potential pathogens may reach the lung by aspiration from the pharynx [59], inhalation from the environment via fomites or droplet spread, by contiguous spread through the bronchial tree, or occasionally by blood spread or by direct spread from an adjacent site [44].

While pneumococcal adherence to isolated oropharyngeal cells may be informative about colonization of the non-ciliated areas of the nasopharynx, relatively little is known about how the pneumococcus interacts with ciliated respiratory mucosa. Here the bacterium is presented with a much more complicated task, to colonize a surface protected by the mucociliary system. The importance of the mucus layer in host bacterial interactions with ciliated respiratory epithelium has recently been demonstrated by an animal organ culture model [60]. In this study it was demonstrated that *S. pneumoniae* rapidly adhered to mucus, but never to ciliated cells or cilia. Even after attempts were made to remove the mucus coat by washing before bacteria were applied to the model, pneumococci adhered only to small areas where the mucus had not been totally eliminated. These results suggest that the pneumococcus cannot adhere to normal ciliated respiratory mucosa, in common with other respiratory tract pathogens [61, 62]. However, the interactions may be different if the respiratory mucosa is damaged. In a study in which *S. pneumoniae* serotype I was used to infect the tracheal epithelium of mice previously infected with influenza A virus [63], the trachea was removed surgically from animals either before or after infection with influenza A and radiolabelled pneumococci were instilled. Pneumococcal adhesion to infected tracheas was significantly increased 6 days after viral infection. Scanning electron microscopy and transmission electron microscopy showed that pneumococci did not adhere to the epithelium of control animals, but at day 6 after viral infection there had been desquamation of viral-infected cells and pneumococci were observed adhering to the microvilli of basal cells and, to a greater extent, to the exposed basement membrane.

We have studied the interaction of *S. pneumoniae* with the human respiratory mucosa and have demonstrated a number of mechanisms by which pneumococcal colonization and spread may occur. Pneumococcal broth culture filtrates and autolysates of the bacterium perturb human respiratory epithelium *in vitro* by causing ciliary beat slowing and disruption of the epithelial surface [64]. Subsequent experiments showed that the toxin pneumolysin, released by the pneumococcus during autolysis, was responsible for both ciliary slowing and epithelial disruption by these preparations. Treatment of a filtrate with a polyclonal antibody to pneumolysin bound to sepharose completely removed the biological activity against the respiratory mucosa, whilst replacement of recombinant pneumolysin [65] restored activity entirely, without any evidence of enhanced activity due to other factors present in culture filtrates [66]. A concentration of 10 µg/ml pneumolysin caused complete epithelial cell disruption in addition to ciliary stasis, while smaller amounts caused predominantly ciliary slowing and stasis without epithelial disruption: ciliary slowing occurred in the absence of cell ultrastructural changes [64]. Pneumolysin is cytolytic and is known to bind to target cells via cholesterol and insert into the lipid bilayer where toxin molecules are oligomerized and act as transmembrane pores [67]. A recent study of an unrelated toxin, *Pasteurella haemolytica* leukotoxin, which damages cells by the formation of similar transmembrane defects, has shown an electrolyte leak from cells [68]. We would speculate that a similar change may occur when pneumolysin affects ciliary function.

Pneumococcal products are known to stimulate mucus secretion [69], and infection of an organ culture of human nasal turbinate tissue with a type III pneumococcus showed a dense granular collection of bacteria in a thickened gelatinous layer overlying the organ culture [15]. The scanning electron microscopy appearances of this layer were unusual for simple mucus, and it may consist of either abnormal mucus or a mixture of mucus with bacterial products such as capsular material. Bacteria were found in large numbers within this layer, whereas no bacteria were seen adherent to cilia or to the epithelial surface [15]. Formation of an abnormal mucinous layer in the presence of compromised ciliary function could be a novel mechanism of bacterial colonization of the respiratory mucosa.

The polysaccharide capsule of the pneumococcus is clearly essential but not sufficient for virulence of the bacterium [70]. There is emerging evidence that certain pneumococcal protein products also contribute to the disease process. For example, a surface protein is found on clinical isolates of the pneumococcus and inactivation of the gene responsible for this protein leads to reduced or abolished virulence of certain pneumococcal strains [71]. There are a number of other pneumococcal products whose activities suggest a role in disease. These include an IgA1 protease, neuraminidase and hyaluronidase, as well as pneumolysin. In common with many bacteria which colonize and infect mucosal surfaces, the pneumococcus cleaves human IgA1 in the hinge region of the heavy chain [25]. It has been suggested that the neuraminidase decreases the viscosity of lung mucus, and may aid bacterial adherence to the epithelial surface by cleaving cell surface sialic acid residues, thus unmasking potential adhesin receptors for common respiratory pathogens [72]. Hyaluronidase may act as a nutrient-gaining enzyme for the pneumococcus [73]. We have found that tissue is necessary for the growth of pneumococci in organ culture, and supernatant fluids taken from an uninfected organ culture also supply sufficient nutrients for pneumococcal growth [15]. As well as supplying essential nutrients, the respiratory mucosa may fulfil another function. The requirement for *in vitro* growth supplements from blood or blood-derived products for the pneumococcus is well known, but these supplements also act to buffer against the pH changes induced by the organism's metabolism of glucose and to remove hydrogen peroxide produced by the bacterium [74]. As well as supplying growth supplements to the pneumococcus, the respiratory mucosa in organ culture may thus fulfil another function, as it has been suggested that respiratory mucus may have an antioxidant function [75] which could aid pneumococcal growth.

It seems likely that the acquisition of pneumococcal pneumonia could occur via a number of routes. Once the pneumococcus has reached the alveoli the development of pneumonia would depend upon the pathogenic potential of the strain involved, along with host factors including lack of recent exposure to the particular serotype.

Pathogenesis of pneumococcal pneumonia

In contrast to the bacteria that colonize the bronchial tree during chronic infections, pneumococcal pneumonia illustrates a disease caused by a classic invasive pathogen with recognized virulence determinants. Three stages have been recognized in the pathology of pneumococcal pneumonia [44]. The first is called *inflammatory congestion*, in which the affected part of the lung is coloured dark red due to hyperaemia, and begins to fill with fluid and haemorrhagic exudate. The second stage is called *red hepatization*, when the exudate coagulates so that the lung assumes the consistency of liver. In the third stage, *grey hepatization*, the lung becomes yellowish/grey, because the neutrophils outnumber the red cells. When resolution takes place the exudate liquefies and is coughed up or otherwise absorbed [44]. Complete resolution of the inflammation in the lungs usually occurs, with little, if any, residual damage, and it has recently been shown that following infection of a rat lung model with *Streptococcus sanguis* no residual damage occurs, provided that the type II pneumocytes escape unharmed [76].

Pneumococcal capsular polysaccharide plays an important role in pneumococcal disease, and this is predominantly related to protection from host defences. The capsule protects the bacterium against most of the acute-phase host defences [77]. For example, it does not react well with complement or C-reactive protein [78–80] and presents a significant obstacle to opsonization and clearance of pneumococci from the lung [81]. Underlying the capsule coat is the pneumococcal cell wall, which is composed of two major components: an interlinked peptidoglycan network, and covalently attached teichoic acid. In contrast to the capsule, the cell wall is a potent stimulator of the alternate complement pathway and binds the acute phase reactant C-reactive protein [77, 82–84].

The complement system plays a critical role in host defence against the pneumococcus [85]. The complement system is composed of a number of serum proteins, and the terminal components C3–C9 are responsible for most of the biologically significant actions of the system. The pathway C3 through to C9 must first be activated, and bacteria may accomplish this by either the classical or the alternative pathways. Activation of the classical pathway is usually initiated by the formation of an antibody–antigen complex, while the alternative pathway can be activated in the absence of specific antibody to bacteria. The pneumococcal cell wall is particularly potent in this respect. Whichever pathway is used, biologically active products are released that are important in the generation of an inflammatory response, and in the defence of the host against infection. For example, C5a is a potent chemotactic factor causing the directed movement of both neutrophils and monocytes, while C3b is an effective opsonin when fixed to the surface of microorganisms. The pneumococcus is, however, particularly resistant to the bactericidal and bacteriolytic actions of complement [86]. While the membrane attack complex of complement forms on the surface of the pneumococcus, it cannot penetrate the cell wall enough to insert in the cell membrane and cause death of the organism [85].

Components of both the alternative and classical pathways can be found in the secretions and alveolar lining fluids of the normal lung [85], and complement has been shown to play an important role in the clearance of pneumococci [87, 88]. The number of neutrophils appearing in lavage fluid of complement-deficient mice after intratracheal challenge with live pneumococci is lower than the number in normal mice, but some are still present [89], indicating that other mechanisms exist to generate the inflammatory response [77]. Similarly, complement plays a crucial role in the clearance of pneumococci from the bloodstream [85]. When challenged intravenously, normal non-immune guinea-pigs have an initial rapid clearance of pneumococci from their bloodstream to undetectable levels [90]. At 24 h low levels of pneumococci reappear and are again cleared by 48 h. Guinea-pigs depleted of C3 also demonstrate an initial rapid clearance of pneumococci, but not to the same degree as normal animals, and low levels of bacteria persist in the bloodstream. In marked contrast to normal animals, C3-deficient animals then show uncontrolled bacterial multiplication, rising levels of bacteraemia, and die. This pattern is also true in C3-deficient animals that have previously been immunized with intact pneumococci, suggesting that the complement system plays an important role in limiting bacteraemia, even in immune individuals possessing antipneumococcal antibodies.

The instillation of live pneumococci into animal models is known to stimulate a brisk inflammatory response of circulating neutrophils and protein moving into the alveolar spaces [77]. The number of leucocytes appearing in lavage fluid and animal mortality both correlate directly with the number of bacteria in the challenge inoculum [77, 91]. Using a rabbit model, various fractions of the bacterium were tested to investigate their ability to engender an inflammatory response [77]. Of the pneumococcal surface components tested, cell wall preparations had the highest specific activity, rapidly producing abnormalities in bronchial lavage fluid cytochemistry in a dose-dependent manner. The pneumococcal capsule was also active, but the inflammatory response to it was delayed, with a peak occurring at 24 h, rather than at 4 h with cell wall components. Studies of subcomponents of the pneumococcal cell wall indicated that both the teichoic acid and peptidoglycan subcomponents were active [77]. Only extensive degradation of the cell wall components by trichloracetic acid was effective in completely removing their inflammatory potential [77].

The mechanism by which bacterial cell wall components elicit inflammation in the rabbit lung, and also in an animal model of meningitis [92], relates to both complement-mediated and complement-independent host responses [93]. Products of arachidonic acid metabolism, in particular the lipoxygenase pathway, are thought to play an important role in this inflammatory process and inhibitors of prostaglandin metabolism can reduce inflammation [77]. Even components of the cell wall released by the action of the penicillin are capable of eliciting such inflammation and it has been suggested that *in vivo* treatment of patients with highly lytic antibiotics can for this reason be associated initially with increased inflammation and worsening of their general condition, despite death of the invading organism [77].

We have used a rat model to show that a protein toxin of the pneumococcus (pneumolysin) can induce an inflammatory response in the rat lung which is identical histologically to that produced by whole bacteria [91]. Pneumolysin is a thiol-activated toxin and is a member of a family of similar toxins produced by diverse Gram-positive bacteria [67]. Previous work has suggested that pneumolysin can induce inflammation in tissues. The toxin has been shown to cause ocular inflammation in animals [94], and has been suggested as a possible cause of cellulitis in pneumococcal infections [95]. There is substantial evidence *in vitro* that pneumolysin has the potential to induce inflammation such as has been shown in the rat lung, but this study [91] was the first demonstration of this potential *in vivo*. Pneumolysin has a wide range of complex dose-related interactions with macrophages and monocytes, polymorphonuclear leucocytes, and lymphocytes [96–99]. The toxin has been shown to be able to activate the classic complement pathway [100], independent of specific pneumococcal antibodies. Thiol-activated toxins have also been shown to cause the generation of leukotrienes from polymorphonuclear leucocytes [101]. Although the role of pneumolysin in human infections is unknown, the fact that pneumolysin is produced in significant amounts in these situations is suggested by the appearance of antibodies in the serum of such patients [102]. Pneumolysin is an intracellular toxin released on lysis of the organism, and it has recently been demonstrated that pneumococcal autolysin, the factor responsible for autolysis of the bacterium, may be a further virulence determinant of the pneumococcus [103]. Although the mechanisms underlying pneumococcal virulence are likely to be complex and multifactorial, lysis of the organism will be accompanied by release of potentially toxic factors, including both cell wall components and pneumolysin, which could stimulate and enhance the inflammatory process leading to the histological picture seen *in vivo*. The acute-phase protein, C-reactive protein, plays an important protective role against fatal pneumococcal infection [104, 105]. It is an interesting, but unexplained, observation that a continuous stretch of amino acids in C-reactive protein has homology with two non-contiguous regions within pneumolysin [70].

Providing the animal survived, the inflammation induced by both whole pneumococci and pneumolysin resolved completely, without any residual structural abnormality [91]. The mortality rate of the illness did not relate to the histological features in the rat lung, and no animals died after pneumolysin injection despite them developing lobar pneumonia. Death is likely to result from systemic spread of bacteria rather than from lung disease. In a mouse model of pneumococcal pneumonia in which 10^6 –10^7 virulent pneumococci were instilled into the nose of an anaesthetized animal, bacterial growth in the lung over the first 24 h of infection was accompanied by the appearance of pneumococci in the blood, although the numbers did not increase over this period and no animals died. Between 24 and 48 h there was explosive growth of bacteria in the blood, reflected by high bacterial counts in the spleen, liver and brain and leading to death of the animal [70].

Treatment and prevention

In contrast to antibiotic treatment of chronic infection of the bronchial tree (described below), the affected pneumonic lung was often previously healthy, and antibiotic treatment of acute infections is relatively straightforward. Barriers to penetration of antibiotic to the site of infection that develop during chronic disease are not present, and the host defences may be relatively intact. The antibiotic of choice in the treatment of pneumococcal infections is penicillin, as it is more active against the pneumococcus than ampicillin or amoxycillin [44]. However, the causative organism of community-acquired pneumonia is usually unknown at presentation and a combination of intravenous cefuroxime and erythromycin will cover most likely pathogens. Currently, relatively penicillin-resistant organisms are estimated to constitute only 1–3% of clinical isolates of pneumococci in North America [106], but resistance has become a serious problem in certain parts of the world such as South Africa and Spain, and may relate to common use of antibiotics for trivial illness. Some strains with high-level penicillin resistance are also resistant to a wide range of other antibiotics and, should these strains become widespread, there are obvious implications for the empirical treatment of community-acquired pneumonia.

There has been considerable interest in developing an effective vaccine in order to prevent pneumococcal pneumonia. Vaccination is much less likely to be successful in bronchial infections, first because most infections occur in the context of failure of host defence mechanisms rather than through the high pathogenic potential of one or more bacterial virulence determinants and, secondly, organisms such as non-typable *H. influenzae* have been found to have diverse genotypes by multilocus enzyme electrophoretic studies [107]. They have therefore great heterogeneity in their major outer membrane proteins and lipopolysaccharide, and elicit antibodies of many different specificities.

Although there is full agreement that pneumococcal pneumonia is well worth preventing, there is controversy about the ability of the vaccine currently available to provide adequate immunity in most of those patients at special risk. The vaccine is a complex polyvalent preparation based on capsular polysaccharide from a range of pneumococcal types covering over 80% of bacteraemic pneumococcal infection in the USA [44]. It has been shown to be effective in controlled trials involving young men [108] and in situations where epidemics occur in isolated or crowded populations [44]. Unfortunately no such clear evidence exists in groups that are at high risk for pneumococcal pneumonia such as the elderly or those with chronic disease (who are at particular risk). At present the evidence is conflicting [44], but it has been shown that the antibody response to some capsular polysaccharides is lower in an elderly bronchitic population than in healthy young adults [109].

The current vaccine contains only 23 of the possible serotypes, and there is therefore a need to survey continually the prevalent serotypes causing disease. Conjugation with a protein antigen may enhance the immunogenicity [110] and hence the efficacy of the vaccine. Mice immunized with pneumolysin alone are partly (but significantly) protected from subsequent pulmonary challenge with the intact organism [111]. More recently, a genetically engineered pneumolysin-negative mutant was found to be more rapidly cleared from the bloodstream, and was significantly less virulent in mice than its pneumolysin-positive wild-type parent. The virulence of the mutant was restored by reinstating its ability to produce the toxin [112]. Taken together with the observation described above (that pneumolysin injected into the rat lung produces a lobar pneumonia identical to that produced by intact bacteria), there is good evidence that pneumolysin contributes to pneumococcal pathogenicity. It is common to all pneumococci and has excellent antigenicity [113], and could therefore be a candidate protein for a future pneumococcal vaccine.

Recurrent acute respiratory infection

Some chronic respiratory infections begin as recurrent episodes of acute infection in which the intervening periods become progressively shorter. More commonly, patients presenting with recurrent episodes of acute respiratory infection continue to suffer the pattern of infections with normal periods between. In a prospective study of nearly 500 patients presenting to a respiratory clinic for infective problems [114], patients with this pattern notably included most of the patients with immune deficiency – in contrast to those expectorating infected sputum persistently (daily) (in whom, paradoxically, very few immune deficiencies were found).

The most frequent immune deficiency in those presenting with recurrent acute infections was selective IgA deficiency (usually without associated IgG subclass deficiency), and this was almost always associated with a history of recurrent viral-type infections and normal periods of varying length. In contrast, almost 75% of patients suffering recurrent bacterial pneumonias were found to have panhypogammaglobulinaemia. This underlines the importance of investigating all patients with recurrent acute and chronic respiratory infection to ascertain whether they have one of the treatable causes of repeated infections, or have repeated allergic or aspiration episodes masquerading as infection. A suggested flow chart for the investigation of adults is shown in Table 6.1 and, if well organized, this can be performed in a day investigation unit over 1 or 2 days. This list is designed for investigation of adult onset symptoms – the rarer immune disorders are (relatively) more frequent in infants and children than in adults and therefore the tests for these disorders assume greater importance and the order of investigations may need to be altered.

Chronic respiratory infection

There is a struggle between the microorganism and its human host which goes back through the evolution of both. The microorganism has the capacity to divide rapidly and thus adapt rapidly – it will therefore always tend to have an 'evolutionary advantage' over its human host. In contrast, the defences of the human respiratory tract have been adapted from those which formerly defended the foregut (from which the respiratory tract is derived). These facts underlie much respiratory disease and it is not surprising that 80% of primary care consultations for respiratory disease in the UK are concerned with infection [115]. A microbe's best strategy for survival is persistence (invasion being suicidal if it results in death or treatment of the host), and much can be learnt about microbial mechanisms for achieving persistence from conditions in which microorganisms colonize and chronically infect their host. An important model for this in the respiratory tract is the disease bronchiectasis [116], defined as irreversible dilatation of a bronchus or bronchi, which is an important cause of chronic bronchial sepsis – the persistent expectoration of purulent infected (as opposed to eosinophilic) sputum. It represents an ideal parasitic state for the bacterium in the previously sterile bronchial tree. Sinusitis, often associated with bronchiectasis, represents a similar, and in some respects a more accessible, condition to study. Both provide an ideal model in which to ask basic questions about the nature of host–bacterial interactions in the respiratory tract [1].

Table 6.1 'Fast track' investigation of the cause of recurrent acute and chronic respiratory infection

Blood

- Differential white cell count and IgE (to exclude allergy)
- IgG, A, M and IgG subclasses
- *Aspergillus* precipitins
- Rheumatoid factor and antinuclear antibodies
- Alpha-1 antitrypsin

Sputum

- Differential white cell count (to exclude eosinophilic bronchitis requiring corticosteroid therapy)
- Culture and sensitivities
- AAFB smear and culture

Chest radiographs (PA and lateral)

Sinus radiographs (to detect sinus fluid)

Immediate hypersensitivity skin tests (to detect allergy and investigate allergic bronchopulmonary aspergillosis)

Thin section CT scan thorax (to detect bronchiectasis)

Fibreoptic bronchoscopy (to exclude mechanical causes, e.g. foreign body, bronchial stenosis)

Sweat electrolyte excretion (± intranasal trans-epithelial potential difference) to exclude cystic fibrosis

Nasal mucociliary clearance (NMCC)

Ciliary beat frequency (if NMCC > 30 min) ± ciliary ultrastructure to exclude primary ciliary dyskinesia

Barium swallow with videofluoroscopy (to detect aspiration)

Respiratory muscle function (if aspiration or ineffective cough suspected)

Seminal analysis (to investigate associated infertility)

Tests for conditions associated with bronchiectasis (see Table 6.2)

Blood tests for rarer immune deficiencies

- Functional antibody
- Secretory IgA on saliva and sputum
- Neutrophil tests
  - Chemotaxis
  - Attachment and internalization (phagocytosis) of particles
  - Microbial killing
  - Metabolic (oxidative) function
- Monocyte tests
  - Chemotaxis
  - Attachment and internalization (phagocytosis) of particles
  - Microbial killing
  - Metabolic (oxidative) function
- Cellular immunity tests (delayed hypersensitivity skin tests, lymphocyte markers, macrophage markers)
- Alveolar macrophage function (on cells obtained at bronchoalveolar lavage)

Bronchiectasis

Bronchiectasis is commonly misunderstood in Europe and the USA as no longer constituting a medical problem since antibiotics and vaccines were introduced to control and prevent childhood infections affecting the respiratory tract. It is true that the florid, suppurative, often localized type of typically saccular bronchiectasis usually following severe lung infection (and associated with expectoration of large volumes of foul sputum and finger clubbing) is now uncommon, but an insidiously progressive cylindrical type of bronchiectasis is now well recognized and is typically associated with a history of wheezy bronchitis or asthma in childhood, a remission in the teens and then 'triggering' of persistent purulent sputum by a viral-type illness. This modern bronchiectasis is often associated with chronic rhinosinusitis and marked (disproportionately great) tiredness with lack of concentration (Table 6.2).

A number of questions need to be asked of chronic respiratory infection if the underlying mechanisms for its development are to be understood and logical treatment developed. Such questions need to be asked not only in the model provided by human bronchiectasis and sinusitis, but also in an experimental model that allows manipulation not possible in the human disease.

Table 6.2 Conditions associated with bronchiectasis

- Purulent rhinosinusitis
- Rheumatoid arthritis
- Ulcerative colitis
- Diffuse panbronchiolitis
- Infertility (in cystic fibrosis, primary ciliary dyskinesia, Young's syndrome)
- Alpha-1 antitrypsin deficiency
- Yellow nail syndrome
- Primary lymphoedema (± hypogammaglobulinaemia)
- Chronic lymphatic leukaemia (± IgM deficiency)
- Acute lymphoblastic leukaemia
- Connective tissue disorders
- Coeliac disease
- Vasculitis

Pathogenesis of bacteria associated with chronic respiratory infection

Bronchiectasis provides the answer to this because the bacteria found in sputum and bronchial secretions in the disease are uncapsulated, non-typable *H. influenzae*, strains of *S. pneumoniae*, *Moraxella catarrhalis*, and mucoid *Pseudomonas aeruginosa*. These bacteria may be regarded as non-virulent by criteria of tissue invasiveness and in some instances may be regarded as non-pathogenic, but this derives from a misunderstanding, equating 'virulence' with 'pathogenicity'. In fact, although non-virulent (i.e. not invading tissue) these bacterial isolates can be shown to cause local damage in the respiratory tract (i.e. to be pathogenic). In an experimental model of bronchiectasis in the rat the isolates of bacteria from the human disease can cause bronchiectasis as long as they are viable and persist within the bronchial tree [117].

The paradox of the human disease is that the bacteria associated with it are not virulent and the patients rarely suffer from immune deficiency, so the reason for the bronchial damage appears at first glance to be obscure. However, there are clues to the mechanisms involved because the disease is the inflammatory end result of several known causes (Table 6.3), although over 60% is idiopathic in the UK. A feature common to all patients is inability to clear bronchial mucus as rapidly as normal

Table 6.3 Causes of bronchiectasis

Congenital
- Bronchial wall components defective
- Associated with other congenital abnormalities
- Pulmonary sequestration

Mechanical obstruction
- Intrinsic
  - Foreign body in bronchial lumen
  - Mucus inspissated in bronchus
  - Stenosis (e.g. post-tuberculous)
  - Tumour
- Extrinsic
  - Lymph node
  - Tumour

Inflammation
- Aspiration
  - Refluxed gastric contents
  - Dysphagia
  - Caustic chemicals
- Inhalation
  - Host/caustic gases
  - Drugs/vehicles

Granulomas and fibrosis
- Tuberculosis (including atypical)
- Sarcoidosis
- Fibrosing alveolitis

Excessive immunological response
- Allergic bronchopulmonary aspergillosis
- Complication of lung transplantation

Deficient immune response
- Primary
  - Panhypogammaglobulinaemia
  - Selective immunoglobulin deficiencies
- Secondary
  - Malignancy (leukaemia, lymphoma)

Defects of mucus clearance
- Genetic
  - Primary ciliary dyskinesia (± Kartagener's syndrome)
  - Cystic fibrosis
- Acquired
  - Young's syndrome
  - Secondary ciliary dyskinesias – asthma or toxic

Post-infective
- Bacterial
- Viral
- Protozoan

Idiopathic (> 60% of cases in the UK)

persons [118]. Hence, inhaled microorganisms will tend to spend longer within the bronchial tree and this may be crucial to the pathogenesis of the disease.

These microorganisms are able to exert significant direct damage to respiratory epithelial defences by a number of mechanisms. and the extra time they spend within the respiratory tract because of diminished mucus transport may allow such mechanisms full reign. These mechanisms include inhibition of ciliary function [64, 66, 119–125], inhibition of mucociliary transport [126, 127], alteration of respiratory epithelial ion transport [128], and stimulation of mucus secretion [129–131]. That these mainly *in vitro* mechanisms are relevant to disease *in vivo* is suggested by the fact that the microbial exotoxins responsible can be shown to be active in *in vivo* models [127] and are present within secretions of patients with bronchiectasis in sufficient concentrations for the relevant effect [132].

With longer sojourn in the bronchial tree because of reduced mucus transport it becomes increasingly likely that such bacterial exotoxins will damage the respiratory epithelium and, in turn, further delay their clearance.

In organ culture experiments using *H. influenzae* as infecting organisms, scanning and transmission electron microscopy suggest that most bacteria are found within the mucus layer [62]. Although the bacteria damage the epithelial cells and subsequently adhere to these damaged cells, the latter are extruded into the overlying mucus. Bacteria are also found sticking to exposed collagen. These findings accord with those of Ramphal *et al.*, who used a model involving *P. aeruginosa* infection [61]. There may be an advantage conferred by fimbriae for adherence to mucus [133].

The host's response to persistent intraluminal bacteria

Persistent bacteria stimulate both a non-specific neutrophil host response and a specific cellular immune response. The chemoattraction of neutrophils from the circulation across the bronchial wall into the lumen can be demonstrated by cell labelling [134] and by histological techniques. The magnitude of this cell traffic is such that in severe bronchiectasis approximately 50% of circulating neutrophils leave the body by this route – making the potential for tissue damage by neutrophil proteinases and oxidants considerable [37, 135]. Indirect microbe-stimulated but host-mediated damage may be responsible for considerable bronchial wall destruction – deforming it and reducing its epithelial mucosal clearance mechanisms even further.

A cellular immune response can be identified within the bronchial wall by appropriate immunohistochemical techniques – in both human bronchiectasis [136] and the experimental model [117] of the disease. The increase in lymphocyte population is predominantly in the CD8+ population, but both antigen-processing cells and mature macrophages are seen in increased numbers. These cells can be shown to be activated with respect to several markers. Whether this cellular immune response has any directly damaging effect on the host bronchus is debatable but it is conceivable that cytokine production could regulate neutrophil traffic across the bronchial wall.

'Vicious circle' hypothesis for the pathogenesis of bronchiectasis

From the evidence cited above it can be seen that a 'vicious circle' of events may occur once the first-line sinobronchial mucus clearance mechanism is damaged (Figure 6.1). Normally, oropharyngeal bacterial flora are inhaled into the bronchial tree and are cleared by the mucociliary clearance mechanism which keeps it sterile. If some insult, such as direct damage from a viral infection, or an inherited predisposition to respiratory infection by way of a genetic abnormality affecting mucus clearance (e.g. cystic fibrosis), compromises mucus transport the inhaled bacteria will remain in the bronchial tree long enough to exert the directly damaging effects described. This damage will reduce their clearance further and predispose to microbial colonization of bronchial mucus. The ensuing host response is unable to eliminate the bacterial colonists and amplifies, causing chronic inflammatory damage to 'bystander' normal lung. The result is a progressive deterioration in lung function and in severe cases leads to the requirement for lung transplantation, or death.

This series of events illustrates the parasitic state achieved by apparently non-virulent bacteria within the respiratory tract. The initiating events and predisposing factors are largely unknown and require much further study to enable therapy to be aimed earlier in the chain of events.

Clinical management of chronic respiratory infection

This is again well illustrated by bronchiectasis.

Diagnosis

The initial step requires a high index of suspicion in any person persistently coughing up mucopurulent or purulent sputum. Such patients should undergo imaging by high-resolution, thin-section computed tomography (CT) scanning because the sensitivity of plain chest radiography in making the diagnosis is less than 50%.

Once the presence of bronchiectasis is proved, a search for the cause should be carried out along the lines of the investigations in Table 6.1 because certain causes (e.g. hypogammaglobulinaemia, cystic fibrosis) require specific treatment in addition to that for the bronchiectasis.

Assessment of disease activity

Whether or not a cause is found (more than 60% of cases in the UK are idiopathic) an assessment of the activity of the inflammatory process should be made using, for instance, indium-111 granulocyte scanning [137] which images the magnitude and site of neutrophil traffic including the paranasal sinuses, the lungs and, in the subgroup of patients with ulcerative colitis, the large intestine. This measure of inflammatory activity, besides indicating the present state of disease (CT scanning images damage already inflicted on the bronchial tree which is probably irreversible)

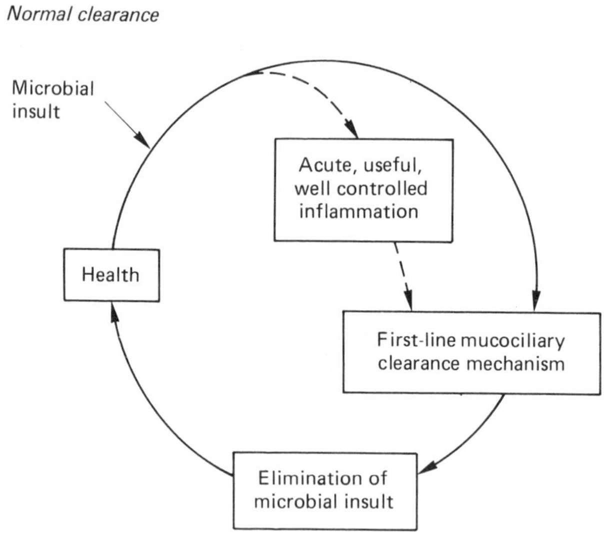

a

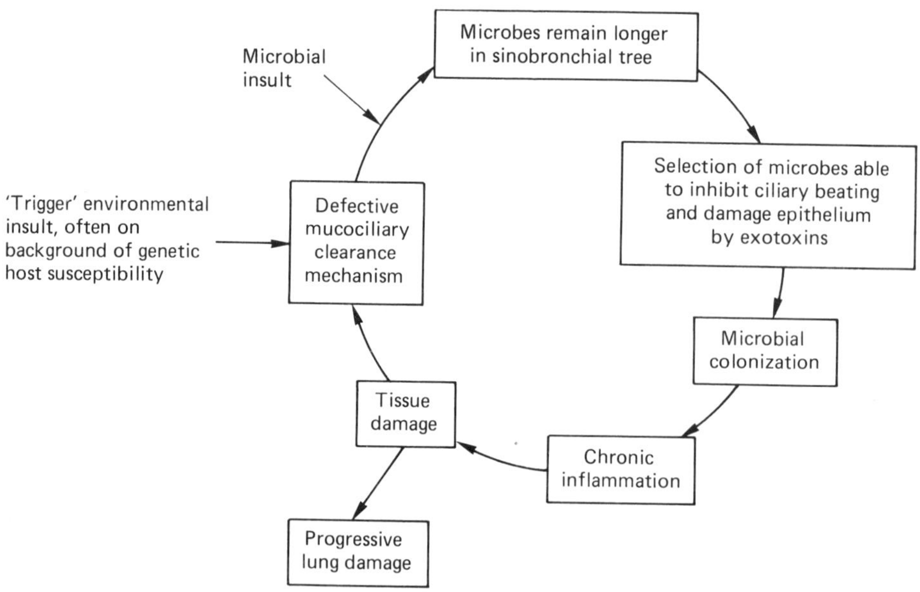

b

Figure 6.1 Pathogenesis of bronchiectasis based on data derived from human and experimental models: (a) Normal clearance; (b) 'vicious circle' of chronic inflammation following defective mucus clearance. (From Cole PJ. Host microbial interactions in chronic suppurative lumg disease. *Eur J Intern Med* 1992, with permission)

requiring treatment, may also provide a prognostic guide because areas of high-intensity granulocyte traffic may be seen in parts of the lung as yet unaffected. This may be of great importance in assessing a patient for surgery because inflammatory activity outside the surgically resectable area of CT-imaged bronchiectasis would suggest the likelihood of recurrence of disease after resection. Finally, indium-111 scanning provides a criterion against which efficacy of treatment regimens can be judged and the regimen modified subsequently.

Present treatment

Prevention

At present this consists of vaccination against childhood exanthema (especially whooping cough and measles) and prompt antimicrobial treatment of respiratory infections.

Treatment of established bronchiectasis

The general framework for treatment is shown in Table 6.4.

More specifically, treatment consists of adequate *postural physiotherapy* (to move mucus from distal airways where retention will favour worsening of bronchiectasis), *bronchodilatation* (because most patients have some reversibility of their air flow obstruction), local *inhaled corticosteroid* (to assist in bronchodilatation and as a local anti-inflammatory agent), and appropriate *antimicrobial therapy* (to achieve bactericidal concentrations within the bronchial secretions) to overcome the barriers to access of drugs into secretions. It is important to treat posterior nasal discharge (which may worsen lower airway hyperreactivity and act as a source of inhaled infection) and to suspect and prevent aspiration of refluxed gastric contents, or less commonly aspiration due to dysphagia from a number of neuromuscular causes.

Antimicrobial therapy is almost always based on empiricism rather than logic, the aim being to eliminate the bacteria colonizing the bronchial tree. Antibiotics penetrate poorly into secretions, and for this reason bactericidal concentrations may not always be achieved. Subminimal inhibitory concentrations of antibiotics in the infected secretions may be beneficial by influencing bacterial properties such as adherence and exotoxin production. The longer and medium-term outcome of antimicrobial therapy needs consideration because a definite strategy is required if the patient is to understand the aim and therefore pursue the means. Initial clearance of infected secretions may have one of several outcomes, each requiring a different treatment strategy. These outcomes probably depend mainly on how capable residual defences are of keeping the sinobronchial tree sterile: where damage is trivial the defences may maintain the patient infection-free until the next viral infection causes recurrence; where damage is less than trivial sputum often gradually becomes purulent again (over several weeks); and where serious damage is present purulent sputum may recur a few hours after discontinuing antibiotics. In these varying circumstances antibiotics may be needed only for use after infective exacerbations associated with purulent sputum production at one end of the spectrum but

Table 6.4 Framework for management of established bronchiectasis

Specific treatment for any cause identified (e.g. aspiration)
Management of the bronchiectasis
- Curative surgical resection of localized disease with no underlying cause or
- Palliative surgical resection of a 'sump' of pus defying medical treatment
- Control symptoms medically
- Prevent disease progression

Management of associated disease (e.g. purulent rhinosinusitis)
Monitoring control of inflammatory activity of disease
Follow-up to detect:
- Increase in severity of symptoms
- Increase in severity of bronchiectasis, spread of it or appearance of it for the first time in a patient with previous purulent sputum but no imaginable bronchiectasis
- Deterioration in lung or heart function
- Other complications

Revision of treatment according to disease activity
If deterioration defies treatment, consider lung transplantation
Follow-up transplanted patient to detect recurrence of disease in the graft

may be required continuously if damage is severe and recurrence rapid. Gradual recurrence of infection makes it necessary to decide when to treat, but 'pulsed' therapy (for example 2 weeks every 6) may be an answer. Where treatment is to be continuous the inhaled route has obvious advantages but is inconvenient and, because of air flow obstruction and mucus plugging, may not reach peripheral parts of the diseased lung. In practice, antibiotic strategy often has to be individually tailored to the patient.

Future treatment

Ideally, treatment would be preventive. This will require additional causes to be found for idiopathic disease and markers for the susceptible state. Early recognition of these may allow preventative strategies to be developed, for example by preventing trigger factors operating or by neutralizing damaging pathogenic mechanisms.

Somewhat less ideal would be to rectify the basic malfunction of mucus transport. Here prospects are more immediate in that recombinant human DNase has been shown to be effective in reducing the viscoelasticity of purulent sputum *in vitro* [138] (the increased viscoelasticity being largely due to polymerization of DNA released by neutrophils in the bronchial secretions). Clinical trials of this agent show promising, safe results [139].

Other possible therapeutic advances will include development of new antibiotics, but novel approaches may include neutralization of neutrophil proteinases by inhaled α_1-antiproteinase [140] and small molecular weight elastase inhibitors, modulating the movement of neutrophils into inflammatory sites, by drawing on increasing knowledge of cell adhesion molecules, and modulating the cellular immune response in the bronchial wall, which may influence the neutrophil traffic.

Summary

Increasing knowledge of the pathogenic mechanisms underlying acute and chronic respiratory infections is allowing novel approaches to management of the conditions as well as enabling improved conventional treatment.

References

1. Cole P, Wilson R. Host–microbial interrelationships in respiratory infection. *Chest* 1989; **95:** 217s–221s.
2. Clarke S. Respiratory defences. Physical defences. In: *Respiratory Medicine*. Brewis RAL, Gibson GJ, Geddes DM eds. London: Baillière Tindall, 1990; 176–189.
3. Stockley RA. Respiratory defences. Cellular and humeral mechanisms. In: *Respiratory Medicine*. Brewis RAL, Gibson GJ, Geddes DM eds. London: Baillière Tindall, 1990; 189–203.
4. Wanner A. Clinical aspects of mucociliary transport. *Am Rev Respir Dis* 1977; **116:** 73–125.
5. Olver RE, Davis B, Marin MG, Nadel JA. Active transport of sodium and chloride across the canine tracheal epithelium in vitro. *Am Rev Respir Dis* 1975; **112:** 811–815.
6. Dulfano MJ, Adler KB. Physical properties of sputum VII. Rheological properties and mucociliary transport. *Am Rev Respir Dis* 1975; **112:** 341–347.
7. Clarke SW. Physical defences. In: *Respiratory Medicine*. Brewis RAL, Gibson GJ and Geddes DM eds. London: Baillière Tindall, 1990; 176–189.
8. Wilson R. Secondary ciliary dysfunction. *Clin Sci* 1988; **75:** 113–120.
9. Sakakura Y. Changes of mucociliary function during colds. *Eur J Respir Dis* 1983; **64** (Suppl. 128): 348–354.
10. Burgi H. Fibre systems in sputum. *Bull Physiol Path Resp* 1973; **9:** 191–196.
11. Pederson M, Sakakura Y, Winther B, Brofeldt S, Mygind N. Nasal mucociliary transport, number of ciliated cells, and beating pattern in naturally acquired common colds. *Eur J Respir Dis* 1983; **64** (Suppl. 128): 355–364.
12. Wilson R, Alton E, Rutman A *et al.* Upper respiratory tract viral infection and mucociliary clearance. *Eur J Respir Dis* 1987; **70:** 272–279.
13. Baltimore RS, Christie LDC, Walker Smith GJ. Immunohistopathological localisation of *P. aeruginosa* in lungs from patients with cystic fibrosis. *Am Rev Respir Dis* 1989; **140:** 1650–1661.
14. Sykes DA, Wilson R, Greenstone M, Currie DC, Steinfort C, Cole PJ. Deleterious effects of purulent sputum sol on human ciliary function *in vitro*: at least two factors identified. *Thorax* 1987; **42:** 256–261.
15. Feldman C, Read R, Rutman A *et al.* The interaction of *Streptococcus pneumoniae* with human respiratory mucosa *in vitro*. *Eur Respir J* 1992; **5:** 576–583.
16. Jacquot J, Puchelle E, Zahm JM, Beck G, Plotkowski MC. Effect of human airway lysozyme on the *in vitro* growth of type I *Streptococcus pneumoniae*. *Eur J Respir Dis* 1987; 71: 295–305.
17. Burnett D. Immunoglobulins in the lung. *Thorax* 1986; 41: 337–344.
18. Richards CD, Gauldie J. IgA mediated phagocytosis by mouse alveolar macrophages. *Am Rev Respir Dis* 1985; **132:** 82–85.
19. Shen L, Fanger MW. Secretory IgA antibodies synergize with IgG in promoting antibody dependent cell mediated cytotoxicity by human polymorphonuclear cells, monocytes and lymphocytes. *Cell Immunol* 1981; **59:** 75–81.
20. Musher DM, Gorce A, Baughn RE, Birdsall HH. Immunoglobulin A from bronchopulmonary secretions blocks bactericidal and opsonising effects of antibody to non-typable *Haemophilus influenzae*. *Infect Immun* 1984; **45:** 36–40.
21. Koistinen J. Selective IgA deficiency in blood donors. *Vox Sanguis* 1975; **29:** 192–202.
22. Stockley RA, Burnett D, Afford SC. The immunological measurements of free secretory piece and its relationship to local IgA production. *Clin Exp Immun* 1981; **45:** 124–130.
23. Brandtzaeg P, Fellanger I, Gjeruldsen ST. Immunoglobulin M: local synthesis and selective secretion in patients with immun oglobulin A deficiency. *Science* 1968; **160:** 789–791.
24. Bjorkander J, Bake B, Oxelius VA, Hanson LA. Impaired lung function in patients with IgA deficiency and low levels of IgG2 or IgG3. *N Engl J Med* 1985; **313:** 720–724.
25. Plaut AG. The IgA proteases of pathogenic bacteria. *Am Rev Microbiol* 1983; **37:** 603–622.
26. Fick RB, Baltimore RS, Squier SU, Reynolds HY. The immunoglobulin G proteolytic activity of *Pseudomonas aeruginosa* in cystic fibrosis. *J Infect Dis* 1985; **151:** 589–598.
27. Moxon ER, Wilson R. The role of *Haemophilus influenzae* in the pathogenesis of pneumonia. *Rev*

Infect Dis 1991; **13** (Suppl. 6): S518–S527.
28. Bricker J, Mulks M, Moxon ER, Plaut AG, Wright A. Physical and genetic analysis of DNA regions in coding the immunoglobulin A proteases of different specificities produced by *Haemophilus influenzae*. *Infect Immun* 1985; **47:** 370–374.
29. Farley MM, Stephens DS, Mulks MH *et al.* Pathogenesis of IgA1 protease-producing and non-producing *H. influenzae* on human nasopharyngeal organ cultures. *J Infect Dis* 1986; **154:** 752–759.
30. Toews GB, Heart DA, Hansen EJ. Effect of systemic immunisation on pulmonary clearance of *Haemophilus influenzae* type b. *Infect Immun* 1985; **48:** 343–349.
31. Fick RB, Olchowski J, Squier SU, Merrill W, Reynolds HY. Immunoglobulin G subclasses in cystic fibrosis. IgG2 response to *Pseudomonas aeruginosa* lipopolysaccharide. *Am Rev Respir Dis* 1986; **133:** 418–422.
32. Fournier M, Lebargy F, Le Roy Ladurid F, Lenormand E, Parienie R. Intraepithelial T lymphocyte subsets in the airways of normal subjects and of patients with chronic bronchitis. *Am Rev Respir Dis* 1989; **140:** 737–742.
33. Du Bois RM. The alveolar macrophage. *Thorax* 1985; **40:** 321–327.
34. Nathan CF. Secretory products of macrophages. *J Clin Invest* 1987; **79:** 319–326.
35. Campbell EJ. Human leukocyte elastase, Cathepsin G and lactoferrin: family of neutrophil granule glycoproteins that bind to an alveolar macrophage receptor. *Proc Natl Acad Sci USA* 1982; **79:** 6941–6945.
36. Ras G, Wilson R, Todd H, Taylor G, Cole P. The effect of bacterial products on neutrophil migration *in vitro*. *Thorax* 1990; **45:** 276–280.
37. Amitani R, Wilson R, Rutman A *et al.* Effects of human neutrophil elastase and bacterial proteolytic enzymes on human ciliated epithelium *in vitro*. *Am J Respir Cell Mol Biol* 1991; **4:** 26–32.
38. Savill JS, Henson PM, Haslett C. Phagocytosis of aged neutrophils by macrophages is mediated by a novel 'change-sensitive' recognition mechanism. *J Clin Invest* 1989; **84:** 1518–1527.
39. Blume RS, Walff SM. The Chediak–Hegashi syndrome: studies in four patients and a review of the literature. *Medicine (Baltimore)* 1972; **51:** 247–280.
40. Segal AW, Heyworth PG, Codecroft S, Barrowmean MM. Stimulated neutrophils from patients with autosomal recessive chronic granulomatous disease fail to phosphorylate a MR-44,000 protein. *Nature* 1985; **316:** 547–549.
41. Bath JCJL, Boissard CPB, Calder MA, Moffat MAJ. Pneumonia in hospital practice in Edinburgh 1960–1962. *Br J Dis Chest* 1964; **58:** 1–16.
42. MacFarlane JT, Finch RG, Ward MJ, Macrae AD. Hospital study of adult community acquired pneumonia. *Lancet* 1982; **ii:** 255–258.
43. Austrian R. Pneumococcal pneumonia. Diagnostic, epidemiologic, therapeutic and prophylactic considerations. *Chest* 1986; **90:** 738–743.
44. Seaton A, Seaton D, Leitch AG. Pneumonia. In: *Crofton and Douglas's Respiratory Diseases* 4th edn. Seaton A, Seaton D and Leitch AG eds. Oxford: Blackwell Scientific, 1989; 285–345.
45. Austrian R, Gold J. Pneumococcal bacteraemia with especial reference to bacteraemic pneumococcal pneumonia. *Ann Intern Med* 1964; **60:** 759–776.
46. Hook EW, Horton CA, Schaberg DR. Failure of intensive care unit support to influence mortality from pneumococcal bacteraemia. *JAMA* 1983; **249:** 1055–1057.
47. Woodhead MA, MacFarlane JT, Rogers FG, Laverick A, Pilkington R, Macrae AD. Aetiology and outcome of severe community acquired pneumonia. J Infect 1985; 10: 204–210.
48. Woodhead MA. BTS study of severe community acquired pneumonia in the intensive care unit. *Thorax* 1990; **45:** 305.
49. British Thoracic Society. Community acquired pneumonia in adults in British hospitals in 1982–1983: A survey of aetiology, mortality factors and outcome. *Q J Med* 1987; **62:** 195–220.
50. Austrian R. Pneumococcal infections. In: *Bacterial Vaccines*. Germanier R ed. London: Academic Press, 1984; 257–288.
51. Andersson B, Eriksson B, Falsen E *et al.* Adhesion of *Streptococcus pneumoniae* to human pharyngeal epithelial cells *in vitro*: differences in adhesive capacity among strains isolated from subjects with otitis media, septicaemia, meningitis or from healthy carriers. *Infect Immun* 1981; **32:** 311–317.
52. Andersson B, Beachey EH, Tomasz A, Tuomanen E, Svanborg-Eden C. A sandwich adhesin on *Streptococcus pneumoniae* attaching to human oropharyngeal epithelial cells *in vitro*. *Microb Pathog* 1988; **4:** 267–278.
53. Andersson B, Porras D, Hason LA, Svanborg-Eden C. Non-antibody-containing fractions of breast milk inhibit epithelial attachment of *Streptococcus pneumoniae* and *Haemophilus influenzae*. *Lancet* 1985; **i:** 643–644.
54. Andersson B, Dahmen J, Frejd T *et al.* Identification of an active disaccharide unit of a glyconjugate receptor for pneumococci attaching to human pharyngeal epithelial cells. *J Exp Med* 1983; **158:**

559–570.
55. Selinger DS, Reed WP. Pneumococcal adherence to human epithelial cells. *Infect Immun* 1979; **23:** 545–548.
56. Beachey EH. Bacterial adherence: adhesin-receptor interactions mediating the attachment of bacteria to mucosal surfaces. *J Infect Dis* 1981; **143:** 325–345.
57. Niederman MS. Bacterial adherence as a mechanism of airway colonisation. *Eur J Clin Microbiol Infect Dis* 1989; **8:** 15–20.
58. Krivan JC, Roberts DD, Ginsburg V. Many pulmonary pathogenic bacteria bind specifically to the carbohydrate sequence Ga1NAcB1–4Gal found in some glyclolipids. *Proc Natl Acad Sci USA* 1988; **85:** 6157–6161.
59. Johanson WG, Pierce AK, Sandford JP, Thomas GD. Nosocomial respiratory infections with Gram negative bacilli: the significance of colonisation of the respiratory tract. *Ann Intern Med* 1972; **77:** 701–706.
60. Plotkowski MC, Beck G, Jacquot J, Puchelle E. The frog palate mucosa as a model for studying bacterial adhesion to mucus coated respiratory epithelium. *J Comp Path* 1989; **100:** 37–46.
61. Ramphal R, Small PM, Shands JW, Fischlschweiger W, Small PA. Adherence of *Pseudomonas aeruginosa* to tracheal cells injured by influenza infection or by endotracheal intubation. *Infect Immun* 1980; **27:** 614–619.
62. Read RC, Wilson R, Rutman A *et al.* Interaction of non-typable *Haemophilus influenzae* with human respiratory mucosa *in vitro*. *J Infect Dis* 1991; **163:** 549–558.
63. Plotkowski M, Puchelle E, Beck G, Jacquot J, Hannoun C. Adherence of type 1 *Streptococcus pneumoniae* to tracheal epithelium of mice infected with influenza A/PR8 virus. *Am Rev Respir Dis* 1986; **134:** 1040–1044.
64. Steinfort C, Wilson R, Mitchell T *et al.* Effect of *Streptococcus pneumoniae* on human respiratory epithelium *in vitro*. *Infect Immun* 1989; **57:** 2006–2013.
65. Mitchell TJ, Walker JA, Saunders FK, Andrew PW, Boulnois GJ. Expression of the pneumolysin gene in *Escherichia coli*: rapid purification and biological properties. *Biochim Biophys Acta* 1989; **1007:** 67–72.
66. Feldman C, Mitchell TJ, Andrew PW *et al.* The effect of *Streptococcus pneumoniae* pneumolysin on human respiratory epithelium *in vitro*. *Microb Path* 1990; **9:** 275–284.
67. Smyth CJ, Duncan JL. Thiol activated (oxygen labile) cytolysins. In: *Bacterial Toxins and Cell Membranes*. Jeljaszewicz J, Wadstrom T eds. London: Academic Press, 1989; 129–183.
68. Clinkenbeard MD, Mosier BA, Confer AW. Transmembrane poor size and role of cell swelling in cytotoxicity caused by *Pasteurella haemolytica* glucose toxin. *Infect Immun* 1989; **57:** 420–425.
69. Adler KB, Hendles DD, Davis GS. Bacteria associated with obstructive pulmonary disease elaborate extracellular products that stimulate mucus secretion by explants of guinea pig airways. *Am J Pathol* 1986; **125:** 501–514.
70. Boulnois GJ, Mitchell TJ, Saunders K *et al.* Analysis of some putative protein virulence factors of *Streptococcus pneumoniae*. In: *Streptococcal Genetics*. Dunny GM, Cleary PP, Mackay LL eds. American Society for Microbiology, 1991; 83–87.
71. Briles DE, Yother J, McDaniel LS. Role of pneumococcal surface protein A and the virulence of *Streptococcus pneumoniae*. *Rev Infect Dis* 1988; **10:** S372–S374
72. Yamazaki Y, Ebisu S, Okada H. *Eikenella corrodens* adherence to human buccal epithelial cells. *Infect Immun* 1981; **31:** 21–27.
73. Ginsberg I. Streptococcal enzymes and virulence. In: *Bacterial Enzymes and Virulence*. Holger IA ed. Boca Raton, Florida: CRCS Press, 1985; 122–144.
74. Colman G. *Streptococcus* and *Lactobacillus*. In: *Topley and Wilson's Principles of Bacteriology, Virology and Immunity*, *vol.* 2, 8th edn. Parker MT and Collier LH eds. London: Edward Arnold, 1990; 119–159.
75. Cross CE, Halliwell B, Allen A. Antioxidant protection: a function of tracheobronchial and gastrointestinal mucus. *Lancet* 1984; **ii:** 1328–1329.
76. Rhodes JC, Tapsall JW, Lykke AWJ. Alveolar epithelial responses in experimental streptococcal pneumonia. *J Pathol* 1989; **157:** 347–357.
77. Tuomanen E, Rich R, Zach O. Induction of pulmonary inflammation by components of the pneumococcal cell wall. *Am Rev Respir Dis* 1987; **135:** 869–874.
78. Fine DP. Pneumococcal type associated variability in alternate complement pathway activation. *Infect Immun* 1975; **12:** 772–778.
79. Coonrod JD, Jenkins S. Interaction of pneumococcal antigens with complement in rats. *Infect Immun* 1979; **23:** 626–632.
80. Winkelstein JA, Bocchini JA, Schiffman G. The role of capsular polysaccharide in the activation of the alternate pathway by the pneumococcus. *J Immunol* 1976; **116:** 367–370.

81. Ansfield MJ, Woods DE, Johanson WG. Lung bacterial clearance in murine pneumococcal pneumonia. *Infect Immun* 1977; **17:** 195–204.
82. Winkelstein JA, Tomasz A. Activation of the alternative pathway by pneumococcal cell wall teichoic acids. *J Immunol* 1978; **120:** 174–178.
83. Hummell DS, Berninger RW, Tomasz A, Winkelstein JA. The fixation of C3B to pneumococcal cell wall polymers as a result of activation of the alternative complement pathway. *J Immunol* 1981; **127:** 1287–1289.
84. Szu SC, Clarke S, Robbins JB. Protection against pneumococcal infection in mice conferred by phosphocholine binding antibodies: specificity of the phosphocholine binding and relation to several types. *Infect Immun* 1983; **39:** 993–999.
85. Winkelstein JA. Complement and the host's defence against the pneumococcus. *CRC Critical Reviews in Microbiology* 1987: **11:** 187–208.
86. Muschel LH, Fong JSC. Serum bactericidal activity and complement. In: *Comprehensive Immunology.* Day NK, Good RA eds. New York: Plenum Press, 1977; 137–157.
87. Heidrink PJ, Toews GB, Gross GN, Pierce AK. Mechanisms of complement mediated clearance of bacteria from the murine lung. *Am Rev Respir Dis* 1982; **125:** 517–520.
88. Gross GN, Rehm SR, Pierce AK. The effect of complement depletion on lung clearance of bacteria. *J Clin Invest* 1978; **62:** 373–378.
89. Toews GB, Vial WC. The role of C5 in polymorphonuclear leukocyte recruitment in response to *Streptococcus pneumoniae. Am Rev Respir Dis* 1984; **129:** 82–86.
90. Hosea SW, Brown EJ, Frank MM. The critical role of complement in experimental pneumococcal sepsis. *J Infect Dis* 1980; **142:** 903–909.
91. Feldman C, Munro NC, Jeffery PK *et al.* Pneumolysin induces the salient histological features of pneumococcal infection in the rat lung *in vivo. Am J Respir Cell Mol Biol* 1991; **5:** 416–423.
92. Tuomanen E, Liu H, Hengstler B, Zach O, Tomasz A. The induction of meningeal inflammation by components of the pneumococcal cell wall. *J Infect Dis* 1985; **151:** 859–868.
93. Tuomanen E, Hengstler B, Zach O, Tomasz A. The role of complement in inflammation during experimental pneumococcal meningitis. *Microb Pathog* 1986; **1:** 15–32.
94. Johnson MK, Allan JH. Ocular toxin of the pneumococcus. *Am J Ophthalmol* 1971; **72:** 175–180.
95. Peters NS, Eykyn SJ, Rudd AG. Pneumococcal cellulitis: a rare manifestation of pneumococcaemia in adults. *J Infect* 1989; **19:** 57–59.
96. Johnson MK, Boese-Marrazzo D, Pierce WA. Effects of pneumolysin on human polymorphonuclear leukocytes and platelets. *Infect Immun* 1981; **34:** 171–176.
97. Paten JC, Ferrante A. Inhibition of human polymorphonuclear leukocyte respiratory burst, bactericidal activity, and migration by pneumolysin. *Infect Immun* 1983; **41:** 1212–1216.
98. Ferrante A, Rowan-Kelly B, Paten JC. Inhibition of *in vitro* human lymphocyte response by the pneumococcal toxin, pneumolysin. *Infect Immun* 1984; **46:** 585–589.
99. Nandoskar MA, Ferrante A, Bates EJ, Hurst N, Paten JC. Inhibition of human monocyte respiratory burst, degranulation, phospholipid methylation and bactericidal activity by pneumolysin. *Immunology* 1986; **59:** 515–520.
100. Paten JC, Rowan-Kelly B, Ferrante A. Activation of human complement by the pneumococcal toxin pneumolysin. *Infect Immun* 1984; **43:** 1085–1087.
101. Brenn KD, Konig W, Pfeiffer P *et al.* Effect of thiol activated toxins (streptolysin O, alveolysin and theta toxin) on the generation of leukotrienes and leukotriene inducing and metabolising enzymes from human polymorphonuclear granulocytes. *Infect Immun* 1985; **50:** 844–851.
102. Jalonen E, Paton JC, Koskela M, Kerttula Y, Leinonen M. Measurement of antibody responses to pneumolysin – a promising method for the presumptive aetiological diagnosis of pneumococcal pneumonia. *J Infect* 1989; **19:** 127–134.
103. Berry AM, Lock RA, Hansman D, Paten JC. Contribution of autolysin to virulence of *Streptococcus pneumoniae. Infect Immun* 1989; **57:** 2324–2330.
104. Mold C, Nakayama S, Holzer TJ, Gewurz H, DuClos TW. C-reactive protein is protective against *Streptococcus pneumoniae* in mice. *J Exp Med* 1981; **154:** 1703–1708.
105. Yother J, Volanakis JE, Briles DE. Human C-reactive protein is protective against fatal *Streptococcus pneumoniae* infection in mice. *J Immunol* 1982; **128:** 2374–2376.
106. Henderson FW, Gilligan PH, Waite K, Goff DA. Nasopharyngeal carriage of antibiotic resistant pneumococci by children in group day care. *J Infect Dis* 1988; **157:** 256–263.
107. Musser JM, Barenkamp SJ, Granoff DM, Selander RK. Genetic relationships of serological nontypable and serotype B strains of *Haemophilus influenzae. Infect Immun* 1986; **52:** 183–191.
108. Austrian R, Douglas RM, Schiffman G *et al.* Prevention of pneumococcal pneumonia by vaccination. *Trans Assoc Am Phys* 1976; **89:** 184.
109. Musher DM, Luchi MJ, Watson DA, Hamilton R, Baughn RE. Pneumococcal polysaccharide vac-

cine in young adults and older bronchitics: determination of IgG responses by ELISA and the effect of absorption of serum with non-type-specific cell wall polysaccharide. *J Infect Dis* 1990; **161:** 728–735.

110. Lin KT, Lee CJ. Immune response of neonates to pneumococcal polysaccharide protein conjugates. *Immunology* 1982; **46:** 333–342.
111. Paten JC, Lock RA, Hansman DJ. Effect of immunisation with pneumolysin on the survival time of mice challenged with *Streptococcus pneumoniae*. *Infect Immun* 1983; **40:** 548–552.
112. Berry AM, Yotcher J, Briles DE, Hansman D, Paten JC. Reduced virulence of a defined pneumolysin negative mutant of *Streptococcus pneumoniae*. *Infect Immun* 1989; **57:** 2037–2042.
113. Lock RA, Paten JC, Hansman D. Comparative efficacy of pneumococcal neuraminidase and pneumolysin as immunogens protective against *Streptococcus pneumoniae*. *Microb Pathog* 1988; **5:** 461–467.
114. Cole PJ. Host-microbe relationships in chronic respiratory disease. In: *Recent Advances in Infection*. Reeves D, Geddes AM eds. Edinburgh: Churchill Livingstone, 1989; 141–151.
115. Morell DC. Expressions of morbidity in general practice. *BMJ* 1971; **2:** 454–458.
116. Cole PJ. Bronchiectasis. In: *Textbook of Respiratory Medicine*. Brewis RAL, Gibson GJ, Geddes DM eds. London: Baillière Tindall, 1990; 726–759.
117. Lapa e Silva JR, Guerreiro D, Noble B, Poulter LW, Cole PJ. Immunopathology of experimental bronchiectasis. *Am J Respir Cell Mol Biol* 1989; **1:** 297–304.
118. Currie DC, Pavia D, Agnew JE *et al*. Impaired tracheo-bronchial clearance in bronchiectasis. *Thorax* 1987; **42:** 126–130.
119. Wilson R, Cole PJ. The effect of bacterial products on ciliary function. *Am Rev Respir Dis* 1988; **138:** S49–S53.
120. Wilson R, Pitt T, Taylor G *et al*. Pyocyanin and 1-hydroxyphenazine inhibit the beating of human respiratory cilia *in vitro*. *J Clin Invest* 1987; **79:** 221–229.
121. Steinfort C, Wilson R, Mitchell T *et al*. The effect of *Streptococcus pneumoniae* on human respiratory epithelium *in vitro*. *Infect Immun* 1989; **57:** 2006–2013.
122. Feldman C, Mitchell TJ, Andrew PW *et al*. The effect of *Streptococcus pneumoniae* pneumolysin on human respiratory epithelium *in vitro*. *Microb Pathog* 1990; **9:** 275–284.
123. Wilson R, Roberts D, Cole PJ. Effect of bacterial products on human ciliary function *in vitro*. *Thorax* 1985; **40:** 125–131.
124. Denny FW. Effect of a toxin produced by *Haemophilus influenzae* on ciliated respiratory epithelium. *J Infect Dis* 1974; **129:** 93–100.
125. Johnson AP, Inzana TJ. Loss of ciliary activity in organ cultures of rat trachea treated with lipo-oligosaccharide isolated from *Haemophilus influenzae*. *J Med Microbiol* 1986; **22:** 265–268.
126. Southern PM, Mays BB, Pierce AK, Sanford JP. Pulmonary clearance of *Pseudomonas aeruginosa*. *J Lab Clin Med* 1970; **76:** 548–559.
127. Munro NC, Barker A, Rutman A *et al*. The effect of pyocyanin and 1-hydroxyphenazine on *in vivo* tracheal mucus velocity. *J Appl Physiol* 1989; **67:** 316–323.
128. Stutts KJ, Schwab JH, Chen MG, Knowles MR, Boucher RC. Effects of *Pseudomonas aeruginosa* on bronchial epithelial ion transport. *Am Rev Respir Dis* 1986; 134: 17–21.
129. Adler KB, Hendley DD, Davis GS. Bacteria associated with obstructive pulmonary disease elaborate extracellular products that stimulate secretion by explants of guinea pig airways. *Am J Pathol* 1986; **125:** 501–514.
130. Somerville M, Rutman A, Wilson R, Cole PJ, Richardson PS. Stimulation of secretion into human and feline airways by *Pseudomonas aeruginosa* proteases. *J Appl Physiol* 1991; **70:** 2259–2267.
131. Somerville M, Taylor GW, Watson D *et al*. Release of mucus glycoconjugates by *Pseudomonas aeruginosa* rhamnolipids into feline trachea *in vivo* and human bronchus *in vitro*. *Am J Respir Cell Mol Biol* 1992; **6:** 116–122.
132. Wilson R, Sykes DA, Watson D, Rutman A, Taylor GW, Cole PJ. Measurement of *Pseudomonas aeruginosa* phenazine pigments in sputum and assessment of their contribution to sputum sol toxicity for respiratory epithelium. *Infect Immun* 1988; **56:** 2515–2517.
133. Barsum W, Wilson R, Read RC *et al*. Interaction of fimbriate and non-fimbriate clinical isolates of non-typable *Haemophilus influenzae* with human respiratory tract mucus *in vitro*. *Thorax* 1992; **47:** 859.
134. Currie DC, Saverymuttu SH, Peters AM *et al*. Indium-111-labelled granulocyte accummulation in respiratory tract of patients with bronchiectasis. *Lancet* 1987; **i:** 1335–1339.
135. Sykes DA, Wilson R, Greenstone M, Currie DC, Steinfort C, Cole PJ. Deleterious effects of purulent sputum sol on human ciliary function *in vitro*: at least two factors identified. *Thorax* 1987; **42:** 256–261.
136. Lapa e Silva JR, Jones JAH, Cole PJ, Poulter LW. The immunological component of the cellular

inflammatory infiltrate in bronchiectasis. *Thorax* 1989; **44:** 668–673.
137. Currie DC, Peters AM, Garbett ND *et al*. Indium-111-labelled granulocyte scanning to detect inflammation in the lungs of patients with chronic sputum expectoration. *Thorax* 1990; **45:** 541–544.
138. Shak S, Capon DJ, Hellmiss R *et al*. Recombinant human DNase reduced the viscosity of cystic fibrosis sputum. *Proc Natl Acad Sci USA* 1990; **87:** 9188–9192.
139. Aitken ML, Burke W, McDonald G *et al*. Effect of inhaled recombinant human DNAse on pulmonary function in normal and cystic fibrosis patients: Phase 1 study. *Am Rev Respir Dis* 1991; **143** (Suppl.): A298.
140. McElvaney NG, Hubbard RC, Birrer P *et al*. Aerosol alpha-1-antitrypsin treatment for cystic fibrosis. *Lancet* 1991; **337:** 392–394.

7

Cystic fibrosis

D.M. Geddes and M.E. Hodson

The past 5 years have seen an enormous increase in understanding of the molecular biology of cystic fibrosis (CF). The gene has been identified and characterized, and the link between CF mutations and protein dysfunction is rapidly being worked out. Similarly the normal and disordered function of the protein is becoming clearer as is its role in epithelial ion transport. It should soon be possible to understand how the CF gene causes disease and this in turn should lead to new forms of treatment.

The CF gene

Before 1989 linkage analysis had assigned the CF locus to the long arm of chromosome 7, band q31 [1–4]. Thereafter various novel gene cloning strategies were used to pinpoint the CF gene [5]. The key approach used was the combination of chromosome walking and jumping. *Walking* consists of comparing known DNA with libraries derived from different tissues so that by matching segments along the gene a complete picture is built up. *Jumping* involves circularizing a segment of DNA so that two distant parts can be brought together. Chromosome jumping, as pioneered by Collins [6] proved to be particularly powerful as it allows the production of a number of additional starting points for chromosome walks and also circumvents blocks caused by unclonable sequences.

A total of 2–3 × 10^5 base pairs were cloned [2] before the end of the gene was found. Thereafter sequences were accumulated and a picture of the gene built up. Several transcribed and conserved sequences were identified, one of which, spanning about 250 000 base pairs, corresponded to the CF gene.

Finally, 18 additional clones were isolated and although none corresponded to the length of the observed transcript a consensus sequence was derived from the overlapping regions. Together these clones span about 6.1 Kb and contain an open reading frame for a protein of 1480 amino acids. The nucleotide sequence allowed deduction of the amino acid sequence and prediction of the protein structure (see below).

Detection of mutation

This required detailed comparison of nucleotide sequences in cDNA from patients with CF and unaffected individuals. A striking difference of a three-base deletion was found which would result in the loss of a phenylalanine residue at position 508. This mutation was present on 68% of CF chromosomes but was not found in any of 198 normal chromosomes ($P\ 10^{-57.5}$).

Haplotype analysis was carried out to explore the nature of the CF mutations further [7]. There was a close association between the position 508 deletion and the most common haplotype, and the existence of at least seven other less common haplotypes suggest there may be as many (or more) further mutations. Subsequent analysis of different populations of patients with CF have shown the frequency of this major mutation to be 75.8% in the USA, 74.4% in the UK [8], 49% in Spain, 43% in Italy [9] and 30.3% in Ashkenazy families [10]. At least 100 different mutations have now been identified.

Tissue distribution

In order to find out where the gene is expressed Riordan *et al.* [11] looked for the relevant mRNA in a range of different cells. RNA gel-blot hybridization with the first isolated cDNA clone (10-1) was used to assess the presence of the RNA transcript of the gene. A prominent band about 6.5 Kb in size was seen in T84 colonic carcinoma cells and similar strong signals were detected in pancreas and primary cell cultures from nasal polyps. The hybridization band intensity allows an estimate of the amount of RNA and suggests that the CF gene transcripts made up about 0.01% of total mRNA in the T84 cells. Similar mRNA was seen in lung, colon, sweat glands, placenta, liver and parotid glands, although the signal was weaker in these tissues. Transcripts were not detectable in brain, adrenal gland, skin fibroblast or lymphocyte cell lines.

It seems, therefore, that the CF gene is expressed in tissues affected by CF and not in those such as brain and adrenal gland which are spared by the disease. Furthermore, the amount and size of the transcripts were the same for CF and control tissues, which is consistent with CF mutations being subtle changes at the nucleotide level.

Predicted protein structure and function

The 1480 amino acid predicted from the DNA sequence has a molecular mass of about 168 000 Da and contains a number of repeated motifs to which possible functions can be given. There are 12 hydrophobic helices capable of spanning the cell membrane and two nucleotide (ATP) binding folds likely to be situated in the cytoplasm. A further putative cytoplasmic domain (labelled the R domain) is in the centre of the polypeptide and contains sequences which could be phosphorylation sites for protein kinases A and C. The 508 deletion occurs in one of the nucleotide binding folds and could therefore interfere with ATP-mediated alterations in protein configuration.

This protein structure is similar to P-glycoprotein which confers multiple drug resistance to some human cancer cells, perhaps by exporting the drug from the cell. It is also similar to a number of well characterized bacterial membrane proteins [12]. These have membrane transport functions dependent on ATP. Another similar protein is associated with chloroquine resistance in the malarial parasite and yet another is responsible for export of a mating pheromone in yeast. On these grounds it appeared likely that the CF-gene-related protein resides in the cell membrane and is associated with transmembrane transport.

Insertion of the wild type CF gene into a number of cell systems has been associated with the appearance of chloride channel function. These findings, together with an ingenious experiment in which specific mutations were induced in the gene in order to alter the charges of the membrane spanning part of the protein and so alter anion permeability, all show that Cystic Fibrosis Transmembrane Regulator (CFTR) proteins has a chloride channel function. It is, however, not yet clear whether this is the only or even the main function of the protein. Over-expression of the related P glycoprotein also induces chloride channel activity while this latter protein has a well established second function as a transporter of macromolecules across the cell membrane.

Antibodies to CFTR have shown its presence in the airway epithelium and submucous glands sweat ducts, gut and pancreatic ducts – all of which are affected by CF. More surprising are the findings that CFTR is present in the collecting tubule of the kidney. The protein is chiefly localized in the plasma membrane but is also demonstrable in association with some intracellular membranes.

The way in which the CF mutation alters the ion transporting properties of the cell is unclear. The chloride channel activity of CFTR could explain the impaired chloride permeability of affected epithelia in CF but does not account for the increased sodium transport in the airways (see below). While it is possible that chloride impermeability itself leads to changes in sodium transport, there are two more likely hypotheses. The first suggests that CFTR exports a macromolecule from the cell and that failure of this export results in the build up of a toxic substance which has widespread effects on ion transport [13]. The second hypothesis suggests that CFTR in the membranes of intracellular organelles facilitates the synthesis of macromolecules destined for the plasma cell membranes; changes in CFTR could alter such macromolecules and so change the ion transport properties of the cell membrane.

Ion transport

For many years abnormalities of ionic concentration of body fluids have been reported in CF. The best known are the high levels of sodium and chloride ions in sweat but there have also been suggestions of a relative deficiency of water in some secretions. Recently there has been an explosion of interest in the transport of ions across epithelial cells in CF and abnormalities have been found in the sweat glands, airways, pancreas and gut; uniting the clinically affected organs by a common defect. The main ions studied have been sodium and chloride and research has focused on their passage through selective ion channels, the control of these channels by cAMP and calcium and the overall effect of these ionic movements in terms of electrical current, potential differences and water flux. It is likely that the CF gene-associated protein modifies the control of ion transport either directly or indirectly by facilitating the export of some controlling factor from the cell (see above). This chapter will concentrate solely on the respiratory epithelium: ion transport in sweat duct [14], secretory coil [15], pancreatic ductal cells [16] and gut [17] in CF have been recently discussed elsewhere.

The key findings in CF airway epithelia have been a raised transepithelial potential difference, an increase in sodium flux from the lumen across the apical cell membrane and a relative impermeability of this apical membrane to chloride ions. Human airways normally absorb sodium from the lumen with little net chloride movement, and it is likely that the increased sodium flux is the most important abnormality in CF and is responsible for the high negative charge. This is supported by the finding that amiloride, a specific blocker of apical sodium channels lowers the potential difference by 80% and abolishes the difference in surface charge between normal airways and those in CF. In spite of the central importance of sodium transport, the chloride channel and its control has been more extensively studied.

In summary, the apical cell membrane in CF is almost completely impermeable to chloride ions and manipulations that open the chloride channels in normal airways, such as increases in cAMP or activity of protein kinases A or C, have no effect in CF. In contrast, elevation of free intracellular calcium opens chloride channels in CF but perhaps only at supraphysiological levels. Interestingly, when a patch of apical membrane is excised from the cell the CF and normal chloride channels are similar, suggesting that control mechanisms may be defective, rather than the channel itself. In contrast, studies of the sodium channel and its control are few, although one preliminary report suggested that the CF sodium channel is open longer than normal.

The finding that CFTR has chloride channel activity can explain the chloride impermeability of CF. The channel concerned is relatively small (7ps) and is regulated by cAMP. Interestingly, when the nucleotides ATP and UTP are applied to the apical surface of the cell chloride secretion is activated in CF, perhaps via purinergic receptors [18]. The excess sodium transport is difficult to link with the known functions of CFTR and possible mechanisms have been discussed above.

Pathogenesis

The link between abnormal ion transport and bacterial infection has not yet been elucidated but there are at least three possible explanations [19]. The first is that the increased sodium flux acts as an osmotic pump and removes excess water from the airway lumen. In support of this are the findings that airway surface liquid in CF is relatively dry and that amiloride increases airway liquid in sheep. In theory, such dehydration could reduce mucociliary clearance in CF, although clearance studies *in vivo* have given conflicting results. Recently, however, nebulized amiloride has been shown to improve clearance in CF. The second possibility is that the increased negative charge on the airway surface may modify mucus properties or bacterial adherence. There is as yet little supporting evidence but amiloride has been shown to affect mucus rheology. The third explanation is that other ions, in particular sulphate, are also affected by the ion transport abnormality. Mucus and cell surface glycoproteins have been shown to have abnormally high sulphation levels in CF and this could alter bacterial adherence or mucociliary clearance.

Diagnosis

Prenatal diagnosis

Prenatal diagnosis of CF by analysis of DNA obtained from chorionic villus sampling has been available since 1986 [20] based on comparing the fetal and parental pattern of markers around the CF locus. This approach requires DNA from a previously affected child and requires both parents to be fully informative (and means that the CF-bearing chromosome can be identified), conditions which are met in 85% of cases [21, 22]. Identification of the ΔF 508 mutation present in 78% of CF chromosomes in the UK [23], now permits screening by direct gene analysis [8, 24] and if both parents are heterozygous for ΔF 508 DNA from a previously affected child is not required. Studies of linked markers remain important in other families and the number of non-informative families is decreasing with the identification of new and more closely linked DNA markers such as KM 19 and XV2C [7, 25].

The introduction of the rapid and sensitive polymerase chain reaction [26] has enabled DNA to be obtained from buccal epithelial cells in mouth-wash samples [27] and from old Guthrie cards of children who have died [27, 28]. Fibroblasts from affected children who have died have also been stored frozen for use in future prenatal diagnosis [29].

Partly informative couples who elect to embark on a further pregnancy may be faced with the decision of whether to abort a fetus which has a 50% chance of being a normal carrier and 50% chance of having CF. Amniocentesis with microvillar enzyme assays enables further screening to be offered to such couples [30], but the optimal time of sampling for this measurement is at 17 weeks' gestation and some couples may find a second trimester abortion unacceptable. In addition, the technique carries a 2% false-positive and a 4% false-negative rate. This technique is a useful adjunct to genetic screening in appropriate cases but is no longer useful as a routine test.

Neonatal screening

Neonatal screening for CF is not widely practised, although a number of screening studies have been carried out using the immunoreactive trypsin (IRT) assay on dried blood spots because serum IRT levels are high in CF during the first year of life. This may be due to back-leakage of enzymes as the pancreatic ducts become blocked in the early stage of pancreatic damage [31]. The screening protocol involves an initial test at 5–8 days of age followed by a second test at 3–7 weeks if the first is positive. If the second test is positive a sweat test is performed together with a full clinical assessment. Retesting rates in most studies are 0.37–0.8% [32–35] but have been as high as 5% [36]. False-negative rates usually reported are 3–8% [33, 34], but have been as high as 23% [36].

The potential advantages of neonatal screening for CF are that earlier diagnosis and institution of appropriate treatment may improve the prognosis of an affected child, and that genetic counselling can be offered to parents before a further pregnancy is planned. The value of early diagnosis to an affected child is uncertain [37], but two reports suggest that infants diagnosed on screening develop fewer chest infections and have better weight gain in the first 2 years of life [35, 38]. It is possible, however, that the groups of patients in these studies are not comparable, particularly as recent evidence suggests that screening is picking up considerable numbers of otherwise undiagnosed patients with milder disease [34]. With regard to genetic counselling, neonatal screening will identify only one in four couples at risk of having an affected child in their next pregnancy, so its potential benefit is considerably lower than with that of population screening of carriers.

While IRT assay offers a simple and effective method of neonatal diagnosis of CF, genetic advances now mean that more than 50% of neonates (those homozygous for the F 508 mutation) can be reliably diagnosed by DNA analysis, specimens for which can also be obtained from dried blood spots [27]. Future neonatal screening programmes may therefore use DNA studies instead of, or in combination with, IRT assays.

Carrier detection

The cloning of the CF gene and characterization of the most common mutation have immediate implications for the identification of carriers of a mutant CF gene. As a result a number of pilot projects are already under way to assess the feasibility and benefits of population screening. There are three main questions to be answered: how informative is population screening? who should be screened? what would be the gains and losses of such a programme?

The results of screening programmes depend upon the number of abnormal mutations and their frequency in the population studied. The 508 mutation is present in about 75% of cases of CF in USA and UK, but is much less frequent in Southern European and Ashkenazy Jewish populations and there are so far about 100 abnormal mutations identified. This means that screening for the 508 mutation would at best detect only 75% of carriers and therefore only 50% of couples at risk. Screening for all known mutations would increase the pick-up rate but this would be much more complex and expensive.

Screening could involve the whole population or selected subgroups such as those with a family history of CF. There are very strong arguments for restricting screening to such high-risk subgroups, at least to begin with: in the first place the tests will be much more informative because the abnormal mutation in the family is usually known, and secondly such families have some knowledge of CF and so counselling is simpler and decisions about prenatal diagnosis and possible termination of pregnancy are better informed. Even in such families screening tests will not always give clear-cut results but only an estimate of probabilities [39].

The most important issue is the balance of benefit and loss to the community and to the carriers who are detected in a screening programme. In theory CF could be eliminated, so reducing suffering and expense, but this is most unlikely. The median survival in CF is 25 years and rising and many parents do not want to terminate an affected pregnancy, particularly when the prospects of new treatments are good. The issues of false-positive results and the stigma of being an identified carrier have also to be considered.

At present carrier detection should be offered only to those with a family history of CF. It is most unlikely that screening programmes will make a major impact on the incidence of new cases of CF, most of whom are born to parents with no family history, for at least the next 10 years.

Routine diagnosis

The sweat test remains central to the diagnosis of CF after full clinical assessment [40]. When performed by experienced personnel and combined with repeat tests using fludrocortisone suppression where necessary, errors are few, but false-positive and false-negative results cause diagnostic problems. Measurement of nasal potential difference has recently been introduced as an additional diagnostic technique for equivocal cases [41–44]. The technique is based on measurement of airway transepithelial potential difference, which is significantly raised in patients with CF. The test is simple to do and well tolerated in most age groups, although it has proved difficult in 2–5-year-old children. Nasal potential difference should not be measured during upper respiratory tract infections (when it is known to be lowered) or in the presence of nasal polyps which exhibit a lower potential difference than normal nasal epithelium. Excluding these two factors, the sensitivity and specificity of the technique are comparable to the sweat test and it is a useful additional diagnostic test.

The recent genetic advances provide another way of confirming the diagnosis which will become increasingly accurate as more mutations are identified. DNA analysis has not yet been used for routine diagnosis.

Pulmonary infection

Microbiology

The main cause of morbidity and mortality in CF is bacterial lung infection, the bacteria most frequently involved being *Haemophilus influenzae, Staphylococcus aureus, Pseudomonas aeruginosa* and *Pseudomonas cepacia*. Infection with *H. influenzae* is often intermittent and, while it may produce acute exacerbations of pulmonary infection, its contribution to chronic lung damage is not as clearly defined as that of the other organisms mentioned [45].

Staphylococcus aureus

Chronic colonization with *S. aureus* is common in children with CF, but intermittent infection also occurs. The reported prevalence of *S. aureus* in the sputum of patients with CF varies from 29% to 72% [45–47] and decreases with age. Advanced lung damage due to staphylococcal infection alone may occur before pseudomonal colonization and before anti-staphylococcal antibiotics were available it was responsible for most of the morbidity and mortality in CF [45]. Some centres use prophylactic anti-staphylococcal antibiotics from the time of the initial diagnosis or from the onset of bacteriologically proven staphylococcal infection [48]. While lower incidences of staphylococcal colonization have been reported with prophylactic treatment [49], there may be a higher incidence of pseudomonal colonization [50]. The restricted use of anti-staphylococcal antibiotics in some centres is claimed to have reduced the incidence of pseudomonal colonization [48]. These issues require further evaluation.

The presence of methicillin-resistant *S. aureus* in the sputum of patients with CF is increasing, but its prevalence is low at around 3% [51] and causes little change in clinical condition.

Pseudomonas aeruginosa

Infection of the airways with *P. aeruginosa* is responsible for most of the pulmonary damage in CF (Table 7.1) The incidence of pseudomonal colonization rises with age and is 70–90% in most adult patient populations [49]. The source of initial colonization may be the environment or cross-infection from another CF patient, and the importance of the latter has been the subject of much recent interest. The observation of an increased rate of acquisition of *P. aeruginosa* in the sputum of a population of Danish patients in whom regular hospital admissions resulted in increased patient contact raised initial concern [50] and subsequent segregation of colonized and non-colonized patients reduced the rate at which colonization was acquired [51]. Suggestions that contamination of inanimate objects in hospital was an important factor [52] have not been confirmed by others [53]. Transient acquisition of new strains in patients sharing hospital rooms has been reported [53]. A number of epidemiological studies in which pseudomonal strain types were studied by serological, and more recently genetic, techniques have demonstrated that siblings with CF usually share strain types [54–57], but that this is uncommon for unrelated patients. It is prolonged, intimate contact that therefore appears important for cross-infection: segregation of colonized and non-colonized patients in clinics and during hospital admission is probably unnecessary.

Initial colonization is usually with non-mucoid strains. The emergence of mucoid strains, which genetic studies now suggest are derived from the existing non-mucoid strains [48], and the development of the host immune response are factors correlated with a worsening prognosis [58].

Bacterial production of toxins and proteases may be important in initial lung damage, but in later stages most lung damage results from neutrophil enzymes and oxidative processes [59].

Pseudomonas cepacia

P. cepacia, a ubiquitous organism, is a relatively new pathogen in CF. Colonization is more common in those with poor pulmonary function [60–62], but occurs with a worrying frequency in patients in whom pulmonary function remains good [63]. The observation of a greater prevalence of the organism and the association of initial colonization with a hospital admission led to concern about cross- infection and precautions taken against this have reduced the incidence of colonization in some centres [64]. In the UK, the incidence appears stable at present [48]. This organism was first reported to produce severe progressive respiratory failure associated with

Table 7.1 Antibiotics used for treatment of pseudomonal infection in CF

Antipseudomonal penicillins or cephalosporins (i.v.)

- Carboxypenicillins
  Carbenicillin
  Ticarcillin
- Ureodipenicillins
  Mezlocillin
  Azlocillin
- Third-generation penicillins
  Ceftazidime
  Cefsuladine
- Aztreonam
- Imipenem
- Temocillin
- Others
  Ciprofloxacin can be given orally or intravenously. Colomycin is given by nebulizer

Aminoglycosides (i.v.)

- Gentamicin
- Tobramycin
- Netilmicin
- Amikacin

high fever, leucocytosis and a high erythrocyte sedimentation rate [60]. However, subsequent studies have shown that serious infection is rare and that colonization usually causes little change in clinical state or prognosis.

Other pulmonary infections

Viral infections

Patients with CF do not have an increased incidence of proven viral infections compared with their normal siblings [65–67]. The frequency of viral infections in CF is, however, closely associated with pulmonary deterioration. Whether this is due directly to viral infection, to viral–bacterial interaction or a combination of the two remains to be clarified.

Mycobacterial infection

The incidence of mycobacterial infection in CF populations where routine sputum examination for acid-fast bacilli is performed has been reported as 3–11% [68, 69]. Organisms reported include *Mycobacterium tuberculosis* in 17-43% of cases, and opportunistic mycobacteria in the remainder. The diagnosis is often not suspected clinically. Night sweats, which are unusual in patients with CF, may be a warning symptom. Most cases respond to appropriate chemotherapy, but occasional fatalities are reported [65, 66].

Aspergillus fumigatus

The incidence of allergic bronchopulmonary aspergillosis is increased in CF. This is an allergic reaction, not an infection, and responds to treatment with steroids.

Treatment of pulmonary infection

The aim of treatment of pulmonary infection is to reduce the progression of lung damage. Physiotherapy is important, but greater clinical improvement may be achieved with appropriate antibiotic therapy [70]. Antimicrobial therapy has a central role, but other drug treatments aimed at suppressing the host immune response may be beneficial and clinical improvement has been reported following long-term alternate-day prednisolone therapy [71]. The value of inhaled steroids is being assessed.

There are many unresolved issues regarding appropriate antibiotic therapy. These include controversy about which antibiotics should be used, whether single or combined treatment is appropriate, what duration of therapy is best, which dosing schedules and means of delivery should be adopted and what significance should be attached to the results of *in vitro* antibiotic sensitivity assays [72]. A recent review of controlled antibiotic trials in CF concluded that placebo-controlled trials have failed to prove benefit for antibiotic therapy in acute exacerbations, suggesting that other treatment methods such as physiotherapy and improved nutritional care may be equally important. While treatment of infective exacerbations results in short-term clinical improvement in terms of pulmonary function tests and weight gain, the long-term benefit remains to be determined and there is no clear definition of what constitutes an infective exacerbation requiring antibiotic treatment [48]. Although trials have shown no advantage from combination antibiotic therapy, concern about later emergence of resistant strains persuade most clinicians to use two drugs. Acquired antibiotic resistance is often short-term but becomes a greater problem in patients receiving frequent antibiotic courses [72]. The need to prescribe antibiotic treatment according to *in vitro* bacterial sensitivities is not established and clinical improvement often occurs when patients are treated with antibiotics to which their infecting organisms are resistant *in vitro* [72]. This issue is the subject of ongoing clinical trials. One reason may be that subinhibitory doses of many antibiotics can reduce the production of pseudomonal toxins and proteases [73].

It is current practice to give two antibiotics to take full advantage of synergy. This is usually an antipseudomonal penicillin or cephalosporin paired with an aminoglycoside (see Table 7.1). Ticarcillin has been compared with carbenicillin [74], azlocillin and carbenicillin [75], tobramycin with gentamicin [76, 77], and ceftazidime with carbenicillin and gentamicin [78]. No difference in clinical response was demonstrated. The choice of antibiotics should therefore be decided by excluding those to which the patient is allergic and those to which the patient's organisms are resistant. It would then be appropriate to choose the cheapest available antibiotic combination. It is the authors' practice not to use piperacillin as a proportion of patients with CF have had febrile reactions following its use. Indications for treatment are an acute exacerbation of symptoms as indicated by cough, sputum or breathlessness, together with a deterioration in chest radiograph, FEV_1, FVC or oxygen saturation. It is essential to continue the treatment for at least 10–14 days; some patients appear to benefit from slightly longer courses of treatment. Drugs may be given in hospital or at home and the use of a long line is preferable to a short cannula which may need to be repositioned a number of times during the course of treatment. Patients requiring this access can benefit from the use of an implanted intravenous device [79].

Home administration of intravenous antibiotics is increasing in both adults and children [80, 81]. It reduces costs, is preferred by many patients and the incidence of complications is extremely low. Use of implantable venous access devices has increased the availability of access [82]. The availability of ciprofloxacin has enabled some infective exacerbations due to *P. aeruginosa* to be treated orally, but organisms frequently acquire resistance to this drug [83].

In addition to the short-term benefit of treating acute infectious exacerbations, long-term benefit may be achieved by regular or continuous antibiotic administration. An improved prognosis has been reported in patients treated with intravenous antibiotic courses at 3-monthly intervals regardless of the patient's clinical condition [50] and this policy is practised in some centres. Continuous aerosol antibiotic therapy, which is performed at home, is of clinical benefit in reducing the frequency of acute infective exacerbations and also improves lung function [84, 85].

Physiotherapy

There have been no major changes in physiotherapy techniques for CF over the past few years and established treatment is highly effective. Present treatment combines the forced expiration technique [86–88], interspersed with controlled diaphragmatic breathing and thoracic expansion exercise, with gravity-assisted postural drainage and coughing. Interspersing the technique with pauses for controlled breathing and relaxation reduces fatigue and prevents hypoxia during therapy [89]. During acute infective exacerbations patients often require assistance with postural drainage, but when well can achieve equally effective sputum clearances when performing postural drainage themselves [86]. Chest percussion is not an essential part of treatment if other techniques are performed effectively [90].

Some centres advocate the use of periodic application of a face mask with positive expiratory pressure (PEP mask) during physiotherapy with the proposed advantages that it can be performed in a sitting position, does not require an assistant and is associated with less oxygen desaturation [91]. Others have shown no advantage of the PEP mask over correctly performed standard treatment as described above [90] and it is not widely used.

The effect of exercise combined with standard physiotherapy in aiding sputum expectoration has recently been evaluated and was found to have no significant effect on daily sputum production [92]. While it has other benefits and should be encouraged, exercise is not a substitute for any part of the current physiotherapy regimens.

Haemoptysis and bronchial artery embolization

Minor episodes of haemoptysis are common in CF, occurring in over 60% of patients [46], but these usually settle with medical management including appropriate antibiotic therapy and correction of any clotting disorders. Bronchial artery embolization for life-threatening massive haemoptysis, which without intervention carries a high mortality rate [93], is occasionally required. Results reported in two recent series [94, 95] give immediate success rates of 55–84% with one embolization, increasing to 88–95% after a second embolization when required. Later severe recurrences, which have been reported in more than 50% of patients, have been treated by repeat embolization with a success rate of 89% [95]. Side effects are usually limited to transient chest pain and pyrexia which can be treated symptomatically. Patients requiring bronchial artery embolization have a higher mortality rate than matched controls during the following 3 months, for which haemoptysis is a contributing cause in one-third [95].

Congestive heart failure

Patients with end-stage respiratory failure may develop right ventricular failure as a result of vasoconstriction in the pulmonary circulation due to hypoxia. It is treated in the conventional way with oxygen therapy together with diuretics and potassium supplements. Some patients appear to benefit from long-term low-concentration oxygen but there are few controlled trials available in patients with CF. It is very difficult to persuade an adolescent or young adult to take 15 hours of oxygen a day except when they are very sick. A few patients who have end-stage disease and are awaiting transplantation have benefited from use of a nasal ventilator [96, 97].

Heart–lung transplantation

The first two successful heart–lung transplants for CF were performed in 1985 [98–100] and now more than 90 patients with CF have received heart–lung transplants in the UK (including two heart–lung and liver transplants) [99–101]. The first patient transplanted is alive and well more than 6 years after transplantation. The actuarial survival at 1 year is 63–69%. Most early deaths are due to bleeding, infection, adult respiratory distress syndrome and multisystem failure. Although the long-term prognosis of these patients is unknown, the results so far are encouraging and give new hope to CF patients with advanced pulmonary disease. Unfortunately, the number of donor lungs available will never satisfy demand in spite of recent advances in lung preservation techniques providing an increase in the number of donors from more distant locations [98, 100] and patients accepted for heart–lung transplantation continue to die while on the waiting list. Careful selection of patients is therefore important.

Assessment for transplantation

The major indication for heart–lung transplantation in CF is deteriorating chronic respiratory failure which is assessed by lung function studies (usually FEV_1 and FVC less than 40% predicted), blood gases, oxygen desaturation at rest and on exercise, the patient's level of exercise tolerance and frequency of admission for intravenous antibiotics (Table 7.2). The optimum time for transplantation is when the prognosis is only a few months but before the patient becomes moribund. This is, however, difficult to judge as the rate of clinical decline is very variable. Relative

Table 7.2 Selection criteria for heart–lung transplantation in CF

Indications
- Deteriorating chronic respiratory failure

Major contraindications
- Psychological disturbance
- Poor treatment compliance
- Age > 50 years
- Weight 50% predicted
- Hepatic cirrhosis*
- Portal hypertension*
- Previous pleurectomy
- ? Multiple resistant *S. aureus*
- Systemic corticosteroid therapy

Minor contraindications
- Psychological disturbance
- Poor treatment compliance
- Age > 50 years
- Weight 75% predicted
- Creatinine clearance 700 ml/min
- Diabetes
- Other pleural therapy
- Mycobacterial or *Aspergillus* infections

*Possible heart, lung and liver transplant

contraindications include major psychosocial problems usually associated with a history of poor compliance, poor nutritional state, pleural adhesions, renal failure, advanced liver disease and systemic corticosteroid therapy. Nutrition can be improved with dietary advice in some patients while others require insertion of a feeding gastrostomy. Computed tomography scanning identifies pleural adhesions. As previous pleurectomy presents a major risk, the role of limited abrasion pleurodesis for patients with recurrent pneumothorax who may later be considered for transplantation is being assessed. Good renal function is necessary because of the use of cyclosporin for immunosuppression. Malabsorption needs to be assessed with faecal fat studies to help in appropriate dosing of oral cyclosporin after surgery. Patients with severe liver disease or portal hypertension can be considered only for combined heart–lung and liver transplantation. Diabetes is not a contraindication. Cardiac assessment is needed as the recipient's heart is now frequently transplanted into another patient (domino procedure). Steroid therapy should be withdrawn if at all possible but in any case reduced below 10 mg per day, as it may interfere with healing of the tracheal anastomosis.

Full microbiological screening is important. Antibiotic sensitivities need to be known for postoperative treatment and infection with *Aspergillus fumigatus* (which may cause postoperative opportunistic infection) or *Mycobacterium tuberculosis* must be treated first. Successful heart–lung transplantation has been performed in patients with methicillin-resistant *S. aureus* infection, which is not therefore a contraindication, but particular care is needed not to contaminate areas needed for continuation of the transplant programme.

Management of terminal illness in patients awaiting heart–lung transplantation can be difficult as decisions have to be made regarding withdrawal of active treatment and whether ventilatory support should be considered. Most centres do not consider that intubation and formal ventilation are appropriate for these patients, but the value of non-invasive nasal ventilation for patients awaiting heart–lung transplantation is now being assessed [96].

The operation

The operation preferred in the UK is heart and lung transplantation with retransplantation of the recipient's heart into another patient. Double lung transplantation is being assessed in the USA.

Following transplantation lung function improves progressively over a period of months towards normal values [19], patients gain weight and finger clubbing resolves. Late complications, the frequency and prognosis of which are not yet known, include recolonization with *Pseudomonas*, malignancy secondary to immunosuppression and obliterative bronchiolitis. The latter is a serious clinical problem which is probably a manifestation of chronic rejection [99, 100]. It presents insidiously with cough and breathlessness associated with a decline in FEV_1/FVC with the chest radiograph showing little change. Affected patients are treated with increased immunosuppression but this is usually of little benefit and lung function continues to decline – a further lung transplant is the only treatment. Lymphoproliferative disorders, which are most commonly of the B cell type and are positive for Epstein–Barr virus nuclear antigen respond to a reduction in immunosuppression combined with intravenous acyclovir. One T-cell lymphoma responded to a reduction in immunosuppression alone [99, 100].

Future improvements in transplantation should come from improved patient selection, increasing the supply of donor organs and improving the management of late complications, particularly obliterative bronchiolitis.

Nutritional care

Energy balance

Undernutrition is a very common problem in patients with CF and is associated with a poorer prognosis [102]: its correction is therefore central to the clinical management of these patients. It arises for three main reasons: inadequate energy intake, energy losses via the gastrointestinal tract and increased energy requirements.

Energy intake

Patients with CF require an energy intake 120–150% that of normal individuals to maintain their weight and need appropriate dietary advice on how to achieve this. A recent comparison of two patient populations in Boston and Toronto [103] demonstrated that patients in the Boston population had lower body weights and a poorer prognosis attributable to worse pulmonary disease. The only significant difference in clinical management of these groups was in the fat content of the diet, which was high in the Toronto group. It is now recommended that patients with CF should have a high-calorie diet with no fat restriction, combined with adequate pancreatic supplementation to prevent steatorrhoea, because the consumption of energy-rich fatty foods helps to maintain a high calorie intake. Medical causes contribute to reduced food intake in CF, particularly acute respiratory exacerbations during which the patients may feel anorectic and be too breathless to eat. If infections are frequent and recurrent, then weight lost may not be fully regained between infections.

Gastrointestinal energy loss

Gastrointestinal energy losses due to malabsorption result from deficiency of pancreatic enzymes, reduced pancreatic bicarbonate secretion rendering the duodenal contents more acid (thus denaturing pancreatic lipase and encouraging precipitation of bile salts), and to excessive abnormal intestinal mucus which may further interfere with absorption [103].

Increased energy consumption

In patients with pulmonary infection increased energy requirements result from the increased work of breathing, but resting energy expenditure has also been shown to be elevated in patients with mild pulmonary disease [102]. Studies *in vitro* have also shown increased oxygen consumption in CF tissues [104]. It is possible that the basic defect in CF involves increased energy consumption, but this has yet to be fully evaluated.

Vitamin deficiencies

Although deficiencies of fat-soluble vitamins are often seen at the time of diagnosis, supplementation is now standard practice and clinically overt signs of deficiency of vitamins A, D and E are rare. A recent report describes asymptomatic conjunctival sclerosis, which was associated with severe night blindness in three patients with CF, suggesting that supplementation is not always adequate [105]. Vitamin E deficiency often manifests itself with evidence of haemolytic anaemia in newly diagnosed infants. In adults, in whom deficiency is rare with adequate supplementation, its manifestations are predominantly neurological and include diminished tendon reflexes, ataxia, muscle weakness and ophthalmoplegia [106–108]. This is often associated with the presence of advanced hepatic disease, and bile salt supplementation can improve vitamin E absorption in these patients [108].

Essential fatty acid deficiency

Clinical features of essential fatty acid deficiency may be observed in undiagnosed infants but are rare in older patients [102]. Low plasma levels of essential fatty acids are usually, but not always, restricted to patients with pancreatic insufficiency [109]. Recently interest has been focused on the possible connection of increased fatty acid metabolism with the basic defect in CF [109], but more work is needed to evaluate this fully. There is presently no convincing evidence of the clinical value of routine supplementation.

Nutritional management

Current nutritional care centres around provision of a high-calorie diet without fat restriction together with adequate pancreatic enzyme supplementation and supplementation with fat-soluble vitamins. Most nutritional problems arise later in the course of the disease when chest infections become more frequent and energy demands are therefore higher. Short-term use of intravenous total parenteral nutrition may be beneficial during an infective episode but weight gain is frequently not maintained [102]. Nasogastric feeding also has short-term benefits but few patients find that they can continue this at home because of problems with nasal irritation and maintaining placement of the tube [102]. Most recent approaches involving the use of nocturnal administration of feeds by gastrostomy [110, 111] or jejunostomy [112] tubes have achieved better results in terms of nutritional gain. Gastrostomies can be inserted endoscopically under local anaesthesia and are generally well tolerated by patients. Whether such improvements in nutrition improve the prognosis in terms of respiratory disease is a point yet to be clarified [102].

Pancreatic enzyme replacement

Adequate doses of pancreatic enzyme supplements control steatorrhoea in most patients and improved results have been obtained with the introduction of enteric-coated encapsulated microsphere preparations [113, 114].

New preparations containing more lipase activity have the advantage of reducing the number of capsules taken, but are otherwise no more effective than other enteric-coated microsphere preparations [115]. In patients who continue to have steatorrhoea the addition of oral H_2 receptor blockers such as cimetidine to reduce duodenal pH may be beneficial [116]. Bile acid supplementation with taurine has also been used but with no confirmed benefit [117].

Other organ systems

Distal intestinal obstruction syndrome

Distal intestinal obstruction syndrome (or meconium ileus) equivalent occurs in 16% of CF patients (usually those with known pancreatic insufficiency) and may be recurrent [46]. Conventional treatment has involved rehydration, oral and rectal *N*-acetylcysteine or gastrografin, enzyme replacement and attention to diet. This is successful in most cases. A recent advance has been the use of a balanced intestinal lavage solution which contains polyethylene glycol to minimize transmucosal fluid flux [118]. Following prophylactic antiemetics 5–6 litres of fluid is administered at a rate of 750–1000 ml/h either orally or via a nasogastric tube. Reports of its use so far indicate that it is an effective treatment with few side-effects [118, 119].

Liver

The incidence of liver disease in CF as defined by clinical hepatomegaly, abnormal biochemical liver function tests or both, has recently been reported in two large series as 24% (age range 16–45 years [120]) and 40% (age range 4–19 years [121]). Associated splenomegaly is reported in the latter series in 9% of patients. The incidence of ascites and oesophageal varices varies between series, possibly because of differences in patient age groups, from one patient with ascites in a population of 153 to 2.6% with bleeding oesophageal varices in a population of 233 in the adult series. However, bleeding oesophageal varices have been reported in as many as 10% of one group of teenagers [117]. These complications are treated in the conventional way. Symptoms of upper abdominal pain are reported in up to 56% of patients with hepatosplenomegaly [121], but liver disease is otherwise asymptomatic.

The variation in occurrence and severity of CF liver disease and the observation that cirrhosis may develop in patients with normal fat absorption indicates that factors additional to intrahepatic biliary obstruction are involved in its pathogenesis. One study [121] reported a very high incidence (96%) of distal common bile duct in CF patients with liver disease compared with none in a control group without liver disease but another study reported an incidence of only 3.5% [120]. A number of patients with distal biliary strictures and symptoms of upper abdominal pain have been treated with surgical bypass with complete relief of symptoms [121]. The early results of liver transplantation for CF are encouraging [122].

As the prognosis of CF patients improves with advances in antibiotic therapy and heart–lung transplantation, the incidence of symptomatic liver disease is likely to increase and will command more clinical attention.

Ursodeoxycholic acid has been shown to produce clinical and biochemical improvement when administered to adult patients with chronic cholestatic liver disease [123]. Preliminary studies have already been carried out in CF patients, with encouraging results [124]; however, the results of treating patients for long periods of time are still awaited.

Joints

Joint symptoms are reported to occur in 9% of CF patients [46, 125]. These are usually associated with infective exacerbations of chest disease, are not accompanied by abnormal physical signs and are treated symptomatically with minor analgesics and non-steroidal anti-inflammatory agents. Hypertrophic pulmonary osteoarthropathy has been reported.

Diabetes mellitus

The incidence of diabetes mellitus in CF is around 10% [46]. Most patients can be treated by dietary management with or without oral hypoglycaemic agents, but about one-third require insulin. Microvascular complications have been reported.

Pregnancy and lactation

Improved survival in CF has resulted in increasing numbers of pregnancies. Spontaneous abortion is no higher than in the general population but shortened gestation and increased perinatal mortality are significantly more common. Maternal complications in pregnancy include poor weight gain, congestive heart failure and worsening of lung function, which does not always return to pregravid values. Intravenous antibiotics have been used during all stages of pregnancy and no cases of fetal congenital abnormalities have been reported. Successful breast feeding may be possible. In general the outcome of these pregnancies has been excellent although poor maternal lung function and nutrition increase the risks [126, 127].

ENT

Sinusitis as a radiological diagnosis is almost universal in patients with CF, and many patients have evidence of active infection [128, 129]. Active infection should be treated by vigorous antibiotic therapy and medication given to improve nasal drainage. Some patients will need antral lavage or Caldwell–Luc surgery. There is a high incidence of nasal polyps in patients with CF; many of these can be successfully treated medically [130], but others may require surgery.

Psychological factors

As increasing numbers of patients survive into adult life, more interest is being focused on their social and psychological status. Many uncontrolled reports suggest few psychological problems in this patient group, an observation recently supported by a controlled study of the psychological assets of adults with CF compared with their healthy peers [131]. Psychological management has been well reviewed by Hodson *et al.* [76, 77].

Survival

In 1938, 80% of babies died within their first year of life [132]. In recent years there has been a significant improvement to survival which is probably due to a combination of factors including better paediatric care, advances in physiotherapy, nutrition, antibiotics and the establishment of special centres for the care of these patients. Survival to the age of 20 in the UK is reported as 49.5% [133]; figures for the USA and Canada are 43% and 55% respectively [103]. Later survival has been reported from Melbourne [134], and Toronto [103] where special clinics care for most CF individuals living in that area. There are about 6000 patients with CF in the UK, of whom 2000 are adults. It is estimated that about 150–200 CF patients reach 16 years of age each year. This increasing number of patients with multisystem and life-threatening disease is a specific challenge for the physicians who take over their care from paediatricians.

Future treatment approaches

Amiloride

Recent advances in knowledge of the epithelial ion transport abnormalities in CF have led to interest in drugs which modify these more basic defects rather than treating the resulting disease. Amiloride, which selectively blocks sodium absorption across the epithelial cell apical membrane, is presently being evaluated as a treatment. Oral administration does not achieve sufficiently high levels at the airway surfaces and interest has centred on its use as inhaled therapy. Studies of mucociliary clearance using radiolabelled inhaled particles in patients with CF have shown that a single dose of nebulized amiloride improves mucociliary clearance and cough clearance, presumably by increasing the depth of the periciliary fluid layer [135]. The effect lasts up to 80 min. Longer-term administration of twice-daily nebulized amiloride over a 3-week period increases the effect of a single dose [136]. In a recent pilot study of the overall clinical benefit of long-term nebulized amiloride in CF, it was administered four times daily for 6 months [137]. Compared with a control period, the patients on treatment demonstrated a slower rate of decline in lung function and improvements in sputum viscosity and elasticity. No toxic effects were noted and further evaluation of the treatment has been recommended. One problem with this study is that in both treated and untreated groups the rates of decline in lung function were higher than is usually observed in clinical practice. Two possible reasons for this are that the preceding treatment with intravenous antibiotics in all patients gave them an unrepresentatively high baseline or that withdrawal of all other respiratory treatment, including oral and inhaled antibiotics and bronchodilators, was responsible. Future studies with amiloride need to evaluate its benefit in addition to treatment already established to be of benefit.

One problem with amiloride is its short duration of action and the need for frequent dosing, which is inconvenient and may cause poor compliance. If it is shown to be of value as a regular treatment, then either longer acting preparations need to be developed or other drugs with a similar effect but longer duration of action evaluated. Therapeutic benefit may also become possible with bradykinin, which is capable of inducing chloride secretion in CF tissue *in vitro* via a receptor-mediated elevation of intracellular calcium [138].

Gene therapy

The most exciting prospect for treatment is to insert a copy of the normal gene for CFTR into the airway epithelium and so cure the defect. This works *in vivo* in a number of cell systems and could be applied to humans if an efficient delivery system can be designed. A number of vectors are being explored, including liposomes, receptor-mediated endocytosis and (most promisingly) viral vectors.

Retroviruses may not be suitable because of difficulties of reaching the airway stem cell and uncertainties about control of expression and safety. Adenoviruses have therefore received the most attention and preliminary results are encouraging. Adenoviruses are tropic for the respiratory epithelium and can be disabled and modified to carry human genes. This vector has been administered into the tracheae of live rats and expression of a human gene by the rat airways has been demonstrated which lasts for up to 1 week [139]. Much more work needs to be done to establish safety (to assess the risks of over-expression) and to determine whether repeated administration will be ineffective due to antibody formation.

Anti-inflammatory approaches

There is overwhelming evidence that the inflammatory processes directed against the colonizing organisms in the lungs not only fail to eradicate the organisms but actually cause local tissue damage. The failure to eradicate the organisms is due partly to the fact that local conditions appear to favour colonization and growth, partly to various defences employed by the bacteria (e.g. alginate production and microcolony formation), and partly to the products of inflammation themselves. In particular the proteolytic enzymes released by inflammatory cells may break down some immune products and so render these immune processes ineffective. For example, neutrophil elastase [140] cleaves chemotactic factors, breaks down some complement components, and inactivates immunoglobulins. In this way an inflammatory response can be considered as excessive in that it inhibits its own antimicrobial actions. At the same time many inflammatory mediators may damage local host tissues and set up a cycle of chronic inflammatory damage and scarring. This damage favours further bacterial growth as local mechanisms of bacterial inhibition and clearance are themselves impaired or destroyed. While many mediators are released during airway inflammation recent attention has focused on neutrophil elastase and free radicals.

A number of ways of countering this inflammatory damage have been proposed. These range from relatively specific therapy directed at proteolytic enzymes such as α1-antitrypsin to more general anti-inflammatory drugs, both steroidal (e.g. prednisolone) and non-steroidal (e.g. ibuprofen). The evidence in favour of these drugs is discussed below. The same logic can be extended to antioxidants such as gluthathione and to immune therapy with drugs such as methotrexate, azathioprine, or cyclosporin A, but these agents have not yet been evaluated in CF. For all of these anti-inflammatory and anti-immune approaches there are risks of uncontrolled infection.

Prednisolone

Corticosteroids, powerful anti-inflammatory drugs with some immunosuppressive properties, can be used to treat any co-existing bronchospasm and to assist mucociliary clearance. Prednisolone has therefore been frequently used as part of the treatment of CF but in low doses for short periods partly because of the risks of long-term side-effects and partly because of the possibility that it might worsen the respiratory infection.

In 1985 Auerbach *et al.* [71] reported a double-blind trial in which children with CF and relatively mild lung disease received prednisolone (2 mg/kg) or placebo on alternate days for 4 years. Prednisolone was associated with better lung function and weight, fewer hospital admissions and less evidence of immune activity as judged by lower IgG levels. Surprisingly, this relatively high-dose therapy was associated with few side-effects.

This study led to considerable interest, as well as some scepticism about the apparent freedom from side-effects, and a large multicentre double-blind study was set up comparing placebo with 1 mg/kg and 2 mg/kg of prednisolone. The patients were monitored every 3 months and an interim analysis of results was performed every 6 months by an unbiased ombudsman. After nearly 3 years the interim analysis showed an unacceptable level of side-effects (glucose intolerance, cataract, growth retardation) in the 2 mg/kg group and this part of the trial was abandoned [141]. Until the final results are available chronic prednisolone treatment cannot be recommended. An alternative approach using chronic inhaled corticosteroids is also being evaluated but has not yet been reported. The inhaled route is likely to cause fewer side-effects but has the theoretical disadvantage that the airways most affected by inflammation are likely to be the most difficult to reach.

Ibuprofen

This drug, in common with many other non-steroidal anti-inflammatory agents, acts by inhibiting arachidonic acid metabolism and so interfering with the production of prostaglandins and leukotrienes at sites of inflammation. Preliminary studies in animals have shown some evidence of protection of the lungs from chronic inflammatory damage [142] and clinical trials are now in progress.

α_1-Antitrypsin

This is the most important of a number of antiproteases which protect the lungs from proteolytic enzymes. While its deficiency was originally associated with lung disease in the form of emphysema, it is now clear that low circulating levels also predispose to bronchiectasis. Furthermore, in chronic pulmonary inflammation its amount, although normal, appears to be inadequate to balance the amount of proteolytic enzyme released. Replacement α_1-antitrypsin therapy may be valuable in the deficiency state, and considerable progress has already been made in investigating this form of therapy. Human α_1-antitrypsin can be prepared from donor blood and both infusions and aerosol delivery have been shown to provide normal levels in the lung epithelial lining fluid in α_1-antitrypsin deficient subjects. Furthermore, the α_1-antitrypsin gene has been cloned and bacterial insertion may eventually provide a pure source of the human antiprotease.

Preliminary studies in CF [143] have shown:

1. Normal levels of α_1-antitrypsin in epithelial lining fluid.
2. High levels of neutrophil elastase in epithelial lining fluid which swamp the α_1-antitrypsin activity.
3. Aerosol α_1-antitrypsin elevates the levels in epithelial lining fluid three- to sixfold

and the levels remain approximately twice normal 12 h after administration.

4. Neutrophil killing of *Pseudomonas* is inhibited by epithelial lining fluid from CF patients (presumably because of the excess neutrophil elastase) but returns to normal following aerosol treatment with α_1-antitrypsin.

Both the theory and these preliminary studies suggest a possible role for α_1-antitrypsin in modifying the airway inflammation and enhancing bacterial killing in CF. There are not, however, as yet any supporting clinical data. Furthermore, *Pseudomonas* colonization occurs in CF before there is gross inflammation and this treatment might only be appropriate for the more severely affected patients, in whom many other factors contribute to their deterioration.

An alternative antiprotease is secretory leukoprotease inhibitor. This is probably a less important system than α_1-antitrypsin but is also subject to much current investigation.

DNase

Uninfected sputum consists of a complex mixture of glycoproteins, water and electrolytes. When sputum becomes infected a large number of additional substances derived from bacteria and from the host's inflammatory response change its physical and chemical properties. In particular DNA, which is derived chiefly from neutrophils, is found in relatively high levels and makes the sputum more viscous and difficult to clear from the lungs.

The gene from DNase 1, the predominant enzyme responsible for the breakdown of DNA, has been cloned and recombinant human DNase (RhDNase) is now available. This enzyme has been studied for its possible benefit in liquefying CF sputum and convincingly reduces the viscosity of sputum derived from chronically infected subjects in a time- and dose-dependent way [144]. The preliminary data are encouraging and clinical studies have begun in the hope that it will be possible to improve sputum clearance at least during infectious exacerbations and so limit the duration of severity of the illness. Even more exciting would be the possibility of improving lung function by removing inspissated secretions or preventing the long-term decline of lung function with chronic use.

These possibilities must be set against the history of DNase therapy, which is in no way new. Bovine pancreatic DNase has been available for 40 years and has been subjected to a number of trials. While benefits have been claimed for its use as an aerosol treatment for pneumonia and CF, the evidence to support any clinical benefit is slight [145, 146]. A well designed trial of bovine DNase in purulent bronchitis showed lessening of sputum viscosity but no benefit in terms of lung function or other clinical parameters [147]. Similarly, a trial in CF showed improved viscosity but clinical benefit was only reported in four of the ten patients who took part. The author of this study claimed a major benefit of DNase especially in more seriously ill patients but the treatment never caught on and so cannot have been dramatically successful. The fact that the DNase was of bovine rather than human origin may not matter as the studies quoted above showed similar results with enzymes from either source. Perhaps the most important problem with earlier trials of DNase was inadequate aerosol technology.

In summary, DNase therapy is logical and merits further study. It will, however, be important for the relatively inexpensive bovine DNase to be compared with the very expensive recombinant human form.

Ethical considerations

The more fundamental treatments such as gene and ion transport therapy will take many years to develop and their assessment will raise new ethical issues. They will, at least in theory, be most likely to benefit the patient if they are given very early, and ideally should be started before the lungs become colonized by bacteria and before vicious cycles of inflammatory damage begin. Indeed, it may well be that these treatments will prove relatively ineffective once the lungs are damaged because in this situation persistent bacterial growth is a consequence of the damage and its secondary effect on lung clearance mechanisms rather than due to the genetic defect itself. These arguments are particularly worrying as there is a natural preference to try out new treatments on those with the most severe disease who are most in need of new drugs and who may therefore be ready to accept the attendant risks.

If it is accepted that presymptomatic patients are the most likely to benefit then difficult ethical issues must be raised. Will it be justifiable to give new treatments to children for many years in order to see whether lung disease is delayed or prevented? In the past when CF was almost fatal in early life this approach would have been more easily accepted than today, when 80% of patients with CF survive to the age of 20 and many are almost free of symptoms. If the prognosis continues to improve then these issues will become even more difficult, particularly with entirely new treatments such as gene therapy. In this situation a short-term safety record would not be reassuring and a long-term safety record could be obtained only by long-term studies in humans.

Nevertheless, in spite of the formidable scientific and ethical difficulties, the future has never looked brighter for people with CF. Not only are a number of entirely new treatments which may prevent lung damage being very actively researched, but progress in transplantation is giving new hope to those with end-stage disease. For those in between conventional treatment is leading to an ever better outlook.

References

1. Tsui L-C, Buchwald M, Barker D. Cystic fibrosis locus defined by a genetically linked polymorphic DNA marker. *Science* 1985; **230:** 1054–1057.
2. Knowlton RG, Cohen-Haguenauer D, Van Cong N *et al*. A polymorphic DNA marker linked to cystic fibrosis is located on chromosome 7. *Nature* 1985; **318:** 380–382.
3. White R, Woodward, Leppert M *et al*. A closely linked genetic marker for cystic fibrosis. *Nature* 1985; **318:** 382–384.
4. Wainwright BJ, Scambler PJ, Schmidtke RJ *et al*. Localisation of cystic fibrosis locus to chromosome 7 cen-q22. *Nature* 1985; **318:** 384.
5. Rommens JM, Lanuzzi MC, Kerem B *et al*. Identification of the cystic fibrosis gene: chromosome walking and jumping. *Science* 1989; **245:** 1059–1065.
6. Collins FS, Drumon ML, Cole JL *et al*. Construction of a general human chromosome jumping library, with application to cystic fibrosis. *Science* 1987; **235:** 1046.
7. Kerem B-S, Rommens JM, Buchanan JA *et al*. Identification of the cystic fibrosis gene: genetic analysis. *Science* 1989; **245:** 1073–1080.

8. McIntosh I, Raeburn JA, Curtis A *et al*. First trimester prenatal diagnosis of CF by direct gene probing. *Lancet* 1989; **ii:** 972.
9. Estivill X, Chillon M, Casals T *et al*. 508 gene deletion in cystic fibrosis in southern Europe. *Lancet* 1989; **ii:** 1404.
10. Lemne WK, Feldman GL, Kerem B. Mutation analysis for heterozygote detection and prenatal diagnosis of CF. *N Engl J Med* 1990; **322:** 291–296.
11. Riordan JR, Rommens JM, Kerem B *et al*. Identification of the cystic fibrosis gene: cloning and characterisation of complementary DNA. *Science* 1989; **245:** 1066–1073.
12. Higgens C. Protein joins transport family. *Nature* 1989; **301:** 103.
13. Ringe D, Petski GA. A transport problem? *Nature* 1990; **346:** 312–313.
14. Reddy MM, Quinton PR. Altered electrical potential profile of human reabsorptive sweat duct cell in CF. *Am J Physiol* 1989; **257:** C722–C727.
15. Sato K, Sato F. Defective beta adrenergic response of cystic fibrosis sweat glands *in vivo* and *in vitro*. *J Clin Invest* 1984; **73:** 1763–1771.
16. Gray MA, Pollard CE, Harris A *et al*. Recent advances in understanding pancreatic duct cell function: Implications for cystic fibrosis. *Paed Pulm* 1990; (Suppl. 5): 181–183.
17. Hardcastle J, Hardcastle PT, Taylor CJ. *Paed Pulm* 1990; (Suppl. 5): 181–183.
18. Knowles MR, Clarke LL, Boucher RC. Activation by extracellular nucleotides of chloride secretion in the airway epithelia of patients with patients with CF. *N Engl J Med* 1991; **325:** 533–538.
19. Geddes DM, Shiner R. Cystic fibrosis from lung damage to symptoms. *Acta Paediatr Scand* 1989; **363** (Suppl.): 52–57.
20. Farrall M, Law H-Y, Rodech CH *et al*. First trimester prenatal diagnosis of cystic fibrosis with linked DNA probes. *Lancet* 1986; **i:** 1402–1405.
21. Super M, Ivinson A, Schwartz M *et al*. Clinical experience of prenatal diagnosis of cystic fibrosis by use of linked DNA probes. *Lancet* 1987; **ii:** 782–784.
22. Schwartz M, Super M, Schmidtke J *et al*. Prenatal diagnosis of cystic fibrosis using linked DNA probes. *Prenat Diag* 1988; **8:** 619–624.
23. Watson E, Williamson R, Brueton LE *et al*. Genetic counselling for cystic fibrosis based upon mutation/haplotype analysis. *Lancet* 1990; **ii:** 190–191.
24. Halley DJJ, Von Damme NHM, Deelan WH *et al*. Prenatal detection of major cystic fibrosis mutation. *Lancet* 1989; **ii:** 972.
25. Estivill X, Farrall M, Scambler J. A candidate for the cystic fibrosis locus isolated by selection for methylation-free islands. *Nature* 1987; **326:** 257–263.
26. Saiki RV, Gelfand DH, Stoffel S *et al*. Primer-directed enzymatic amplification of DNA with a thermostable DNA polymerase. *Science* 1988; **239:** 487–491.
27. Williams C, Weber L, Williamson R *et al*. Guthrie spots for DNA-based carrier testing in cystic fibrosis. *Lancet* 1988; **ii:** 693.
28. McIntosh I, Strain L, Brock DJH. Prenatal diagnosis of cystic fibrosis where single affected child has died: Guthrie spots and microvillar enzyme sampling. *Lancet* 1988; **ii:** 1085.
29. Curtis A, Strain L, Mennie M *et al*. First-trimester prenatal diagnosis of cystic fibrosis using fibroblasts from a deceased index child to establish haplotypes. *Prenat Diagn* 1988; **8:** 625–628.
30. Brock EH, Clarke HAK, Barron L *et al*. Prenatal diagnosis of cystic fibrosis by microvillar enzyme assay on a sequence of 258 pregnancies. *Hum Genet* 1988; **78:** 271–275.
31. Durie PR, Forster G. Pathophysiology of the exocrine pancreas in cystic fibrosis. *J R Soc Med* 1989; **2** (Suppl. 16): 2–10.
32. Adrianssens K, Janssens H, Van Soom H. Two tier screen for cystic fibrosis. *Lancet* 1981; **i:** 833.
33. Wilken B, Brown ARD, Urwin R *et al*. Cystic fibrosis screening by dried blood spots trypsin assay: results in 75,000 newborn infants. *J Paediatr* 1983; **102:** 383–387.
34. Ryley HC, Deam SM, Williams J *et al*. Neonatal screening for cystic fibrosis in Wales and the West Midlands: I. Evaluation of immunoreactive trypsin test. *J Clin Pathol* 1988; **41:** 726–729.
35. Bowling FG, Cleghorn G, Chester A *et al*. Neonatal screening for cystic fibrosis. *Arch Dis Child* 1988; **63:** 726–729.
36. Roberts G, Stanfield M, Black A *et al*. Screening for cystic fibrosis: a four year regional experience. *Arch Dis Child* 1988; **63:** 1438–1443.
37. Colten HR. Screening for cystic fibrosis. Public policy and personal choices. *N Engl J Med* 1990; **322:** 328–329.
38. Wilken B, Chalmers G. Reduced morbidity in patients with cystic fibrosis detected by neonatal screening. *Lancet* 1985; **ii:** 1319–1321.
39. Beaudet AL. Carrier screening for CF. *Am J Hum Genet* 1990; **47:** 603–605.
40. Littlewood JM. An overview of the management of cystic fibrosis. *J R Soc Med* 1986; **79** (Suppl. 12): 55–63.
41. Knowles MR, Carson JL, Collier AM *et al*. Measurement of nasal transepithelial elective potential

difference in normal human subjects *in vivo*. *Am Rev Respir Dis* 1981; **124:** 484–496.
42. Hay JG, Geddes DM. Transepithelial potential difference in cystic fibrosis. *Thorax* 1985; **40:** 493–496.
43. Alton EWFW, Hay JG, Munro C *et al*. Measurement of nasal potential difference in adult cystic fibrosis, Young's syndrome and bronchiectasis. *Thorax* 1987; **42:** 815–817.
44. Alton EWFW, Currie D, Logan-Sinclair R *et al*. Nasal potential difference: a clinical diagnostic test for cystic fibrosis. *Eur Respir J* 1990; **3:** 922–926.
45. Hoiby N. *Haemophilus influenzae, Staphylococcus aureus, Pseudomonas cepacia* and *Pseudomonas aeruginosa* in patients with cystic fibrosis. *Chest* 1988; **94:** 975–1015.
46. Penketh ARL, Wise A, Mearns MB *et al*. Cystic fibrosis in adolescent and adults. *Thorax* 1987; **42:** 526–532.
47. Bauernfeind A, Horl G, Przyklenk B. Microbiologic and therapeutic aspects of *Staphylococcus aureus* in cystic fibrosis patients. *Scand J Gastroenterol* 1988; **23** (Suppl. 143): 99–102.
48. Govan JRW, Glass S. The microbiology and therapy of cystic fibrosis lung infections. *Rev Med Microbiol* 1990; **1:** 19–28.
49. Neijens HJ. Strategies and perspectives in treatment of respiratory infections. *Acta Paed Scand Suppl* 1989; **363:** 66–73.
50. Pedersen SS, Jensen T, Hoiby N *et al*. Management of *Pseudomonas aeruginosa* lung infection in Danish cystic fibrosis patients. *Acta Paed Scand* 1987; **78:** 395–404.
51. Hoiby N, Pedersen SS. Estimated risk of cross-infection with *Pseudomonas aeruginosa* in Danish cystic fibrosis patients. *Acta Paed Scand* 1989; **78:** 395–404.
52. Zimakoff J, Hoiby N, Rosendal K *et al*. Epidemiology of *Pseudomonas aeruginosa* infection and the role of contamination of the environment in a cystic fibrosis clinic. *J Hosp Infect* 1983; **4:** 31–40.
53. Speert DP, Campbell ME. Hospital epidemiology of *Pseudomonas aeruginosa* from patients with cystic fibrosis. *J Hosp Infect* 1987; **9:** 11–21.
54. Kelly NM, Fitzgerland MX, Tempany E *et al*. Does *Pseudomonas* cross infection occur between cystic fibrosis patients? *Lancet* 1982; **ii:** 688–690.
55. Grothues D, Koopman V, van der Haart H *et al*. Genome finger printing of *Pseudomonas aeruginosa* indicates colonisation of cystic fibrosis siblings with closely related strains. *J Clin Microbiol* 1988; **26:** 1973–1977.
56. Speert DP, Campbell ME, Farmer SW *et al*. Use of a pilin gene probe to study molecular epidemiology of *Pseudomonas aeruginosa*. *J Clin Microbiol* 1989; **27:** 2589–2593.
57. Wolz CE, Kiosz G, Ogle JW *et al*. *Pseudomonas aeruginosa* cross-colonization and persistence in patients with cystic fibrosis: Use of a DNA probe. *Epidem Infect* 1989; **102:** 205–214.
58. Van Bever HP, Gigase PL, de Clerck LS *et al*. Immune complexes and *Pseudomonas aeruginosa* antibiotics in cystic fibrosis. *Arch Dis Child* 1988; **63:** 1222–1228.
59. Doring G, Albus A, Hoiby N. Immunologic aspects of cystic fibrosis. *Chest* 1988; **94** (Suppl. 2): 1095–1135.
60. Isles A, Maclusky I, Corey M *et al*. *Pseudomonas cepacia* infection in cystic fibrosis. An emerging problem. *J Paed* 1984; **104:** 206–210.
61. Tablan OC, Chorba TL, Schidlow DV *et al*. *Pseudomonas cepacia* colonisation in patients with cystic fibrosis, risk factors and clinical outcome. *J Paed* 1985; **107:** 382–387.
62. Lewin LO, Byard PJ, Davis PB. Effects of *Pseudomonas cepacia* colonisation on survival and pulmonary function in cystic fibrosis patients. *J Clin Epidemiol* 1990; **43:** 125–131.
63. Thomassen MJ, Demko CA, Klinger JD *et al*. *Pseudomonas cepacia* colonisation among patients with cystic fibrosis. A new opportunist. *Am Rev Respir Dis* 1985; **131:** 791–796.
64. Thomassen MJ, Demko CA, Doershuk CF *et al*. *Pseudomonas cepacia*: decrease in colonisation in patients with cystic fibrosis. *Am Rev Respir Dis* 1986; **134:** 669–671.
65. Efthimiou J, Smith MJ, Hodson ME *et al*. Fatal pulmonary infection with *Mycobacterium fortuitum* in cystic fibrosis. *Br J Dis Chest* 1984; **78:** 299–302.
66. Efthimiou J, Taylor P, Hodson ME *et al*. Importance of viruses and *Legionella pneumophila* in respiratory exacerbations of patients with cystic fibrosis. *Thorax* 1984; **39:** 150–154.
67. Wang EL, Prober CG, Manson B *et al*. Association of respiratory viral infections with pulmonary deterioration in cystic fibrosis. *N Engl J Med* 1984; **311:** 1653–1658.
68. Smith MJ, Efthimiou J, Hodson ME *et al*. Myocbacterial isolations in young adults with cystic fibrosis. *Thorax* 1985; **39:** 369–375.
69. Hjelle L, Petrini B, Kallenius G *et al*. Prospective study of mycobacterial infections in patients with cystic fibrosis. *Thorax* 1990; **45:** 401–402.
70. Regelmann EW, Elliot GR, Warwick WJ *et al*. Reduction of sputum *Pseudomonas aeruginosa* density by antibiotics improves lung function in cystic fibrosis more than do bronchodilators and chest physiotherapy alone. *Am Rev Respir Dis* 1990; **141:** 914–921.
71. Auerbach HS, Williams M, Kilpatrick JA *et al*. Alternate day prednisolone reduces morbidity and improves pulmonary function in cystic fibrosis. *Lancet* 1985; **ii:** 686–688.

72. Geddes DM. Antimicrobial therapy against *Staphylococcus aureus, Pseudomonas aeruginosa* and *Pseudomonas cepacia. Chest* 1988; **94:** 140S–143S.
73. Grimwood K, To A, Rabin HR *et al.* Inhibition of *Pseudomonas aeruginosa* exoenzyme expression by subinhibitory antibiotics concentrations. *Antimicrob Agents Chemother* 1989; **33:** 41–47.
74. Penketh ARL, Hodson ME, Batten JC. Ticarcillin compared with carbenicillin in the treatment of exacerbations of bronchopulmonary infection in cystic fibrosis. *Br J Dis Chest* 1983; **77:** 179–184.
75. Penketh ARL, Hodson ME, Gaya H, Batten JC. Azlocillin compared with carbenicillin in the treatment of bronchopulmonary infection due to *Pseudomonas aeruginosa* in cystic fibrosis. *Thorax* 1984; **39:** 299–304.
76. Hodson ME, Norman AP, Batten JC (eds) *Emotional and Social Aspects of Treatment in Cystic Fibrosis.* London: Baillière Tindall, 1983; 242–259.
77. Hodson ME, Wingfield HJ, Batten JC. Tobramycin and carbenicillin compared with gentamicin and carbenicillin in the treatment of infection with *Pseudomonas aeruginosa* in adult patients with cystic fibrosis. *Br J Dis Chest* 1983; **77:** 71–77.
78. British Thoracic Society Research Committee. Ceftazidime compared with gentamicin and carbenicillin in patients with cystic fibrosis, pulmonary *Pseudomonas* infection an an exacerbation of respiratory symptoms. *Thorax* 1985; **40:** 358–363.
79. Stead RJ, Skypala I, Hodson ME. Enteric coated microsplens of pancreatin in the treatment of cystic fibrosis. Comparison with a standard enteric coated preparation. *Thorax* 1987; **42:** 533–537.
80. David JT. Intravenous antibiotics at home in children with cystic fibrosis. *J R Soc Med* 1989; **82:** 130–131.
81. Kuzenko JA. Home treatment of pulmonary infections in cystic fibrosis. *Chest* 1988; **94:** 1625–1655.
82. Ball ABS, Duncan FR, Foster FJ *et al.* Long term venous access using a totally implantable drug delivery system in patients with cystic fibrosis and bronchiectasis. *Respir Med* 1989; **83:** 429–431.
83. Hodson ME, Butland RJA, Roberts M *et al.* Oral ciprofloxacin compared with conventional intravenous treatment for *Pseudomonas aeruginosa* infection in adults with cystic fibrosis. *Lancet* 1987; **i:** 236–237.
84. Hodson ME, Penketh ARL, Batten JC. Aerosol carbenicillin and gentamicin treatment of *Pseudomonas aeruginosa* infection in patients with cystic fibrosis. *Lancet* 1981; **ii:** 1137–1139.
85. Hodson ME. Antibiotic treatment. Aerosol therapy. *Chest* 1988; **94** (Suppl.): 156S–163S
86. Pryor JA, Webber BA, Hodson ME *et al.* Evaluation of the forced expiration technique as an adjunct to postural drainage in treatment of cystic fibrosis. *BMJ* 1979; **ii:** 417–418.
87. Webber BA, Hofmeyr BA, Morgan MDL *et al.* Effects of postural drainage incorporating the forced expiration technique on pulmonary function in cystic fibrosis. *Br J Dis Chest* 1986; **80:** 353–359.
88. Sutton PP, Parker RA, Webber BA *et al.* Assessment of the forced expiration technique, postural drainage and directed coughing in chest physiotherapy. *Eur J Respir Dis* 1983; **64:** 62–68.
89. Pryor JA, Webber BA, Hodson ME. Effects of chest physiotherapy on oxygen saturation in patients with cystic fibrosis. *Thorax* 1990; **45:** 77.
90. Hofmyer J, Webber BA, Hodson ME. Evaluation of positive expiratory pressure as an adjunct to chest physiotherapy in the treatment of cystic fibrosis. *Thorax* 1986; **41:** 951–954.
91. Falk M, Kelstrup M, Andersen JR *et al.* Improving the ketchup bottle method with positive expiratory pressure, PEP, in cystic fibrosis. *Eur J Respir Dis* 1984; **65:** 423–432.
92. Salh W, Bilton D, Dodd M *et al.* Effect of exercise and physiotherapy in aiding sputum expectoration in adults with cystic fibrosis. *Thorax* 1989; **44:** 1006–1008.
93. Holselaw DS, Grand RJ, Shwachmann H. Massive haemoptysis in cystic fibrosis. *J Paediatr* 1970; **76:** 829.
94. Cohen AM, Doershuk CF, Stern RC. Bronchial artery embolisation to control haemoptysis in cystic fibrosis. *Radiology* 1990; **175:** 401–405.
95. Sweezy NB, Fellows KE. Bronchial artery embolisation for severe haemoptysis in cystic fibrosis. *Chest* 1990; **97:** 1322–1326.
96. Hodson ME, Madden BP, Steven MH *et al.* Non invasive mechanical ventilation for cystic fibrosis patients – a potential bridge to transplantation. *Eur Respir J* 1991; **4:** 524–527.
97. Hodson ME, Madden BP, Steven MH, Tsang VT, Yacoub MH. Non-invasive mechanical ventilation for cystic fibrosis patients – a potential bridge to transplantation. *Eur Respir J* 1991; **4:** 524–527.
98. Jones K, Higgenbottom T, Wallwork J. Successful heart-lung transplantation for cystic fibrosis. *Chest* 1988; **93:** 644–645.
99. Yacoub MH, Banner NR. Recent developments in lung and heart-lung transplantation. In: *Transplantation Reviews, Vol 3.* Morris P, Tilne NL eds. Philadelphia: WB Saunders, 1990; 1–29.
100. Yacoub MH, Fitzgerald M, Radley-Smith R. Combined heart and lung transplantation for cystic fibrosis and subsequent 'domino' cardiac transplantation. *J Heart Transplant* 1990; **9:** 459–467.
101. Scott J, Higenbottom T, Hutter J *et al.* Heart lung transplantation for cystic fibrosis. *Lancet* 1988; **ii:**

192–194.
102. Durie PR, Pencharz PB. A rational approach to the nutritional care of patients with cystic fibrosis. *J R Soc Med* 1989; **82** (Suppl. 16): 11–20.
103. Corey M, McLaoughlin FJ, Williams M *et al.* A comparison of survival, growth and pulmonary function in patients with cystic fibrosis in Boston and Toronto. *J Clin Epidemiol* 1988; **41:** 583–591.
104. Stutts MJ, Knowles MR, Gatzy JT. Oxygen consumption and oubain binding sites in cystic fibrosis nasal epithelium. *Paediatr Res* 1986; **20:** 1316–1320.
105. Vernon SA, Neugebauer MAZ, Brimlow G *et al.* Conjunctival xerosis in cystic fibrosis. *J R Soc Med* 1989; **82:** 46–47.
106. Cynamon HA, Milor DE, Valenstein E *et al.* Effects of vitamin E deficiency on neurological function in patients with cystic fibrosis. *J Paediatr* 1988; **113:** 637–640.
107. Elias E, Muller DPR, Scott J. Effects of vitamin E deficiency on neurological function in patients with cystic fibrosis. *J Paediatr* 1981: **113:** 637–640.
108. Sitrin MD, Lieberman F, Jansen WE *et al.* Vitamin E deficiency and neurologic disease in adults with cystic fibrosis. *Ann Intern Med* 1987; **107:** 51–54.
109. Standvik B. Relation between essential fatty acid metabolism and gastrointestinal symptoms in cystic fibrosis. *Acta Paed Scand Suppl* 1989; **363:** 58–65.
110. Levy LD, Durie PR, Rencharz PB. Effects of long-term nutritional rehabilitation on body composition and clinical status in malnourished children and adolescents with cystic fibrosis.*J Paed* 1985; **107:** 225–250.
111. Shepherd RW, Holt TL, Thomas BJ *et al.* Nutritional rehabilitation in cystic fibrosis. Controlled studies of effects on nutritional growth retardation, body protein turnover and course of pulmonary disease. *J Paed* 1986; **109:** 788–794.
112. Boland MP, Stoski DS, MacDonald ME . Chronic jejunostomy feeding with a non-elemental formula in undernourished patients with cystic fibrosis. *Lancet* 1986; **i:** 232–234.
113. Haymans HSA. Gastrointestinal dysfunction and its effects on nutrition in cystic fibrosis. *Acta Paed Scand Suppl* 1989; **363:** 74–79.
114. Stead RJ, Davidson TI, Duncan FR, Hodson ME, Batten JC. Use of a totally implantable system for venous access in cystic fibrosis. *Thorax* 1987; **42:** 149–150.
115. Robinson PJ, Olinsky A, Smith AL *et al.* High compared with standard dose lipase pancreatic supplements. *Arch Dis Child* 1989; **64:** 143–145.
116. Zentler-Munro RL, Fine DR, Batten JC *et al.* Effects of cimetidine on enzyme inactivation, bile acid precipitation and lipid solubilisation in pancreatic steatorrhoea due to cystic fibrosis. *Gut* 1985; **26:** 892–901.
117. Sinaasappel M. Hepatobiliary pathology in patients with cystic fibrosis. *Acta Paed Scand Suppl* 1989: **363:** 45–51.
118. Cleghorn GJ, Stringer DA, Forstner GG *et al.* Treatment of distal obstruction syndrome in cystic fibrosis with balanced intestinal lavage solution. *Lancet* 1986; **i:** 8–9.
119. Davidson AC, Harrison AK, Geddes DM. Treatment of distal intestinal obstruction syndrome in patients with cystic fibrosis. *Thorax* 1986; **41:** 732.
120. Nagel RA, Westaby D, Javaid A *et al.* Liver disease and common bile duct abnormalities in adults with cystic fibrosis. *Lancet* 1989; **ii:** 1422–1425.
121. Gaskin KJ, Waters D, Howman-Giles R *et al.* Liver disease and common bile duct stenosis in cystic fibrosis. *N Engl J Med* 1988; **318:** 340–346.
122. Mieles LA, Orenstein RM, Toussant RM, Selby R, Gordon RD, Starzi TW. Outcome after liver transplantation for cystic fibrosis. *Paed Pulm* 1991; (Suppl. 6): 130–131.
123. Cotting J, Lentzt MJ, Reichen J, Effects of ursodeoxycholic acid treatment on nutrition and liver function in patients with cystic fibrosis and longstanding cholestasis. *Gut* 1990; **31:** 918–921.
124. Colombo C, Castellani MR, Assaisso ML, Givnta A. Ursodeoxycholic acid therapy in cystic fibrosis. *Paed Pulm* 1990 (Suppl. 15): 76–78.
125. Dixey J, Redington AN, Butler RC *et al.* The arthropathy of cystic fibrosis. *Ann Rheum Dis* 1988; **47:** 218–223.
126. Cohen LF, Sant'Agnese PA, Friedlander J. Cystic fibrosis and pregnancy. A national survey. *Lancet* 1980; **ii:** 842–844.
127. Palmer J, Dilloon-Baker C, Tecklin JS *et al.* Pregnancy in patients with cystic fibrosis. *Ann Intern Med* 1983; **99:** 596–600.
128. Cuyler J, Monaghan A. Cystic fibrosis and sinusitis. *J Otolaryngol* 1989; **18:** 173–175.
129. Shapiro E, Milmoe G, Wald E, Rodman J, Rowen A. Bacteriology of the maxillary sinus in patients with cystic fibrosis. *J Infect Dis* 1982; **4:** 209–214.
130. Chalton R, Mackay I, Wilson R *et al.* Double blind placebo controlled trial of betamethasone nasal drops for nasal polyposis. *BMJ* 1985; **291:** 788.

131. Shepherd SL, Hovell MF, Harwood IR *et al.* A comparative study of the psychological assets of adults with cystic fibrosis and their healthy peers. *Chest* 1990; **97:** 1310–1316.
132. Andersen DH. Cystic fibrosis of the pancreas and its relation to celiac disease. A clinical and pathological study. *Am J Dis Child* 1938; **56:** 344–399.
133. British Paediatric Association Working Party on Cystic Fibrosis. Cystic Fibrosis in the United Kingdom 1977–85: an improving picture. *BMJ* 1988; **297:** 1599–1602.
134. Phelan P, Hey E. Cystic fibrosis mortality in England and Wales and in Victoria, Australia 1976–80. *Arch Dis Child* 1984; **59:** 71–83.
135. Kohler D, App E, Schmitz-Schumann M *et al.* Inhalation of amiloride improves the mucociliary and the cough clearances in patients with cystic fibrosis. *Eur J Respir Dis* 1986; **69** (Suppl. 146): 319–326.
136. App EM, King M, Helfesreider R *et al.* Acute and long term amiloride inhalation in cystic fibrosis lung disease. *Am Rev Respir Dis* 1990; **141:** 605–612.
137. Knowles MR, Church NJ, Waltner WE *et al.* A pilot study of aerosolised amiloride for the treatment of lung disease in cystic fibrosis. *N Engl J Med* 1990; **322:** 1189–1194.
138. Boucher RC, Cheng EHC, Pardison AM *et al.* Chloride secretory response of cystic fibrosis human airway epithelia: Preservation of calcium but not protein kinase C- and A-dependent mechanisms. *J Clin Invest* 1989; **84:** 1424–1431.
139. Rosenfeld MA, Siegfried W, Yoshimura K *et al.* Adenovirus-mediated transfer of a recombinant alpha I antitrypsin gene to the lung epithelium *in vivo*. *Science* 1991; **252:** 431–443.
140. Berger M. Inflammation in the lung in cystic fibrosis. *Clin Rev Allergy* 1991; **9:** 119–142.
141. Rosenstein BJ, Eigen H. Risks of alternate day prednisolone in patients with CF. *Pediatrics* 1991; **87:** 245–246.
142. Konstan MW, Vargo KM, Davis PB. Ibuprofen attenuates the inflammatory response to *Pseudomonas aeruginosa* in a rat model of chronic pulmonary infection: implications for antiinflammatory therapy in cystic fibrosis. *Am Rev Respir Dis* 1990; **141:** 186–192.
143. McElvaney NG, Hubbard RC, Birrer P *et al.* Aerosol alpha I antitrypsin treatment for cystic fibrosis. *Lancet* 1991; **337:** 392–394.
144. Shak S, Capon DJ, Helmis R, Marsters SA, Baker CL. Recombinant human DNase I reduces the viscosity of cystic fibrosis sputum. *Proc Natl Acad Sci USA* 1990; **87:** 9188–9192.
145. Spier R, Whiebsky E, Paine JR. Aerosolised pancreatic dornase and antibiotics in pulmonary infections. *JAMA* 1961; **178:** 878–886.
146. Liebermann J. Dornase aerosol: Effects on sputum viscosity in cases of cystic fibrosis. *JAMA* 1968; **205:** 312–313.
147. Elmes PC, White JC. Deoxyribonuclease in the treatment of purulent bronchitis. *Thorax* 1953; **8:** 295–300.

8

Human immunodeficiency virus infection and the lung

J. Wiggins and J. Collins

Introduction

The advent of the epidemic of human immunodeficiency virus (HIV) infection has increased the workload of lung specialists throughout the world. Individuals infected by the virus develop impaired cellular immunity and are prone to infections and malignant disease of the lungs. These complications are very common [1] and are often the presenting feature leading to a diagnosis of the acquired immunodeficiency syndrome (AIDS). While the lungs are a ready portal for entry of infection and more susceptible than other organs, the greater frequency with which the lungs are affected in HIV-related disease is due to a number of factors; the immune mechanisms in the lung may be more depressed than in other parts of the body and HIV-induced factors may cause specific adverse effects on lung defences [2].

The currently recognized ways in which the lungs are affected by HIV include a variety of secondary infections and the development of malignancies, interstitial pneumonia, non-specific pneumonitis and the adult respiratory distress syndrome (ARDS). The malignancies include Kaposi's sarcoma and non-Hodgkin's lymphoma. The incidence of Kaposi's sarcoma is much higher in HIV-related disease in homosexuals than in other groups infected. This difference is unexplained but may suggest that a sexually transmitted factor is involved in its pathogenesis [3]. To date, the results of treatment of malignancies related to HIV infection have been disappointing.

Most HIV-related lung infections are caused by a limited range of organisms, particularly *Pneumocystis carinii* and mycobacteria. However, a very wide variety of other organisms have been reported to cause pulmonary infections in this disease. These include pyogenic bacteria, viruses (especially cytomegalovirus and herpes simplex), parasites and fungi (especially *Candida* species, *Histoplasma* and *Coccidioides*).

The purpose of this chapter is to review the diagnosis, clinical features and management of the pulmonary complications of HIV infections.

Diagnosis of pulmonary complications of HIV infection

It is now generally accepted that for optimal practice a specific diagnosis of any HIV-related lung complication should be made and that empirical treatment is seldom advisable. It is not usually possible to reach a firm diagnosis on the basis of the history and physical examination alone and a wide range of investigations is commonly used for the assessment of these problems. Non-invasive tests include measurement of CD4 lymphocyte counts and CD4/CD8 lymphocyte ratios, chest radiographs, skin tests, gallium lung scans, assessment of arterial oxygenation and lung function. Non-invasive protocols are particularly useful in the investigation of outpatients [4]. More invasive investigations used include sputum induction, fibreoptic bronchoscopy with bronchoalveolar lavage and transbronchial lung biopsy: open lung biopsy is seldom necessary or justifiable.

Non-invasive investigation

Chest radiography

A number of radiological patterns have been found associated with the lung disorders that occur in individuals infected by HIV [5]. These include a normal chest radiograph, diffuse reticulonodular shadowing, focal consolidation, hilar adenopathy, pleural effusion and pneumothorax. However, all these patterns have at some time been shown to be associated with each of the known lung complications of HIV disease and thus the chest radiograph cannot be relied upon to give a specific diagnosis.

A normal chest radiograph may be seen in cases of infection with *Pneumocystis carinii, Mycobacterium avium intracellulare, Histoplasma* and cytomegalovirus [6, 7]. Computed tomography (CT) has not been widely used in the investigation of HIV-related lung disease but a number of typical abnormal patterns have been reported. Where patients' symptoms are relevant or there are strong grounds for suspecting HIV infection, yet the plain chest radiograph appears normal, CT films may be helpful.

Diffuse reticulonodular infiltrates are usually seen in association with *Pneumocystis carinii* pneumonia, presenting typically as bilateral perihilar diffuse shadowing, disseminated tuberculosis, infection with *Histoplasma* and *Coccidioides* and lymphocytic interstitial pneumonia [8, 9]. More focal abnormalities may be seen with bacterial pneumonias, Kaposi's sarcoma and cryptococcosis.

Hilar lymphadenopathy, with or without other chest radiological abnormalities, tends to be associated with tuberculous infection, Kaposi's sarcoma, disseminated *Mycobacterium avium intracellulare* infection and non-Hodgkin's lymphoma [10]. Pleural effusions, sometimes accompanied by other radiographic abnormalities, occur most frequently in patients with Kaposi's sarcoma, tuberculosis, non-Hodgkin's lymphoma and pyogenic empyema.

Lung function tests

Lung function tests may be helpful in identifying the physiological effects of pulmonary complications associated with HIV infection. Since the range and distribution of complications are wide, it is understandable that their effects on lung function are varied. The most common pattern recognized is of a restrictive ventilatory defect with reduced vital capacity [11]; this is associated with a low arterial oxygen tension and widening of the alveolar-arterial gradient, which is further increased by exercise. This pattern is typical of infection with *Pneumocystis carinii*. These changes are usually accompanied by a reduction of carbon monoxide transfer factor and this has been shown to be a sensitive index of *Pneumocystis* infection [12]. Kaposi's sarcoma has been recognized to cause an obstructive ventilatory defect [13] but this is a non-specific change which may be caused by other conditions.

Pulmonary function tests are generally not used in the routine assessment of HIV-infected patients because of anxieties about cross-infection. The use of filter valves and modified lung function testing equipment [14] may diminish this anxiety, but the modified equipment needs further assessment in practice before it can be recommended for wider use. It has been argued that the safest approach to prevent cross-infection is to assume that all patients, regardless of source, are potentially infectious and to adopt lung function testing methods which obviate the risk of cross-infection.

Gallium-67 scanning

The radionuclide Gallium-67 (^{67}Ga) will accumulate in areas of inflammation. Although the mechanism responsible for this is unknown, gallium scanning has been shown to be highly sensitive for identification of *Pneumocystis carinii* pneumonia (PCP), in which diffuse or parenchymal uptake of the isotope occurs. Unfortunately, the technique is not specific: uptake has also been described in other infectious and non-infectious complications of HIV-related lung disease [15, 16]. The main value of ^{67}Ga scanning is in the assessment of patients with symptoms suggestive of PCP and a normal chest radiograph. Where the ^{67}Ga scan is positive, more invasive lung investigations should be considered.

^{67}Ga may also be taken up by hilar and mediastinal nodes, directing investigation accordingly, whilst focal parenchymal accumulation has been described in *Mycobacterium avium intracellulare infection* [17]. A further potential role of ^{67}Ga is in monitoring treatment responses in PCP [18].

More invasive techniques

Sputum induction

With the exception of patients with bacterial lung infections, most individuals suffering from the pulmonary complications of HIV infection do not spontaneously produce sputum samples. However, sputum expectoration can be induced by the inhalation of an aerosol of 20–30 ml of hypertonic (3–5%) normal saline [19, 20], generated by an ultrasonic nebulizer. The mechanism by which a sputum sample is produced is unknown and may involve stimulation of both mucus secretion and coughing. The technique, which is well tolerated and can be performed in outpatients, is particularly useful in the diagnosis of PCP. Early studies using routine stains (such as Giemsa) showed a diagnostic yield of 55–75% [21, 22]. More recently the use of immunofluorescent antibody techniques has further improved the sensitivity of the technique [23]. These results have been difficult to reproduce and success with sputum induction is dependent on attention to technique, including oral cleansing to avoid sample contamination, close supervision of patient expectoration and meticulous laboratory processing of the samples obtained.

Bronchoscopy

In units where sputum induction has not been successfully introduced, the mainstay of the invasive investigation for pulmonary complications of HIV infection is fibreoptic bronchoscopy with bronchoalveolar lavage and transbronchial lung biopsy. The combination of these procedures has a diagnostic yield for all pathogens of nearly 100% [24]. However, transbronchial biopsy is unsafe in severely hypoxaemic patients and those with bleeding disorders, and is associated with a high incidence of pneumothorax in patients with PCP [24]. The diagnostic yield with bronchoalveolar lavage alone is high, so some units do not perform transbronchial lung biopsy routinely during the bronchoscopic investigation of HIV-related complications [25]. However, bronchoalveolar lavage is less sensitive than biopsy in identifying fungal and mycobacterial infections [26], malignancy, drug toxicity and lymphocytic interstitial pneumonitis. Where bronchoalveolar lavage does not give a diagnosis, the decision to perform a second bronchoscopy with transbronchial biopsy rests upon the assessment of the severity of the disorder and a balance between the risks of investigation and empirical treatment.

Other invasive techniques

The analysis of bronchial washings obtained via catheters passed into the trachea under local anaesthesia may be a useful technique for the investigation of patients suspected of having PCP where bronchoalveolar lavage is not freely available [27]. Percutaneous fine needle aspiration of the lung is associated with an unacceptably high incidence of pneumothorax and is not often used in the investigation of HIV-related infections, although it may be useful in patients with circumscribed lung lesions or mediastinal lymphadenopathy [28].

Open lung biopsy may be considered in the investigation of deteriorating patients in whom bronchoscopy has failed to provide a satisfactory diagnosis. This procedure carries an acceptable morbidity rate and has a high diagnostic yield [29]. However, debate continues as to the advisability of identifying by open biopsy Kaposi's sarcoma, interstitial disorders and the other complications of HIV-related disease because of the increased risk to staff and the poor prospect of producing a sustained and satisfactory improvement in the patient's condition.

Infectious pulmonary complications of HIV infection

Pneumocystis carinii pneumonia

To date, PCP has proved the most common pulmonary complication of HIV-related disease [1]. Infection with this organism was rare before the AIDS epidemic and was generally seen in other immunosuppressed patients. It is extremely rare in non-immunosuppressed individuals, although occasionally clusters have been reported in immunocompetent patients [30]. The taxonomy of this organism is not yet resolved and, although it is often believed to be a protozoan, evidence suggests that it may be a fungus [31].

PCP is the presenting diagnosis in 60% or more of cases of HIV-related lung disease in the USA and Europe [32] and more than 80% of HIV-positive patients have one or more episodes during their lifetime after diagnosis of AIDS [33]. Infection with *Pneumocystis* appears to be less common in African patients [34].

The epidemiology of infection is poorly understood. Primary exposure seems to occur in early life and most young children have serum antibodies to the organism [35]. Thereafter, the organism is thought to become part of the resident flora and most PCP associated with HIV infection is thought to occur from such commensal *Pneumocystis*. However, *Pneumocystis carinii* was not found in lung biopsy specimens taken from non-immunosuppressed individuals dying suddenly [36] and is not present in sputum induced by saline in healthy adults [37]. It is possible that airborne transmission is important, and carriage by healthy intermediaries has been suggested [38].

The most common presenting features of PCP, which may have persisted for several weeks, include fever of variable degree, a non-productive cough and marked breathlessness. The chest radiograph is often normal and there may be no abnormal signs on clinical examination. Less commonly, wheeze and crackles may be audible over the lungs. Haemoptysis is very rare [39]. Physical signs do not correlate with the severity of the disease.

When PCP develops, it is usual for the patient's CD4 lymphocyte count to fall below 200/ml, the median count being less than 100/ml [40]. Other abnormal blood tests include a high serum lactic dehydrogenase, and changes in the serum concentration of this enzyme mirror disease progress [41]. A wide variety of radiographic appearances have been reported, including a clear film, diffuse interstitial shadowing, focal infiltrates, pulmonary nodules, pulmonary cavities and pneumothorax which may be recurrent [42]; pleural effusions seem to be rare.

The initial investigations should include chest radiography, and lung function studies may be helpful as a low carbon monoxide transfer factor, low total lung capacity, arterial oxygen desaturation with a wide alveolar–arterial gradient all point towards the diagnosis of PCP. ^{67}Ga lung scans have been useful in demonstrating lung involvement by PCP, especially where the chest radiograph is normal, and the gallium scan may be positive in *Pneumocystis* infection before clinical features develop [43]. Unfortunately, although this test is highly sensitive, its specificity is low. Currently, where sputum induction techniques are reliable, the diagnosis of PCP can be confirmed in 25–85% of cases. In most units, bronchoalveolar lavage is the most reliable and simplest technique available and will give positive results in 75–95% of cases, while transbronchial biopsy has been reported to give a diagnostic rate of up to 95%. Identification of *Pneumocystis carinii* using the new monoclonal antibody immunofluorescence technique seems likely to replace the earlier silver staining Giemsa and Diffquick.

The mainstay of treatment of PCP remains either co-trimoxazole (trimethoprim-sulphamethoxazole) or pentamidine. These two drugs have similar efficacies (70–95%) and rates of adverse reaction [44, 45]. The adverse reactions to co-trimoxazole, which include fever, rashes and bone marrow dysplasia, occur in about 50% of patients, generally after 7–14 days of therapy [46]. Intravenous pentamidine is associated with potentially serious problems including hypoglycaemia, cardiac arrhythmias, bone marrow dysplasia and severe hypocalcaemia [44, 45]. Fortunately, patients switching from one drug to another because of side-effects do not usually develop toxicity to the second drug. The optimal duration of treatment is not known. Patients with AIDS suffering from PCP may respond to treatment more slowly than patients who have immunosuppression not related to HIV infection [47] and recovery of *Pneumocystis carinii* cysts and trophozoites in patients after 3 weeks' treatment has been demonstrated [44]. As a result, most centres usually treat for 2–3 weeks unless side-effects make it necessary to stop treatment.

Other possible therapies are dapsone in combination with trimethoprim [48, 49] (but dapsone has an unacceptable failure rate when used alone [50]); eflornithine [51]; and primaquine with clindamycin [52]. These drugs have not yet been extensively used but are valuable for patients who fail to respond, or who cannot tolerate standard drugs. Nebulized pentamidine may be effective in milder disease [53], although it is less effective than intravenous pentamidine in patients with more severe disease [54, 55].

The role of corticosteroids in the treatment of PCP is uncertain [56], but high-dose steroid therapy may improve survival of patients with respiratory failure caused by PCP [57, 58]. Recent uncontrolled reports [59] have supported this role and have suggested that the use of corticosteroids does not increase the morbidity associated with the treatment of PCP [60]. A recently published controlled trial has suggested that corticosteroids can prevent early deterioration in patients with moderately severe PCP [61]: earlier studies did not support this finding [62]. Although further trials are needed, it seems reasonable to add corticosteroids to the initial treatment regimen of severely hypoxic patients [63].

Survival from an episode of PCP has improved and is at least 60–90% at many centres, especially for initial episodes [64]. The use of intensive care and assisted ventilation for patients with PCP is still controversial: early reports suggested that the prognosis of patients requiring intensive therapy was so poor that such treatment was soon not offered for patients with respiratory failure due to PCP [65, 66]. However, more recent reports have suggested that the prognosis of this group of patients is improving [67, 68] and, interestingly, this seems to be independent of patient selection and prophylactic treatment for *Pneumocystis* [69]. At present, the use of intensive care for patients with PCP is a subject for careful consideration of individual detail and the availability of resources. It would seem justifiable for initial episodes of PCP early in the course of HIV-related disease.

At present, most centres have vigorous programmes of prophylaxis against PCP with regular inhalation of nebulized pentamidine, which has a long tissue half-life in the lung and produces low systemic drug levels and toxicity [70]. A recent multicentre trial of pentamidine prophylaxis has confirmed the effectiveness of both 150 mg nebulized fortnightly and 300 mg nebulized monthly: a lower dose regimen of 30 mg every 2 weeks was significantly less effective [71]. Nebulized pentamidine is well tolerated, the main problem being bronchospasm which can be diminished by pre-treatment with a beta-agonist [72]. Co-trimoxazole is also effective for prophylaxis [73] but may be associated with a greater incidence of side-effects when used in standard doses. However, a recent study has suggested that low-dose co-trimoxazole three times a week is effective, well absorbed and less costly than usual doses [74]. Patients with CD4 lymphocyte count of < 200/ml should be offered chemoprophylaxis whether or not they have had PCP [75]: its use should also be considered for those with CD4 counts of 200–400/ml.

Bacterial infections

About one-third of AIDS patients at post mortem have evidence of bacterial pneumonia [76], and a similar figure was reported in a clinical study [77]. However, this may be an over estimate because other clinical studies have reported an incidence of only 3–4% [78]. The bacteria commonly responsible for community-acquired infections in HIV-infected subjects are *Streptococcus pneumoniae*, *Haemophilus influenzae*, *Mycobacterium tuberculosis* and *Mycobacterium avium intracellulare* complex. Of the hospital-acquired infections in these patients, staphylococci and aerobic Gram-negative organisms are the most common causes. Community-acquired and nosocomial infections due to *Legionella*, *Nocardia* and *Mycoplasma pneumoniae* may occur.

Tuberculosis

Reactivation of endogenous mycobacterial infection associated with HIV-related disease is an important cause of the recent increased incidence of tuberculosis in Europe and the USA [79], in Africa and developing countries [80]. Tuberculosis is a transmissible, curable and preventable disease and much attention has justly been paid to the management of this complication of HIV infection.

The development of tuberculosis and the clinical features of the disease depend on the HIV-infected patient's residual degree of immunity. Early in the course of HIV infection when immunocompetence is not severely impaired, most cases of tuberculosis in Europe and the USA present with upper lobe cavitatory disease of the traditional pattern [81] and only 15–20% show extrapulmonary features. Most of these patients remain reactive to tuberculin. Later in the course of HIV infection, as immunity becomes progressively more severely compromised, the clinical pattern changes. The tuberculin reaction usually becomes negative and the chest radiograph appearances are more atypical, often with lower zone shadows rather than diffuse disease [82]. Extrapulmonary mycobacterial infection occurs in about 50% of more compromised patients. The atypical features may mislead clinicians and the diagnosis is easily missed [83], although delayed diagnosis cannot always be attributed to atypical features [84]. A high index of suspicion of tuberculous infection should be maintained for all HIV-infected patients [85]. The diagnosis is made using standard techniques, although if made by microscopy it should be confirmed by culture because of the high incidence of non-tuberculous mycobacterial disease.

Treatment for tuberculosis should begin as soon as acid-fast bacilli are identified, and can be modified later on the basis of the culture results. It is recommended that treatment should begin with at least three and preferably four drugs, as many as possible of which should be bactericidal. Treatment for a minimum of 9 months, or 6 months from culture conversion to negative, is advisable [86]. It is possible that tuberculosis has a worse than usual prognosis in HIV-infected individuals, who also seem to suffer greater toxicity from antituberculous drugs.

It is sensible practice to offer tuberculin testing to all newly diagnosed HIV-infected individuals. In the USA those with reaction to 5 tuberculin units (5 TU) of ≥ 5 mm undergo chest radiography, and those with a normal film are offered chemoprophylaxis with isoniazid 300 mg daily for 12 months [87]. Where there is radiological evidence of disease, treatment with a full complement of drugs should be started immediately.

Mycobacterium avium intracellulare complex

Infection with *Mycobacterium avium* and *Mycobacterium intracellulare* (*Mycobacterium avium* complex, MAC) occurs in about 5% of HIV-infected individuals [88, 89]. Infection is associated with more severe immunosuppression and tends to occur later in the course of AIDS. MAC presents as a wasting syndrome with fever, weight loss, cachexia, chronic diarrhoea and abdominal pain. It progresses to an unremitting anaemia with chronic intestinal malabsorption and intrabiliary obstructive jaundice [90].

Treatment of MAC is generally very difficult and unrewarding. The regimen should include ciprofloxacin, rifampicin, ethambutol and amikacin [91]. Although this combination has been shown to reduce sputum colony counts, improve systemic symptoms and reduce the need for blood transfusion, prolonged disease remission is not achieved in most patients [90] and it is debatable whether any treatment other than supportive care should be offered.

Virus infection and HIV

Cytomegalovirus

Most healthy people will have been infected by cytomegalovirus (CMV) by middle age. Reactivation of CMV infection appears to have, in most instances, a trivial effect on the clinical cause of HIV-related disease. CMV can be identified in 40–50% of bronchoalveolar lavage specimens taken during investigation of AIDS-related pneumonitis [1, 92] and in the lungs at *post mortem* of up to 90% of patients dying from AIDS [93]. However, in most instances CMV is likely to be a 'bystander' [94], and the true incidence of CMV pneumonitis is probably less than 1% of cases of pulmonary infections in AIDS patients.

For confirmation of CMV pneumonitis, the following criteria should be fulfilled:

1. The identification of CMV on cultures of bronchoalveolar lavage.
2. The presence of CMV inclusion bodies in cells found in bronchoalveolar lavage fluid or lung biopsies.
3. The absence of other identifiable pathogens.
4. Progressive radiological and clinical deterioration.
5. An improvement on treatment with ganciclovir and foscarnet.

Ganciclovir is probably the first choice for treatment of proven CMV pneumonitis [95], but foscarnet is a possible alternative for patients failing to respond [96].

Fungal infections

Aspergillosis

Contrary to findings in other type of immunosuppressed patients, those with HIV-related disease only rarely suffer infection with *Aspergillus* species [97, 98] and such infection is not regarded as an indicator of AIDS. The most commonly reported form of infection with HIV-related disease is invasive pulmonary aspergillosis, although aspergillomas and pseudomembranous necrotizing bronchial aspergillosis have also been recorded. Treatment with amphotericin may be successful if started early, but the response to therapy is generally poor [98].

Candidiasis

In patients with HIV-related disease, pulmonary candidiasis is an uncommon, late and frequently terminal event, yet *Candida* infections, especially of the oropharynx, are the most common opportunistic infection in such patients after PCP. The diagnosis of lung candidiasis must be based on the demonstration of tissue invasion by *Candida*. Treatment (with amphotericin) is often disappointing and difficult.

Cryptococcosis

Although rarely seen in Europe, 6–13% of AIDS patients in the USA have been reported to suffer clinical cryptococcal infection [99] and the incidence is believed to be much higher in Africa [100]. The presentation with lung infection by this fungus is with fever and cough and the common radiographic appearances include hilar lymphadenopathy, interstitial infiltrates, or both [101]. Pleural effusion may occur [102]. Silent meningitis may co-exist with cryptococcal pneumonia and should be suspected in all patients. The diagnosis is made by the demonstration of cryptococci in secretions, bronchoalveolar lavage, pleural fluid or lung biopsies. Treatment is with intravenous amphotericin. Lifelong maintenance treatment is necessary and fluconazole may be useful in preventing relapses [103]. The prognosis is poor.

Coccidioidomycosis

This, although common in the USA, is rarely seen in HIV patients in Europe, except in those who have come from the USA. It is a late reactivation of previous coccidioidomycotic disease and presents with fever, weight loss and fatigue [104]. The diagnosis is made by identification of coccidioides in sputum samples, bronchoalveolar lavage fluid or lung biopsy. The treatment is with amphotericin.

Histoplasmosis

Chest infection with *Histoplasma capsulatum* in HIV-related disease has mostly been seen as a complication in the USA. It occurs with distal deposition of *Histoplasma* in the lungs and most patients present with fever, cough and breathlessness; about one-half have significant weight loss and about one-third have been reported variously to have splenomegaly, lymphadenopathy and hepatomegaly [105]. The chest radiograph appearance most commonly seen is diffuse reticulonodular shadowing. Diagnosis is established by bone marrow culture. Treatment is with amphotericin and must be maintained for some time after a satisfactory clinical response has been achieved.

Non-infectious pulmonary complications of HIV infection

Kaposi's sarcoma

Kaposi's sarcoma is the main non-infectious pulmonary disorder in AIDS. Before the AIDS epidemic, Kaposi's sarcoma presented as a slowly progressive cutaneous neoplasm which affected the legs of elderly men and spared the lung. The disease is more aggressive in immunosuppressed patients. The relationship between Kaposi's sarcoma and HIV infection is obscure. Concomitant infection with CMV, genetic susceptibility and environmental factors have been proposed as possible explanations [106].

Up to 40% of AIDS patients in hospital may be affected by Kaposi's sarcoma, the respiratory tract being involved in about 20% of cases [107, 108]. However, at present, the incidence of the disease seems to be declining [109]. Systemic spread may be extensive and the degree of lung involvement may not correlate directly with the extent of disease of other organs [110]. The clinical features, which include cough, breathlessness and fever, are non-specific and may mimic an infectious process. Other more specific symptoms include wheeze and stridor, related to endobronchial plaques and haemoptysis. Relevant findings on clinical examination include the typical violaceous skin lesions of Kaposi's sarcoma and signs of pleural effusion.

The radiographic features of pulmonary Kaposi's sarcoma are non-specific and include lung nodules and linear opacities, pleural effusion and hilar lymphadenopathy; appearances mimicking PCP and mass lesions have also been described [111–113]. Pulmonary Kaposi's sarcoma lesions detected at *post mortem* may not have been identified on standard chest radiographs and the nodular and linear opacities seen on radiographs correlate with different pathological appearances. CT scanning may provide additional radiological information [113] but gallium scanning is generally unhelpful.

The diagnosis of pulmonary Kaposi's sarcoma may be difficult because many of its features are non-specific and other diseases can coincidentally affect the lungs in patients with cutaneous Kaposi's sarcoma. The appearances of endobronchial Kaposi's sarcoma at bronchoscopy are characteristic, appearing as raised plaque-like violaceous cherry red lesions. Biopsy may be unnecessary but supplementary histology can sometimes be helpful [114] and, despite the vascularity of the lesions, severe haemorrhage following biopsy is not a problem. Open lung biopsy may be necessary to establish a diagnosis in cases with peripheral parenchymal lesions because transbronchial biopsy rarely provides enough representative material. Cytological examination of pleural fluid and pleural biopsy are not usually helpful [108]

The overall mean survival of patients with cutaneous Kaposi's sarcoma is 12–18 months [115], and the prognosis deteriorates considerably once the pulmonary disease develops [116]. Treatment is with radiotherapy [117] or chemotherapy [100], but neither approach has been shown to be very successful and trials are continuing to find better treatment.

Non-Hodgkin's lymphoma

This is the second most common malignancy associated with HIV infection and its recognition establishes the diagnosis of AIDS. These lymphomas are B-cell tumours but differ from those occurring in individuals without HIV infection in that they show multiple rather than single B-cell clones [118]. The development of this tumour in HIV-infected and in non-infected subjects is clearly related to Epstein–Barr virus infection [119].

Non-Hodgkin's lymphomas in HIV-infected subjects often present with disseminated disease and extranodal involvement [120]. Sites commonly involved are the central nervous system, gastrointestinal tract and the liver. Thoracic involvement is less common although occasionally the disease is confined to the lung. Reported radiographic appearances include parenchymal infiltrates, pleural effusion and mediastinal masses. Diagnosis may be difficult: gallium scans are non-specific and bronchoscopy may be unhelpful; open lung biopsy may be required to confirm clinical suspicions [121]. The prognosis of AIDS-related lymphoma is poor, with a median survival of only 6 months [122]. Treatment is intravenous chemotherapy, and aggressive multidrug regimens have been reported to improve median survival to 20 months in small numbers of patients [123]. Death is often caused by concomitant opportunistic infections.

Lymphoid interstitial pneumonitis

Lymphoid interstitial pneumonitis is characterized histologically by diffuse infiltration with small lymphocytes and plasma cells in the alveolar septa and along lymphatic vessels. In non-HIV-infected patients this disease is usually idiopathic but associations with Sjögren's syndrome, myasthenia gravis and chronic active hepatitis have been described. The disorder is more frequent in HIV-infected individuals, suggesting that its pathogenesis has an immunological basis.

HIV-related lymphoid interstitial pneumonitis has been described in both children [124] and adults [9, 125]: in children, the prognosis is generally favourable although progression to lymphoma has been reported, but the prognosis in adults is more variable. Presenting features include slowly progressive breathlessness and dry cough [126]; some patients may be febrile and the presentation may mimic an infective process; lymphocytosis and hypergammaglobulinaemia are common. The chest radiographic findings include bilateral reticulonodular infiltrates and more diffuse infiltrates similar to those seen in PCP [127]. Because of the similarity with infective processes, invasive investigations (including open lung biopsy) may be necessary to confirm the diagnosis. Treatment is not always necessary in patients with stable disease. Oral corticosteroids, initially in high dose, have been useful in some patients with progressive disease.

Other non-infectious disorders

Lymphocytic alveolitis

The bronchoalveolar lavage fluid obtained from many patients with a variety of HIV-related problems has been found to contain increased numbers of lymphocytes which are predominantly cytotoxic [128]. The cause of this, and its relationship to the development of clinically important lung disease, is unknown.

Disease of the airways

HIV-infected individuals may develop clinically important airways obstruction, independent of smoking habits and previous asthma [129]. In some patients, this may be caused by Kaposi's sarcoma, viral infections, lymphocytic infiltrates and drug hypersensitivity; in others the cause is obscure.

Adult respiratory distress syndrome

This is unusual in HIV-infected individuals. It may follow superadded infection but may occur with no identifiable cause.

Drug reaction

Lung problems caused by drugs used to treat HIV related disorders include pulmonary fibrosis caused by cytotoxic chemotherapy (particularly bleomycin used in the treatment of Kaposi's sarcoma and lymphoma), and hypersensitivity pneumonitis associated with co-trimoxazole therapy.

References

1. Murray JF, Felton CP, Garay S. Pulmonary complications of the acquired immunodeficiency syndrome: report at a National Heart, Lung and Blood Institute workshop. *N Engl J Med* 1984; **310:** 1682–1688.
2. Rankin JA, Collman R, Daniele RP. Acquired immune deficiency syndrome and the lung. *Chest* 1988; **94:** 155–164.
3. Beral V, Peterman TA, Berkelman RL *et al.* Kaposi's sarcoma among persons with AIDS: a sexually transmitted infection? *Lancet* 1990; **335:** 123–128.
4. Leach RM, Davidson AC, O'Doherty MJ *et al.* Non-invasive management of fever and breathlessness in HIV positive patients. *Eur Respir J* 1991; **4:** 19–25.
5. Cohen BA, Pomeranz S, Rabinowitz JG *et al.* Pulmonary complications of AIDS: radiologic features. *Am J Radiol* 1984; **142:** 115–122.
6. Goodman PC, Broaddus VC, Hopewell PC. Chest radiographic patterns in the acquired immune deficiency syndrome. *Am Rev Respir Dis* 1984; **130:** 689–694.
7. Goodman PC, Gamsu G. Pulmonary radiographic findings in the acquired immunodeficiency syndrome. *Postgrad Radiol* 1987; **7:** 3–15.
8. Hopewell PC, Luce JM. Pulmonary involvement in the acquired immunodeficiency syndrome. *Chest* 1985; **87:** 104–112.
9. Solal-Celigny P, Coudere LJ, Herman D *et al.* Lymphoid interstitial pneumonitis in the acquired immunodeficiency syndrome-related complex. *Am Rev Respir Dis* 1985; **131:** 956–960.
10. Stern RG, Gamsu G, Golden JA. Intrathoracic adenopathy: differential features of AIDS and diffuse lymphadenopathy syndrome. *Am J Radiol* 1984;. **141:** 689–692.

11. Murphy PM, Fox C, Travis W *et al.* Acquired immunodeficiency syndrome may present as severe restrictive lung disease. *Am J Med* 1989; **86:** 237–240.
12. Shaw RJ, Roussak C, Forster SM *et al.* Lung function abnormalities in patients infected with the human immunodeficiency virus with and without overt pneumocystis. *Thorax* 1988; **43:** 436–440.
13. Meduri GU, Stover DE, Lee M *et al.* Pulmonary Kaposi's sarcoma in the acquired immunodeficiency syndrome. Clinical, radiographic and pathologic manifestations. *Am J Med* 1986; **81:** 11–18.
14. Denison DM, Cramer DS, Hanson PJV. Lung function testing and AIDS. *Respir Med* 1989; **83:** 133–138.
15. Coleman DL, Hattner RS, Luce JM *et al.* Correlation between gallium lung scans and fibreoptic bronchoscopies in patients with suspected *Pneumocystis carinii* pneumonia and the acquired immunodeficiency syndrome. *Am Rev Respir Dis* 1984; **130:** 1166–1169.
16. Kramer EL, Sanger JH, Garay SM *et al.* Diagnostic implications of Ga-67 chest-scan patterns in human immunodeficiency virus – seropositive patients. *Radiology* 1989; **170:** 671–676.
17. Kramer EL, Sanger JJ, Garay SM. Gallium-67 scans of the chest in patients with acquired immunodeficiency syndrome. *J Nucl Med* 1987; **28:** 1107–1114.
18. Hattner RS, Solitto RA, Golden JA *et al.* Sensitivity and specificity of Ga-67 pulmonary scans for the detection of *Pneumocystis carinii* pneumonia in patients with the acquired immunodeficiency syndrome and pulmonary symptoms. *J Nucl Med* 1984; **25:** 43.
19. Luce JM. Sputum induction in the acquired immunodeficiency syndrome. *Am Rev Respir Dis* 1986; **133:** 513–514.
20. Leigh TR, Parsons P, Hume C *et al.* Induced sputum: a sensitive test for diagnosis of *Pneumocystis carinii* pneumonia in AIDS patients. *Lancet* 1989; **ii:** 205–206.
21. Pitchenik AE, Ganjei P, Torres A *et al.* Sputum examination for the diagnosis of *Pneumocystis carinii* pneumonia in the acquired immunodeficiency syndrome. *Am Rev Respir Dis* 1986; **133:** 226–229.
22. Bigby TD, Margolskee D, Curtis JL *et al.* The usefulness of induced sputum in the diagnosis of *Pneumocystis carinii* pneumonia in patients with the acquired immunodeficiency syndrome. *Am Rev Respir Dis* 1986; **133:** 515–518.
23. Kovacs JA, Ng UL, Masur H *et al.* Diagnosis of *Pneumocystis carinii* pneumonia: improved detection in sputum with use of monoclonal antibodies. *N Engl J Med* 1988; **313:** 589–593.
24. Broaddus VC, Dake MD, Stulbarg MS *et al.* Bronchoalveolar lavage and transbronchial biopsy for the diagnosis of pulmonary infection in the acquired immunodeficiency syndrome. *Ann Intern Med* 1985; **102:** 747–752.
25. Golden JA, Hollander H, Stulbarg MS *et al.* Bronchoalveolar lavage as the exclusive diagnostic modality for *Pneumocystis carinii* pneumonia. *Chest* 1986; **90:** 18–22.
26. Weldon-Linne CM, Rhone DP, Bourassa R. Bronchoscopy specimens in adults with AIDS. Comparative yields of cytology, histology and culture for diagnosis of infectious agents. *Chest* 1990; **98:** 24–28.
27. Martin WR, Albertson TE, Siegel B. Tracheal catheters in patients with acquired immunodeficiency syndrome for the diagnosis of *Pneumocystis carinii* pneumonia. *Chest* 1990; **98:** 29–32.
28. Bottles K, McPhaul LW, Volberding P. Fine needle aspiration in patients with the acquired immunodeficiency syndrome (AIDS): experience in an outpatient clinic. *Ann Intern Med* 1988; **108:** 42-45.
29. Fitzgerald W, Bevelaqua FA, Garay SM. The role of open lung biopsy in patients with the acquired immunodeficiency syndrome. *Chest* 1987; **91:** 659–661.
30. Jacobs JL, Libby DM, Winters RA *et al.* A cluster of *Pneumocystis carinii* pneumonia in adults without predisposing illnesses. *N Engl J Med* 1991; **324:** 246–250.
31. Edman JC, Kovacs JA, Masur H *et al.* Ribosomal RNA sequence shows *Pneumocystis carinii* to be a member of the fungi. *Nature* 1988; **334:** 519–522.
32. Selik RM, Starcher ET, Curran JW. Opportunist diseases reported in AIDS patients: frequencies association and trends. *AIDS* 1987; **1:** 175–182.
33. Murray JF, Garay SM, Hopewell PC. NHLBI workshop summary. Pulmonary complications of the acquired immunodeficiency syndrome: an update. *Am Rev Respir Dis* 1987; **135:** 504–509.
34. Clumeck N, Sonnet J, Taelman H *et al.* Acquired immunodeficiency syndrome in African patients. *N Engl J Med* 1984; **310:** 492–497.
35. Pifer L, Hughes WT, Stagno S *et al. Pneumocystis carinii* infections: evidence for high prevalence in normal and immunosuppressed children. *Paediatrics* 1978; **61:** 35–41.
36. Coleman DL, Luce JM, Wilber JC *et al.* Antibody to the retrovirus associated with acquired immunodeficiency syndrome (AIDS). Presence in presumably healthy San Franciscans who died unexpectedly. *Arch Intern Med* 1986; **146:** 713–715.
37. Leigh TR, Wiggins J, Midgeley J *et al. Pneumocystis carinii*: attempted isolation from induced sputum and bronchoalveolar lavage specimens of non-HIV infected individuals using immunofluo-

rescent stains. *Thorax* 1990; **45:** 304.
38. Giron JA, Martinez S, Walzer PD. Should patients with *Pneumocystis carinii* be isolated? *Lancet* 1982; **ii:** 46.
39. Mascarenhas DAN, Vasundevan VP, Vaidyu KP. *Pneumocystis carinii* pneumonia. Rare cause of haemoptysis. *Chest* 1991; **99:** 251–253.
40. Masur J, Frederick P, Ognibene FP *et al.* CD4 counts as predictors of opportunistic pneumonias in human immunodeficiency virus (HIV) infection. *Ann Intern Med* 1989; **111:** 223–231.
41. Zaman MK, White DA. Serum lactate dehydrogenase levels and *Pneumocystis carinii* pneumonia. *Am Rev Respir Dis* 1988; **137:** 796–800.
42. Beers ME, Sohn M, Swartz M. Recurrent pneumothorax in AIDS patients with pneumocystis pneumonia. *Chest* 1990; **98:** 266–270.
43. Reiss TF, Golden J. Abnormal lung gallium-67 uptake preceding pulmonary physiologic impairment in an asymptomatic patient with *Pneumocystis carinii* pneumonia. *Chest* 1990; **97:** 1261–1263.
44. Wharton JM, Coleman DL, Wofsy CB *et al.* Trimethoprim-sulfamethoxazole or pentamidine for *Pneumocystis carinii* pneumonia in the acquired immunodeficiency syndrome. *Ann Intern Med* 1986; **105:** 37–44.
45. Sattler FR, Cowan R, Nielsen DM *et al.* Trimethoprim-sulfamethoxazole compared with pentamidine for the treatment of *Pneumocystis carinii* pneumonia in the acquired immunodeficiency syndrome. A prospective, noncrossover study. *Ann Intern Med* 1988; **109:** 280–287.
46. Gordin FM, Simon GL, Wofsy CB *et al.* Adverse reaction to trimethoprim-sulfamethoxazole in patients with the acquired immunodeficiency syndrome. *Ann Intern Med* 1984; **100:** 495–499.
47. Kovacs JA, Hiemenz JW, Macher AM *et al. Pneumocystis carinii* pneumonia: a comparison between patients with the acquired immunodeficiency syndrome and patients with other immunodeficiencies. *Ann Intern Med* 1984; **100:** 663–671.
48. Leoung GS, Mills J, Hopewell PC *et al.* Dapsone-trimethoprim for *Pneumocystis carinii* pneumonia in the acquired immunodeficiency syndrome. *Ann Intern Med* 1986; **105:** 45–48.
49. Medina I, Mills J, Leoung G *et al.* Oral therapy for *Pneumocystis carinii* pneumonia in the acquired immunodeficiency syndrome. A controlled trial of trimethoprimsulfamethoxazole versus trimethoprim-dapsone. *N Engl J Med* 1990; **323:** 776–782.
50. Mills J, Leoung G, Medina I *et al.* Dapsone treatment of *Pneumocystis carinii* pneumonia in the acquired immunodeficiency syndrome. *Antimicrob Agents Chemother* 1988; **32:** 1057–1060.
51. Golden JA, Sjoerdsma A, Santi DV. *Pneumocystis carinii* pneumonia treated with alpha difluoromethylornithine. *West J Med* 1984; **141:** 613–623.
52. Toma E, Fournier S, Poisson M *et al.* Clindamycin with primaquine for *Pneumocystis carinii* pneumonia. *Lancet* 1989; **i:** 1046–1048.
53. Montgomery AB, Debs RJ, Luce JM *et al.* Aerosolized pentamidine as sole therapy for *Pneumocystis carinii* pneumonia in patients with acquired immunodeficiency syndrome. *Lancet* 1987; **ii:** 470–483.
54. SooHoo GW, Mohsenifar Z, Meyer RD. Inhaled or intravenous pentamidine therapy for *Pneumocystis carinii* pneumonia in AIDS. A randomised trial. *Ann Intern Med* 1990; **113:** 195–202.
55. Conte JE, Chernoff D, Feigal DW *et al.* Intravenous or inhaled pentamidine for treating *Pneumocystis carinii* pneumonia in AIDS. A random trial. *Ann Intern Med* 1990; **113:** 203–209.
56. Chemel H. *Pneumocystis carinii* pneumonia. The steroid dilemma. *Arch Intern Med* 1990; **150:** 1793–1794.
57. MacFadden DK, Edelson JD, Hyland RH *et al.* Corticosteroids as adjunctive therapy in the treatment of *Pneumocystis carinii* pneumonia in the acquired immunodeficiency syndrome. *Lancet* 1987; **i:** 1477–1479.
58. Montaner JSG, Russell JA, Lawson L *et al.* Acute respiratory failure secondary to *Pneumocystis carinii* pneumonia in the acquired immunodeficiency syndrome. A potential role for systemic corticosteroids. *Chest* 1989; **95:** 881–884.
59. Schiff MJ, Farber BF, Kaplan MH. Steroids for *Pneumocystis carinii* pneumonia and respiratory failure in the acquired immunodeficiency syndrome. A reassessment. *Arch Intern Med* 1990; **150:** 1819–1821.
60. Lambertus MW, Goetz MB, Murthy AR *et al.* Complications of corticosteroid therapy in patients with the acquired immunodeficiency syndrome and *Pneumocystis carinii* pneumonia. *Chest* 1990; **98:** 38–43.
61. Montaner JSG, Lawson LM, Levitt N *et al.* Corticosteroids prevent early deterioration in patients with moderately severe *Pneumocystis carinii* pneumonia and the acquired immunodeficiency syndrome (AIDS). *Ann Intern Med* 1990; **113:** 14–20.
62. Clement M, Edison R, Turner J *et al.* Corticosteroids as adjunctive therapy in severe *Pneumocystis carinii* pneumonia. A prospective placebo controlled trial. *Am Rev Respir Dis* 1989; **139:** A250.
63. Kovacs JA, Masur H. Are corticosteroids beneficial as adjunctive therapy for pneumocystis pneumonia in AIDS? *Ann Intern Med* 1990; **113:** 1–3.

64. Brenner M, Ognibene P, Lack EE *et al.* Prognostic factors and life expectancy of patients with acquired immunodeficiency syndrome and *Pneumocystis carinii* pneumonia. *Am Rev Respir Dis* 1987; **136:** 1119–1206.
65. Wachter RM, Luce JM, Turner J *et al.* Intensive care of patients with the acquired immunodeficiency syndrome: outcome and changing patterns of utilization. *Am Rev Respir Dis* 1986; **134:** 891–896.
66. Schein RM, Fischl MA, Pitchenik AE. ICU survival of patients with the acquired immunodeficiency syndrome. *Crit Care Med* 1986; **14:** 1026–1027.
67. Friedman Y, Franklin C, Rackow EC *et al.* Improved survival in patients with acquired immunodeficiency syndrome, *Pneumocystis carinii* pneumonia and severe respiratory failure. *Chest* 1989; **96:** 862–866.
68. Efferen LS, Nadarajah D, Palat DS. Survival following mechanical ventilation for *Pneumocystis carinii* pneumonia in patients with the acquired immunodeficiency syndrome: a different perspective. *Am J Med* 1989; **87:** 401–404.
69. Wachter RM, Russi MB, Bloch DA *et al.* *Pneumocystis carinii* pneumonia and respiratory failure in AIDS. Improved outcome and increased use of intensive care units. *Am Rev Respir Dis* 1991; **143:** 251–256.
70. Montgomery AB, Debs RJ, Luce JM *et al.* Selective delivery of pentamidine to the lung by aerosol. *Am Rev Respir Dis* 1988; **137:** 477–478.
71. Leoung GS, Feigal DW, Montgomery AB *et al.* Aerosolized pentamidine for prophylaxis against *Pneumocystis carinii* pneumonia. The San Francisco community prophylaxis trial. *N Engl J Med* 1990; **323:** 769–775.
72. Leigh TR, Wiggins J, Gazzard BG *et al.* Effect of terbutaline on bronchoconstriction induced by nebulised pentamidine. *Thorax* 1991; **46:** 122–123.
73. Fischl MA, Dickinson GM, LaVoie L. Safety and efficacy of sulfamethoxazole and trimethoprim chemoprophylaxis for *Pneumocystis carinii* pneumonia in AIDS. *JAMA* 1988; **259:** 1185–1189.
74. Ruskin J, LaRiviere M. Low-dose co-trimoxazole for prevention of *Pneumocystis carinii* pneumonia in human immunodeficiency virus disease. *Lancet* 1991; **337:** 468–471.
75. Centers for Disease Control. Guidelines for prophylaxis against *Pneumocystis carinii* pneumonia for persons with human immunodeficiency virus infection. *Morbid Mortal Weekly Rep* 1989; **38:** 1–8.
76. Marchevsky A, Rosen MS, Chrystal G *et al.* Pulmonary complications of the acquired immunodeficiency syndrome: a clinicopathologic study of 70 cases. *Hum Pathol* 1985; **16:** 659–670.
77. Witt DJ, Craven DE, McCabe WR. Bacterial infections in adult patients with the acquired immunodeficiency syndrome (AIDS) and AIDS-related complex. *Am J Med* 1987; **82:** 900–906.
78. Polsky B, Gold JWM, Whimbey E *et al.* Bacterial pneumonia in patients with the acquired immunodeficiency syndrome. *Ann Intern Med* 1986; **104:** 38–41.
79. Centers for Disease Control. Tuberculosis, final data – United States, 1986. *Morbid Mortal Weekly Rep* 1988; **36:** 817–820.
80. Elliott AM, Luo N, Tembo G *et al.* Impact of HIV on tuberculosis in Zambia: a cross sectional study. *BMJ* 1990; **301:** 412–415.
81. Colebunders RL, Ryder RW, Nzilambi N. HIV infection in patients with tuberculosis in Kinshasa, Zaire. *Am Rev Respir Dis* 1989; **139:** 1082–1085.
82. Pitchenik AE, Rubinson HA. The radiographic appearance of tuberculosis in patients with the acquired immunodeficiency syndrome (AIDS) and pre-AIDS. *Am Rev Respir Dis* 1985; **131:** 393–396.
83. Flora GS, Modilevsky T, Antoniskis D *et al.* Undiagnosed tuberculosis in patients with human immunodeficiency virus Infection. *Chest* 1990; **98:** 1056–1059.
84. Kramer F, Modilevsky T, Waliany AR *et al.* Delayed diagnosis of tuberculosis in patients with human immunodeficiency virus infection. *Am J Med* 1990; **89:** 451–456.
85. Ellner JJ. Tuberculosis in the time of AIDS. The facts and the message. *Chest* 1990; **98:** 1051–1052.
86. American Thoracic Society/Centres for Disease Control. Mycobacterioses and the acquired immunodeficiency syndrome. *Am Rev Respir Dis* 1987; **136:** 492–496.
87. Selwyn PA, Hartel D, Lewis VA *et al.* A prospective study of the risk of tuberculosis among intravenous drug users with human immunodeficiency virus infection. *N Engl J Med* 1989; **320:** 545–550.
88. Zakowski P, Fugiel S, Berlin GW *et al.* Disseminated *Mycobacterium avium-intracellulare* infection in homosexual men dying of acquired immunodeficiency. *JAMA* 1982; **248:** 2980–2982.
89. Horsburgh CJ Jr, Selik RM. The epidemiology of disseminated non-tuberculous mycobacterial infection in the acquired immunodeficiency syndrome (AIDS). *Am Rev Respir Dis* 1989; **139:** 4–7.
90. Jacobson MA. Mycobacterial diseases: tuberculosis and *Mycobacterium avium* complex. *Infect Dis Clin North Am* 1988; **2:** 465–474.
91. Chiu J, Nussbaum J, Bozzette S *et al.* Treatment of disseminated *Mycobacterium avium* complex infection in AIDS with amikacin, ethambutol, rifampicin and ciprofloxacin. *Ann Intern Med* 1990; **113:** 358–361.

92. Miles PR, Baughman RP, Linnemann CC. Cytomegalovirus in the bronchoalveolar lavage fluid of patients with AIDS. *Chest* 1990; **97:** 1072–1076.
93. Welch K, Fukbeiner W, Alepers CE *et al.* Autopsy findings in the acquired immunodeficiency syndrome. *JAMA* 1984; **252:** 1152–1159.
94. Millar AB, Patou G, Miller RF *et al.* Cytomegalovirus in the lungs of patients with AIDS. Respiratory pathogen or passenger? *Am Rev Respir Dis* 1990; **141:** 1474–1477.
95. Masur H, Lane HC, Palestino A *et al.* Effect of PHPG on serious cytomegalovirus disease in eight immunosuppressed homosexual men. *Ann Intern Med* 1986; **104:** 41–44.
96. Jacobson MA, O'Donnell JJ, Mills J. Foscarnet treatment of cytomegalovirus retinitis in patients with the acquired immunodeficiency syndrome. *Antimicrob Agents Chemother* 1989; **33:** 736–741.
97. Blaser MJ, Cohn DL. Opportunistic infections in patients with AIDS: clues to the epidemiology of AIDS and the relative virulence of pathogens. *Rev Infect Dis* 1986; **8:** 21–30.
98. Denning DW, Follansbee ST, Scolaro M *et al.* Pulmonary aspergillosis in the acquired immunodeficiency syndrome. *N Engl J Med* 1991; **324:** 654–662.
99. Kovacs JA, Kovacs AA, Polis M *et al.* Cryptococcosis in the acquired immunodeficiency syndrome. *Ann Intern Med* 1985; **103:** 533–538.
100. Eng RH, Bishurg E, Smith SM *et al.* Cryptococcal infections in patients with acquired immunodeficiency syndrome. *Am J Med* 1986; **81:** 19–23.
101. Miller WJ Jr, Edelman JM, Miller WT. Cryptococcal pulmonary infection in patients with AIDS: radiographic appearance. *Radiology* 1990; **175:** 725–728.
102. Newman TG, Soni A, Acaron S *et al.* Pleural cryptococcosis in the acquired immunodeficiency syndrome. *Chest* 1987; **91:** 459–461.
103. Stern JJ, Hartman BJ, Sharkey P *et al.* Oral fluconazole therapy for patients with acquired immunodeficiency syndrome and cryptococcosis: experience with 22 patients. *Am J Med* 1988; **85:** 477–480.
104. Bronnimann DA, Adam RD, Galgiani JN *et al.* Coccidioidomycosis in the acquired immunodeficiency syndrome. *Ann Intern Med* 1987; **106:** 372–379.
105. Johnson PC, Hamil RJ, Sarosi GA. Clinical review: progressive disseminated histoplasmosis in the AIDS patient. *Semin Respir Infect* 1989; **4:** 139–146.
106. Krown SE. AIDS-associated Kaposi's sarcoma: pathogenesis, clinical course and treatment. *AIDS* 1988; **2:** 71–80.
107. Zibrak JD, Silvestri RC, Rostello P *et al.* Bronchoscopic and radiologic features of Kaposi's sarcoma involving the respiratory system. *Chest* 1986; **90:** 476–479.
108. Garay SM, Belenko M, Fazzini E *et al.* Pulmonary manifestations of Kaposi's sarcoma. *Chest* 1987; **91:** 39–43.
109. Drew WL, Mills J, Hauer LB *et al.* Declining prevalence of Kaposi's sarcoma in homosexual AIDS patients paralleled by fall in cytomegalovirus transmission. *Lancet* 1988; **i:** 66.
110. Ognibene FP, Steis RG, Macher AM *et al.* Kaposi's sarcoma causing pulmonary infiltrates and respiratory failure in the acquired immunodeficiency syndrome. *Ann Intern Med* 1985; **102:** 471–475.
111. Davis SD, Henschke CI, Chamides B *et al.* Intrathoracic Kaposi's sarcoma in AIDS patients: Radiographic–pathologic correlation. *Radiology* 1987; **163:** 495–500.
112. Sivit CJ, Schwartz AM, Rockoff SD. Kaposi's sarcoma of the lung in AIDS patients. Radiographic–pathologic analysis. *Am J Radiol* 1987; **148:** 25–28.
113. Naidich DP, Garay SM, Leitman BS *et al.* Radiographic manifestations of pulmonary disease in the acquired immunodeficiency syndrome (AIDS). *Semin Roentgenol* 1987; **22:** 14–30.
114. Hamm PG, Judson MA, Aranda CP. Diagnosis of pulmonary Kaposi's sarcoma with fibreoptic bronchoscopy and endobronchial biopsy. A report of 5 cases. *Cancer* 1987; **57:** 807–810.
115. Safai B, Johnson KG, Myskowski PL *et al.* The natural history of Kaposi's sarcoma in the acquired immunodeficiency syndrome. *Ann Intern Med* 1985; **103:** 144–150.
116. Ognibene FP, Shelhamer JH. Kaposi's sarcoma. *Clin Chest Med* 1988; **9:** 459–465.
117. Cooper TS, Fried PR, Laubenstein LJ. Initial observations on the effect of radiotherapy on epidemic Kaposi's sarcoma. *JAMA* 1984; **252:** 934–935.
118. Knowles DM, Chamulak GA, Subar M *et al.* Lymphoid neoplasia associated with the acquired immunodeficiency syndrome AIDS. *Ann Intern Med* 1988; **108:** 744–753.
119. Hamilton-Dutoit SJ, Pallosen G, Karkov J *et al.* Identification of EBV-DNA in tumour cells of AIDS-related lymphoma by *in-situ* hybridisation. *Lancet* 1989; **i:** 554–555.
120. Kaplan LD, Abrams DI, Feigal E *et al.* AIDS-associated non-Hodgkin's lymphoma in San Francisco. *JAMA* 1989; **26:** 719–724.
121. Poelzleitner D, Huebsch P, Mayerhofer S *et al.* Primary pulmonary lymphoma in a patient with the acquired immune deficiency syndrome. *Thorax* 1989; **44:** 438–439.
122. Lowenthal DA, Straus DJ, Campbell SW *et al.* AIDS-related lymphoid neoplasia: the Memorial Hospital experience. *Cancer* 1988; **61:** 2325–2337.

123. Bermudez MA, Grant KM, Rodvien R *et al.* Non-Hodgkin's lymphoma in a population with or at risk for acquired immunodeficiency syndrome: indication for intensive chemotherapy. *Am J Med* 1989; **86:** 71–76.
124. Scott GB, Buck BE, Letteman JG *et al.* Acquired immunodeficiency syndrome in infants. *N Engl J Med* 1984; **310:** 76–81.
125. Grieco MH, Chinoy-Acharya P. Lymphocytic interstitial pneumonia associated with the acquired immune deficiency syndrome. *Am Rev Respir Dis* 1985; **131:** 952–955.
126. Morris JC, Rosen MJ, Marchevsky A *et al.* Lymphocytic interstitial pneumonia in patients at risk for the acquired immunodeficiency syndrome. *Chest* 1987; **91:** 63–67.
127. Oldham SA, Castillo M, Jacobson FL *et al.* HIV associated lymphocytic interstitial pneumonia: radiologic manifestations and pathologic correlation. *Radiology* 1989; **107:** 83–87.
128. Guillon JM, Autran B, Denis M *et al.* Human immunodeficiency virus-related lymphocytic alveolitis. *Chest* 1988; **94:** 1264–1270.
129. O'Donnell CR, Bader MB, Zibrak JD *et al.* Abnormal airway function in individuals with the acquired immunodeficiency syndrome. *Chest* 1988; **94:** 945–948.

9

The adult respiratory distress syndrome

M. Messent and T.W. Evans

Introduction

The term adult respiratory distress syndrome (ARDS) defines the condition of severe parenchymal lung injury leading to refractory hypoxaemia in the absence of left ventricular failure and was first described in 1967 [1], although an identical phenomenon was noted during the Second World War and again in the Vietnam conflict complicating non-pulmonary trauma.

ARDS is characterized by non-hydrostatic pulmonary oedema, reduced lung compliance and hypoxaemia and may result from a wide range of serious medical and surgical disorders, directly affecting the lung or arising at a distant (non-pulmonary) site. Furthermore, of those patients with conditions associated with the development of ARDS, only a minority develop the full-blown syndrome [2]. Consequently, there has been a growing awareness that ARDS probably represents the extreme end of a spectrum of lung injury. The simple clinical criteria used to diagnose the condition to date are therefore too broad to allow comparisons of disease severity between different patients and clinical centres. In an effort to overcome this problem, Murray [3] has developed a score for patients with lung injury that takes account of the appearances on chest radiography, pulmonary compliance, degree of hypoxaemia and the use of positive end expiratory pressure (PEEP) in ventilatory support. These parameters are graded for severity, permitting the calculation of an overall score of injury. Although this approach should change the manner in which clinicians currently regard ARDS as a single disease entity and improve the way in which new therapeutic interventions can be assessed, limitations remain, including the omission of a loading factor for the underlying illness which undoubtedly influences prognosis.

The clinical features that define ARDS are attributable to an increase in pulmonary endothelial permeability, but it is now apparent that increased vascular leak occurs in other organs such as the kidney [4] and it seems likely that all capillary beds are influenced to a greater or lesser extent by the disease process. The endothelium is emerging as an important regulatory body in pulmonary [5] and systemic [6] vascular contro. Endothelial damage and loss of integrity has important implications for the development of both ARDS and the syndrome of multisystem organ failure, in which the failure of three or more organ systems is associated with a mortality in excess of 90% [7].

Incidence

In 1972 it was estimated that there were 150 000 cases of ARDS per year in the USA alone [8]. European data are scarce and estimates of incidence vary widely. A recent retrospective study in a single region of the UK found 2.5 cases per 100 000 population [9], suggesting that there are probably 1000–1500 cases of established ARDS in the UK each year. A recent study of ARDS in an island population in which all cases could be easily traced revealed a comparable incidence of about 3.5 per 100 000 population [10].

Aetiology

ARDS is associated with a wide range of clinical conditions, only some of which involve the lung (Table 9.1) and between which there is no obvious connection. The severity of the injury and mortality rate appears to vary according to the predisposing cause. Thus, the risk of developing ARDS after surgery involving cardiopulmonary bypass is 1.31% [11], whilst that associated with sepsis is of the order of 18–23% [12, 13]. The spectrum of lung injury has recently been quantified by Rocker *et al.* in a study of patients with a range of risk factors for ARDS and variable degrees of respiratory failure [14]. The severity of respiratory failure was positively correlated with the leakage of protein from the pulmonary vasculature and markers of neutrophil degranulation. As the clinical parameters of lung damage worsened, the measured protein leak and levels of neutrophil elastase increased. Whether this approach will prove useful in the clinical setting remains to be seen.

Table 9.1 Conditions associated with the adult respiratory distress syndrome

Pulmonary	*Non-pulmonary*
Aspiration	Sepsis
Near drowning	Fat embolism
Smoke inhalation	Hypovolaemia
Direct lung trauma	Head injury
Pneumonia	DIC
	Pancreatitis
	Eclampsia

Prognosis

The mortality rate associated with ARDS remains high [12]; the rate in patients with sepsis and ARDS is 70% and approaches 90% for ARDS complicating aspiration pneumonia [15]. The cause of death is related to the underlying insult, its site and severity, the response to therapy and the incidence of complications. Irreversible respiratory failure is responsible for only 16% of fatalities [7] and the majority of deaths are attributable to multisystem organ failure. Persistent acidaemia (pH less than 7.40), plasma bicarbonate levels below 20 mmol and greater than 10% band forms on the blood film are all associated with an increased incidence of death [15].

Pathology and pathophysiology

At necropsy the lungs from patients with ARDS are heavy, poorly aerated and exhibit a liver-like consistency. The disease process tends to be patchy, some parts of the lung showing no changes at all. The affected areas are infiltrated with neutrophils. Additionally, eosinophilic hyaline membranes may be found in the airways and alveoli, similar to those associated with infantile respiratory distress syndrome (Figure 9.1). Initially, widespread alveolar and interstitial oedema develops and the Type I pneumocytes become denuded and oedematous. The hyaline membrane represents fibrin deposition that eventually becomes polymerized; microvascular emboli consisting of fibrin and platelets and neutrophils are seen. Finally, there is often evidence of a disorganized healing process with interstitial fibroblast proliferation and Type II pneumocyte hyperplasia (responsible for the formation of new Type I pneumocytes). *Post mortem* studie in patients that survive for more than 10 days have shown increased total lung collagen, although before this there is little evidence of fibrosis [16].

In patients who recover, lung function tests reveal a decreased diffusing capacity for carbon monoxide and decreased vital capacity and total lung capacity up to months later; deficiencies that do not correlate with the initial degree of lung injury [17].

Pathophysiology

The poor prognosis of patients with ARDS has provided a considerable impetus to elucidating the mechanisms that initiate pulmonary vascular injury. These seem to depend upon the interaction of activated inflammatory cells, humoral mediators

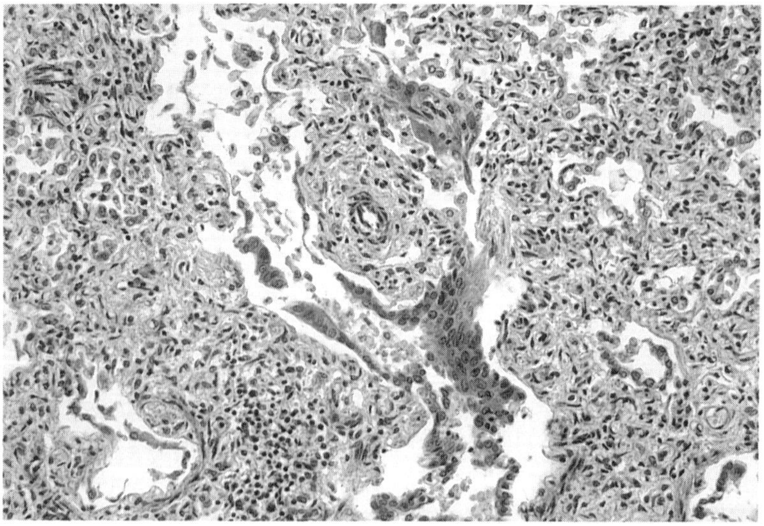

Figure 9.1 Open lung biopsy from a patient with ARDS. Note the dense inflammatory infiltrate

and endothelial cells [18] (Figure 9.2). A better understanding of these mechanisms will determine the development of effective pharmacological interventions. Most recent research has focused on the mechanisms leading to the activation of inflammatory cells (particularly the neutrophil); platelets and other clotting factors [19, 20]. Neutrophil activation is at least partially dependent upon cytokines, potent inflammatory molecules released from macrophages which may themselves directly damage vascular endothelial cells [21]. Platelet activation and sequestration in the lungs of patients with ARDS is also recognized and may be a consequence of, or occur independently of, neutrophil activation [19]. In these circumstances the release of proteolytic enzymes, reactive oxygen metabolites and inflammatory mediators leads, directly or indirectly, to endothelial damage producing the pulmonary oedema and impaired peripheral oxygen uptake that define the clinical syndrome [22]. Platelet microemboli almost certainly exacerbate the pulmonary hypertension seen in ARDS and may contribute directly to the late complication of pulmonary fibrosis through the release of platelet-derived growth factor, which has a potent mitogenic effect on pulmonary fibroblasts [23].

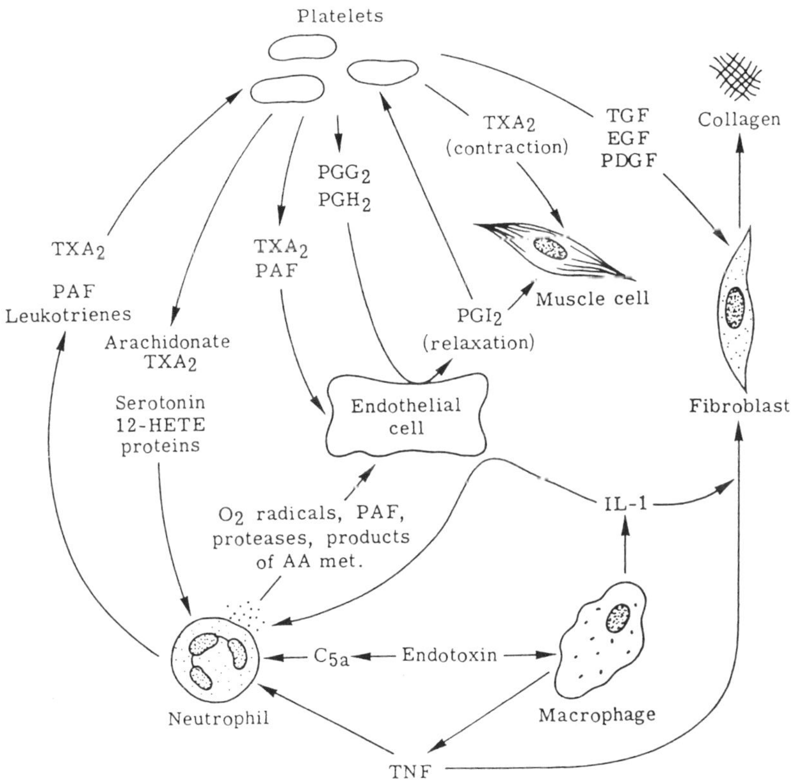

Figure 9.2 Schematic representation of possible mechanisms underlying ARDS. Note the central interaction of inflammatory cells/mediators and the endothelial cell. TNF, Tumour necrosis factor; IL-1, interleukin-1; AA, arachidonic acid; 12-HETE, 12-hydroxyeicosatetraenoate; EGF, epidermal growth factor; PAF, platelet-activating factor; PG, prostaglandins; TGF, transforming growth factor; TXA_2, thromboxane A_2; PGDF, platelet-derived growth factor

Neutrophil activation may occur via a number of disparate pathways including complement and cytokines, specifically tumour necrosis factor (TNF) and interleukin-1 (IL-1), produced by macrophages amongst other cell types. The biological properties of these two agents are remarkably similar and include the induction of pyrexia, hypotension, local tissue necrosis, fibroblast proliferation and endothelial cell activation. The effects of TNF have been shown to mimic closely those of endotoxin *in vivo* [24] and interleukins can induce an ARDS-like syndrome in pigs, effects that are almost certainly induced via neutrophils. High levels of TNF have been isolated in bronchoalveolar lavage fluid obtained from patients with established ARDS [25] and in low doses TNF has been shown to influence pulmonary endothelial cell function in rats [26].

Clinical and experimental data demonstrate that platelets sequester in the pulmonary circulation early in the course of acute oedematous lung injury, possibly due to the release of platelet-activating factor (PAF), leukotrienes, thromboxane and prostanoids produced following endothelial cell damage and neutrophil activation [27]. PAF is possibly the most potent inflammatory mediator of increased vascular permeability in experimental animals [28]. Activated platelets may themselves activate complement and further release products of arachidonic acid metabolism that are chemoattractant and that prime neutrophils. Platelets also produce platelet-derived growth factor and transforming growth factor B, which can directly affect collagen production by fibroblasts in the reparative phase following lung injury. Collagen metabolism may also be affected following the mildest insults to the lung, such as that consequent upon cardiopulmonary bypass surgery [29]. Less work has been carried out to evaluate the effects of blocking the effects of platelet activation, although PAF has been implicated in mediating the increased vascular permeability associated with bleomycin- and endotoxin-induced lung injury in rats [30, 31].

In experimental models and in clinical cases of ARDS there is evidence of free radical formation and their damaging effects [32, 33]. The pulmonary endothelium is attacked by reactive oxygen species generated intracellularly and by those generated by neutrophils and macrophages. This effect is compounded by the high fractional inspired oxygen concentrations (FIO_2) required to support patients with ARDS.

Reactive oxygen species can be formed when a cell becomes hypoxic, following exposure to endotoxin [34] and as a consequence of any mechanism that disrupts the cell wall. These can all lead to xanthine oxidase being formed from the xanthine dehydrogenase. In its modified form this enzyme becomes a free radical generator which disrupts the internal workings of the cell. Endogenous antioxidants are generated in the normal cell via the glutathione system, and superoxide dismutase and catalase. Brigham and co-workers have demonstrated the induction of manganese superoxide dismutase in the face of oxidant stress [35] and it seems likely that tissue damage occurs when these systems are overwhelmed. Adherence of neutrophils to the pulmonary vascular endothelium leads to an oxidative burst and the generation of reactive oxygen into the microenvironment near the pulmonary endothelium. Elastase released by neutrophils also contributes to the formation of xanthine oxidase. The disruption of the cell membrane leads to release of iron and via Fenton reactions to further generation of reactive oxygen species.

Pulmonary physiology

As a result of the inflammatory process the alveolar–capillary membrane becomes highly permeable, allowing the formation of non-hydrostatic pulmonary oedema. This causes an increase in shunt fraction and a fall in lung compliance. Ventilatory dead space increases consequent upon the formation of microemboli and the over-distension of some alveoli.

The fall in lung compliance can be seen if the pressure–volume curves of normal and injured lungs are compared (Figure 9.3). Closing volume remains the same and the fall in functional residual capacity leads to alveolar collapse during tidal ventilation. Shunt is increased because of adverse ventilation ($\dot{V}$) perfusion ($\dot{Q}$) matching, which possibly develops through a loss of hypoxic pulmonary vasoconstriction.

Cardiac performance and oxygen delivery

In patients with ARDS, oxygen delivery (Do_2; Table 9.2) is reduced by hypoxaemia and pulmonary hypertension, which also increases right ventricular afterload and causes interventricular septal shift, thereby impairing left ventricular stroke volume. In patients with sepsis, cardiac contractility may be further diminished by a circulating myocardial depressant factor similar to TNF in terms of molecular size

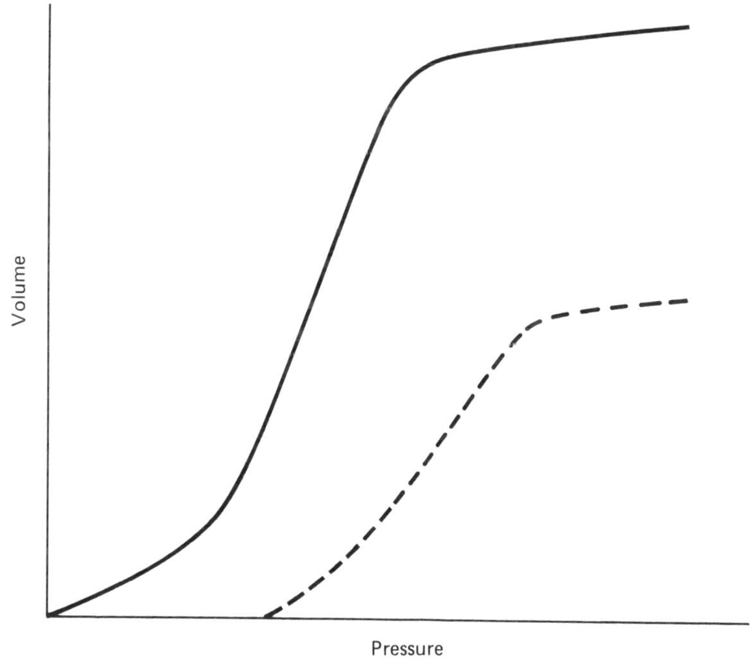

Figure 9.3 Schematic representation of the pressure–volume relationship in normal (—) lungs and the non-compliant lungs of ARDS (- - -)

Table 9.2 Indices used to aid the haemodynamic management of patients with ARDS

Systemic vascular resistance	(MAP–CVP)/cardiac output (SVR)
Pulmonary vascular resistance (PVR)	(MPAP–PAOP)/cardiac output
Oxygen delivery (Do_2)	CI × Sao_2 × Hb × 13.9
Oxygen consumption (Vo_2)	CI × (Sao_2 – Svo_2) × Hb × 13.9

MAP, Mean arterial pressure; CVP, central venous pressure; MPAP, mean pulmonary pressure; PAOP, pulmonary artery occlusion pressure; Sao_2, arterial oxygen saturation; Svo_2, mixed venous saturation; Hb, haemoglobin concentration (g/dl); CI, cardiac index. Note that oxygen dissolved in the plasma has been ignored because it contributes little to oxygen delivery in normobaric conditions

and its effects on the systemic circulation [36, 37]. Inadequate Do_2 is manifest by an inappropriate increase in the oxygen saturation of mixed venous blood (Mvo_2) through diminished oxygen extraction (Vo_2), increased blood lactate levels and evidence of peripheral organ dysfunction. Sepsis also causes a reduction in systemic vascular resistance (SVR) and a loss of peripheral microvascular regulation. Cardiac output is increased, but the heart becomes dilated with decreased ejection fraction and contractility.

Central to the management of patients with ARDS and multisystem organ failure is an understanding of the relationship between Do_2 and Vo_2 (Figure 9.4). Clinical studies of patients with ARDS and sepsis have demonstrated a dependence of Vo_2 on Do_2 at levels of delivery well above the normal (critical) level below which anaerobic metabolism occurs ($Do_{2\,crit.}$, usually considered to be 330 ml/min/m²) [38], suggesting the presence of a covert oxygen debt. In describing this phenomenon, Bihari *et al.* found that those patients who subsequently died displayed the biggest incremental rise in Vo_2 as Do_2 was increased using prostacyclin, suggesting that delivery dependence of oxygen consumption may have important prognostic significance

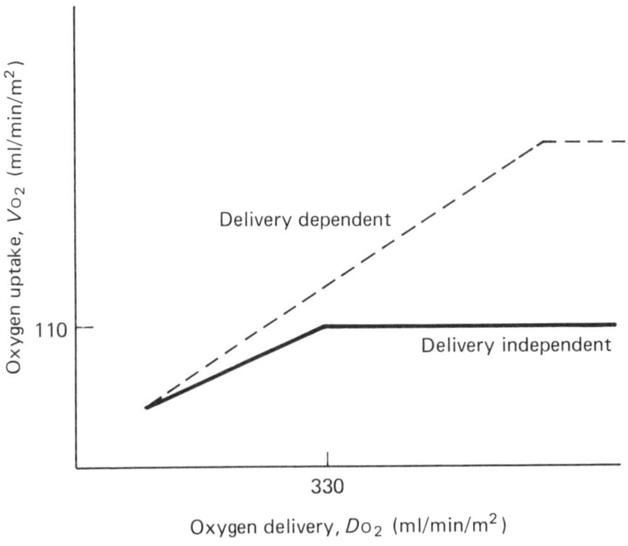

Figure 9.4 Relationship between oxygen delivery and uptake in normal individuals (—) and those with ARDS, as in multi-organ failure (- - -)

[39]. This potentially important phenomenon can be explained in one of three ways: first, a defect in the mitochondrial use of oxygen may occur in such patients; secondly, the increased distance between capillaries and mitochondria consequent upon the presence of interstitial oedema may prevent oxygen uptake; thirdly, some authorities have suggested that the relationship may be wholly attributable to mathematical coupling. Thus, VO_2 can be measured directly by analysis of expired gas or indirectly by calculation in the conventional manner (Table 9.2). In a recent investigation, delivery dependence could be demonstrated only when direct measurements of VO_2 were made; otherwise the study failed to show any abnormality in the relationship between DO_2 and VO_2 in ARDS patients [40].

Clinical features

Dyspnoea following some identifiable precipitating event is usually the first complaint of patients with acute lung injury. The chest radiograph is frequently normal at this early stage, although increased endothelial permeability may be detectable using radioisotopes. Initially there is hypoxaemia with a normal to low arterial carbon dioxide tension ($PaCO_2$), followed by bilateral shadowing indicative of pulmonary oedema on chest radiography. The alveolar oedema increases in intensity, leading to decreased compliance and increased difficulty in breathing. Despite raising the FIO_2, hypoxaemia persists and, if dead space ventilation is markedly increased, $PaCO_2$ rises. In the terminal phase of ARDS the clinical picture is one of refractory and extreme hypoxaemia with elevated $PaCO_2$ despite a high delivered minute volume. This terminal phase is now seen relatively rarely, because a wide range of respiratory support is available; concomitant failure of other organ systems is now the most common cause of death.

Making the diagnosis

ARDS remains a clinical diagnosis of exclusion, with no specific diagnostic physical and/or humoral tests. The chest radiograph, simple lung function tests and arterial gas analysis merely confirm the clinical symptoms and signs outlined above. Computed axial tomography of the lungs is difficult to perform in the critically ill, but has shown that the lungs are not homogeneously affected. Consolidation and alveolar oedema affect the whole lung, but to variable degrees. Dependent areas of lung show large areas of collapse [41] (Figure 9.5). The placement of a balloon-tipped flow-directed pulmonary artery catheter, preferably of the thermodilution type to permit estimations of cardiac output, is essential in distinguishing between high permeability and cardiogenic pulmonary oedema. In ARDS the pulmonary artery occlusion pressure (PAOP) is less than 18 mmHg and pulmonary vascular resistance (PVR) is frequently raised. Interpretation of measurements of PAOP in patients receiving PEEP is a matter of some debate. Some authorities believe that PEEP must be removed, but this may not be possible in the critically ill: in these circumstances it is customary to subtract 50% of the PEEP value from that of PAOP, although it has been demonstrated recently that in severe ARDS the correlation between left ventric-

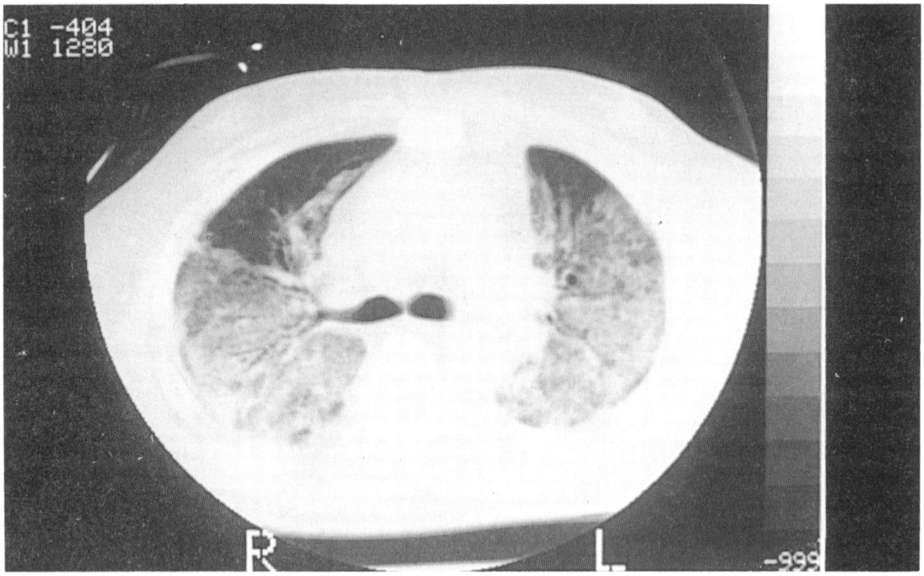

Figure 9.5 Computed axial tomography in ARDS. Note **that only the dependent parts of the lung are** consolidated

ular end diastolic pressure and PAOP is unaffected by PEEP [42].

Radiolabelled albumin and transferrin can be used to demonstrate increased pulmonary vascular permeability in ARDS, although the technique is not widely available [43, 44]. In established ARDS, the degree to which permeability is increased does not correlate with clinical course, nor does it necessarily predict outcome [45].

Management

The management of ARDS involves the provision of respiratory support in conjunction with measures to control the precipitating illness. As already intimated, ARDS appears to be the pulmonary manifestation of a generalized endothelial cell injury: all organs are therefore at risk of failure. Furthermore, the application of supportive measures to one system may place an intolerable burden on a second. It is therefore imperative to consider the patient as a physiological whole when making management decisions.

Respiratory support

Continuous positive airways pressure

Continuous positive airway pressure (CPAP) can be applied to the patient with acute lung injury to reduce the fall in functional residual capacity that is a consequence of pulmonary oedema due to any cause. This has the added benefit of recruiting collapsed alveoli, moving the patient onto the favourable or compliant portion of their pressure–volume curve and thereby reducing the work of breathing (Figure 9.3). Shunt fraction is reduced and oxygenation improves. In order to achieve true CPAP, a tightly fitting face mask is attached to a gas delivery system capable of delivering 80–100 l/min, preferably of varying FIO_2 (Figure 9.6). The high flow thus produced prevents the pressure in the system dropping during the initial (high flow) phase of inspiration. Alternatively, a reservoir bag included in the inspiratory limb of the CPAP circuit obviates the need for high gas flows and reduces gas wastage. The end-expiratory pressure required is variable, but should not exceed 15 cm H_2O. The effectiveness of CPAP can be further enhanced by using the airway pressure-release technique described recently by Downs and Stock [46]. Enhanced alveolar ventilation is achieved by intermittently decreasing the positive airway pressure during expiration. This temporarily reduces functional residual capacity, but increases the elimination of CO_2. If the lung injury progresses, CPAP becomes ineffective and endotracheal intubation and formal mechanical ventilation are required.

Mechanical ventilation

The decision to institute mechanical ventilation should be made on clinical grounds. A high respiratory rate, exhaustion, a laboured or paradoxical pattern of respiration or stupor suggest disordered physiology with low tidal volume and compliance: hypoxaemia, hypercarbia, low maximal inspiratory pressure, increased dead space and low lung volumes ensue. Mechanical ventilation should aim to achieve adequate oxygenation and CO_2. clearance without exacerbating lung injury. A high FIO_2 is often needed to prevent hypoxaemia, but if >0.6 it is associated with decreased pulmonary compliance [47] and oxygen toxicity, although the latter probably occurs with any level above 0.21. Because of adverse changes in V/Q matching, high levels of FIO_2 may do little to increase PaO_2.

Persistent hypoxaemia can be influenced favourably by PEEP, which decreases alveolar collapse, increases functional residual capacity and so improves oxygenation consequent on a reduction of shunt fraction [48]. However, PEEP increases intrathoracic pressure, reduces venous return and causes direct cardiac compression. Cardiac output and therefore DO_2 (Table 9.2) may be diminished even though PaO_2 is raised. The use of PEEP prophylactically has not been shown to influence the clinical course of ARDS [49].

Conventional respiratory support dictates the use of large tidal volumes as physiological dead space is increased, but when in the order of 12–15 ml/kg can lead to

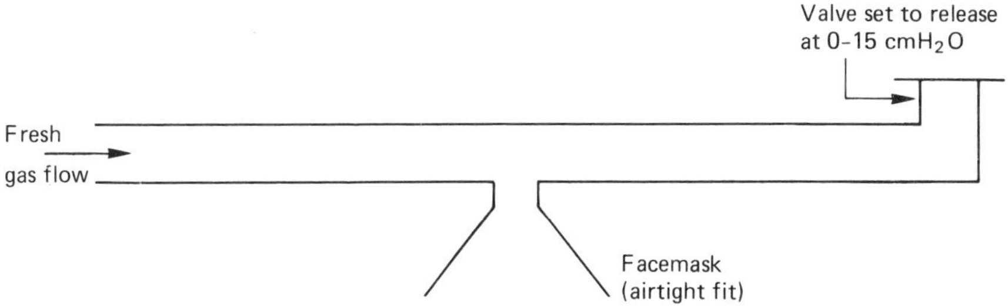

Figure 9.6 CPAP circuit

peak inflation pressures >60 cmH_2O as the patient moves on to the top (flat) portion of their pressure-volume curve (Figure 9.3). High peak airway pressures are associated with barotrauma in the form of pneumomediastinum, pneumothorax and peribronchial and perivascular interstitial emphysema [50]. There is no well-defined safe upper limit to peak airway pressure, although above 50 cmH_2O the incidence of barotrauma increases significantly [51]. Prolonging the inspiratory time even to the point of reversing the inspiratory/expiratory (I:E) ratio (inverse ratio ventilation, IRV) reduces peak airway pressures and promotes alveolar stability, but can lead to stacking of ventilated breaths and gas trapping. New approaches to mechanical ventilatory support have, however, tended to use this approach (Figure 9.7).

Volume-controlled IRV

In this form of ventilation a preset tidal volume is delivered irrespective of adverse changes in compliance. It is associated with a decrease in shunt fraction and therefore improvements in $Pa\text{O}_2$, but overall $D\text{O}_2$ may be diminished due to adverse effects on cardiac output [52].

Pressure-controlled IRV

As there is a limit set to the maximum peak airway pressure, this form of ventilation reduces the risk of barotrauma. The short expiratory phase leads to an increase in mean airway pressure and increases functional residual capacity. Two studies of pressure-controlled IRV [53, 54] have demonstrated significant falls in peak airway pressure and the amount of PEEP required to oxygenate patients with ARDS who had failed to improve using more conventional ventilatory techniques. No cardiovascular compromise was observed, but neither was an improvement in survival [55].

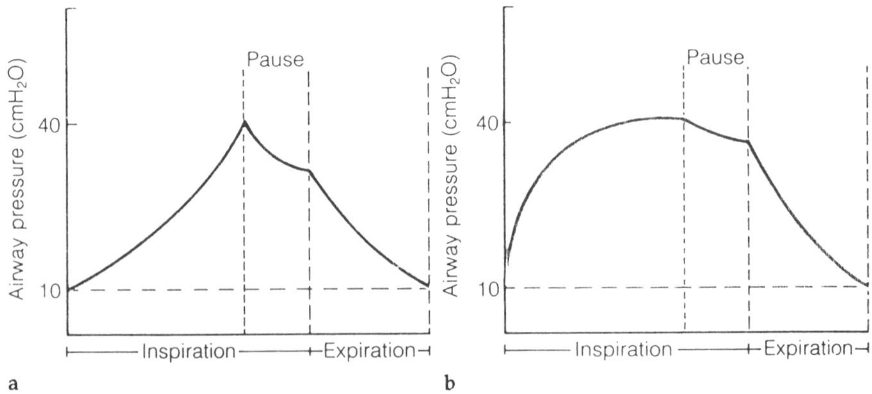

Figure 9.7 (a) The pattern of airway pressure seen with volume-controlled IRV. Note that an inspiratory pause following delivery of the preset tidal volume is included in the cycle. (b) The pattern of airway pressure seen with pressure-controlled inverse ratio ventilation. Note that the airway pressure rapidly rises to equal the pressure control level. Note a positive end-expiratory pressure of 10 cmH_2O in both diagrams

Permissive hypercapnia

The above techniques may reduce barotrauma, but can lead to inadequate oxygenation and CO_2 elimination, normally dependent on the frequency of ventilation. Eliminating CO_2 further depends on increasing tidal volume, leading to rises in peak airway pressure and the incidence of barotrauma. Recently, a technique allowing $Paco_2$ to rise has been advocated [56]. Using pressure-limited ventilation (tidal volumes as low as 5 ml/kg) with synchronized intermittent mandatory ventilation, hypercapnia was well tolerated by patients. However, this is not without risk in certain patient groups (such as those with ischaemic heart disease) and may exacerbate $\dot{V}/\dot{Q}$ mismatch [57]. It remains to be seen if this technique will improve mortality rates.

High-frequency jet ventilation

This technique employs pulses of high-pressure gas administered at supra-physiological frequencies (60–600 breaths/min). Each pulse delivered down the endotracheal tube entrains gas, variations in which determine the FIo_2. The mechanism of gas exchange remains uncertain, but almost certainly involves augmented gas diffusion in the alveoli and small airways. High-frequency jet ventilation offers potential advantages both in terms of improved gas exchange and decreases in peak airway pressure. Unfortunately, a large prospective comparative study [58] published in the early 1980s showed that the technique offered no advantage over conventional therapy although it was effective in achieving oxygenation in patients with ARDS. Interest in the use of this technique in ARDS subsequently waned, but the recent use of ventilatory frequencies approaching lung resonance (about 5 Hz) has proved successful in maintaining lung volume and improving oxygenation in patients with severe ARDS who were failing on conventional treatment [59] (Figure 9.8). Research activity continues into high-frequency oscillation (up to 50 Hz) but as yet these techniques have not been applied clinically.

Extracorporeal support

The deficiencies in conventional mechanical ventilatory support provided the initial spur for trials of extracorporeal membrane oxygenation in patients with ARDS; particularly as evidence accumulated that mechanical ventilation might actually contribute to the pathophysiology of lung injury and substantially influence the course of the disease [60]. Thus, although the role of elevated peak airway pressure in the evolution of barotrauma is generally accepted, the high-volume ventilation required in ARDS (regardless of the associated peak airway pressure) may lead to increased lung microvascular permeability or to exacerbations of pre-existing lung injury [60, 61]. The theoretical attractions of this technique are therefore considerable [62]. Extracorporeal gas exchange has emerged as the blanket term describing all techniques of extracorporeal respiratory support, but the specific approach employed depends upon the desired therapeutic goal (Table 9.3). In true extracorporeal membrane oxygenation, oxygenation is the prime objective and the transfer

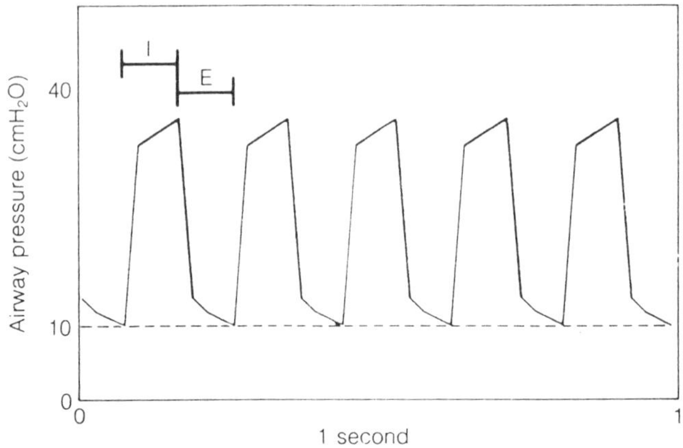

Figure 9.8 High-frequency jet ventilation measured over 1 s at the tip of the endotracheal tube. Frequency is 5 Hz and inspiratory time is 37%. Note that the positive end-expiratory pressure is an intrinsic property of the system and has not been externally applied. I, Inspiration; E, expiration

Table 9.3 Current techniques of extracorporeal gas exchange

Extracorporeal membrane oxygenation
High blood flows required to achieve oxygenation and CO_2 removal
Partial CO_2 removal
Partial removal of CO_2 by low membrane blood flow
Total CO_2 removal
Total removal of CO_2 via membrane (1–2 l flow)

of carbon dioxide (CO_2) occurs as a secondary effect. Blood flow rates in excess of 50% of cardiac output are required. By contrast, the objective in extracorporeal CO_2 removal is to reduce the need for alveolar ventilation; thereby diminishing the potential for further pulmonary injury due to barotrauma. Partial CO_2 removal can be achieved with blood flow rates as low as 0.8–1 l/min passing across only one gas-exchanging membrane, but the total removal of CO_2 usually requires higher flow rates (1–2 l/min) and the use of two membranes in series. This technique provides only 20–30% of total body oxygen requirements, so some ventilatory support is still required. This can be provided in one of three ways: spontaneous ventilation with or without the aid of continuous positive airways pressure (CPAP) (the term extracorporeal lung assist has been used recently to describe this technique); by controlled conventional positive pressure ventilation at low frequency (LFPPV, e.g. 4–6 breaths/min) with positive end-expiratory pressure (PEEP); and by 'apnoeic' intratracheal oxygen insufflation with PEEP.

Compared with conventional therapy in ARDS, extracorporeal gas exchange was unsuccessful in reducing mortality in early controlled trials [63, 64]. This may have reflected patient selection criteria, the severity of the underlying disease and the continued use of conventional ventilatory support which may have exacerbated pre-existing lung damage. The tendency to use this technique as a supportive measure of last resort has been a feature of most studies, and survival figures of around 10%

reported in a recent informal survey in centres in the USA are therefore not surprising [65]: 80% of the patients had received extracorporeal gas exchange for cardiopulmonary failure following cardiac surgery and 17% for ARDS, where the expected mortality with conventional treatment is high. The best results published to date have been from Italy using partial CO_2 removal with LFPPV and venovenous bypass, where a reduction in mortality from 90% to 50% has been claimed [66, 67]. These results are surprisingly good, particularly as the average length of pulmonary insult before the institution of extracorporeal gas exchange in survivors was 7.86 (± 11.7) days. By contrast, in a collaborative extracorporeal membrane oxygenation (veno-arterial) study from the USA, patients with more than 1 week of acute respiratory failure had a less than 4% chance of survival, regardless of treatment modality [63]. Other experience of large series have reported survival rates of 56–70% in up to 100 patients with severe ARDS [68, 69]. The main difficulty of evaluating extracorporeal gas exchange in a scientifically acceptable fashion in respiratory failure is the lack of controlled trials: in the studies published so far, this problem has been addressed by quoting historical control data from the US national study of extracorporeal membrane oxygenation. Nevertheless, partial CO_2 removal and extracorporeal lung assist are emerging as the most successful forms of extracorporeal gas exchange used in ARDS to date (Table 9.4).

The use of extracorporeal support as a bridge to transplantation deserves special comment. Although the results of the multicentre NIH trial in the USA did not demonstrate any difference in overall survival between those treated with extracorporeal membrane oxygenation and those treated conventionally, survival was greater between days 2 and 11 in the former group [63]. Thus, extracorporeal gas exchange may increase the time available to search for suitable donor organs. We have found this approach useful on a number of occasions: although only three of six patients treated left hospital after organ transplantation, all but one survived until organs became available [70, 71]. Prolonged support with extracorporeal gas exchange may lead to irreversible tissue damage, thereby compromising the patient's survival after transplantation, but this is at present impossible to assess. Extracorporeal membrane oxygenation in any form is fraught with complications, including haemorrhage, renal failure, sepsis, multisystem organ failure and thromboembolism; it requires a high input from skilled personnel, making the procedure relatively expensive.

Table 9.4 Current trials of extracorporeal membrane oxygenation

Centre	*No. patients*	*No. survivors*
Marburg	103	54
Berlin	13	8
Dusseldorf	4	1
Milan-Monza	79	36
Stockholm	16	6
Paris	19	6
Salt Lake	19	8
Ann Arbor	11	6
Total	264	125

From [66], with permission

The future of extracorporeal gas exchange in adult respiratory failure is linked to the effectiveness of other new modes of ventilatory support. Although attractive as a means of 'resting' the injured lung and avoiding the damaging effects of mechanical ventilation, the technique is costly, fraught with complications and has not yet been shown to be effective in controlled trials.

Intravascular gas exchange

A miniaturized hollow fibre oxygenator designed to provide pre-pulmonary exchange of oxygen and carbon dioxide in venous blood has recently been developed. This is placed into veins from the confluence of the iliac veins, through the inferior vena cava and right atrium to the superior vena cava. Pure oxygen is drawn through the fibres (under sub-atmospheric pressure to avoid air embolus) whilst anticoagulated (venous) blood flows between them. Oxygen diffuses passively down its concentration gradient to the blood, and carbon dioxide diffuses out. In animal studies, >150 ml/min oxygen can be exchanged, providing approximately 70% of resting oxygen requirements. The need for conventional mechanical ventilatory support is markedly reduced, thus diminishing the danger of barotrauma and reducing the toxic effects of high inspired oxygen concentrations. Blood entering the lungs is oxygenated, which may stimulate the pulmonary repair processes. Initial trials with intravascular oxygen (IVOX) are under way but published experience is so far confined to case reports [72].

Fluid therapy/renal support

The movement of fluid across capillaries is governed by Starling's law:

$$\text{net filtration} = K_f[(P_{mv}-P_{pmv})-\sigma(\pi_{mv}-\pi_{pmv})]$$

where: K_f = capillary filtration coefficient, σ = protein reflection coefficient, P_{mv} = microvascular hydrostatic pressure, P_{pmv} = perimicrovascular pressure, π_{mv} = microvascular osmotic pressure, π_{pmv} = perimicrovascular osmotic pressure.

Fluid and protein leak from the capillary bed to the interstitium in normal lungs, to be cleared by the pulmonary lymphatics. In ARDS the protein reflection coefficient falls, the net filtration becoming dependent upon capillary-to-tissue hydrostatic pressure differences. By reducing P_{mv}, oedema formation is slowed. Fluid restriction therapy applied in ARDS therefore has a rational basis in the underlying pathophysiology, but the use of albumin is of little benefit as far as lung oedema is concerned because the problem lies with σ, the protein reflection coefficient. A negative fluid balance, obtained using fluid restriction, diuretics and ultrafiltration, should lower P_{mv}, but severe fluid restriction causes cardiac output to fall, compounding the already depressed cardiac performance: both factors lower Do_2 further. The nearest clinical approximation to P_{mv} is PAOP, which should be kept at 8–10 mmHg. Fluid management is further complicated by the low compliance of the left ventricle in ARDS [73], which means that the administration of small volumes of fluid can cause precipitous rises in PAOP (P_{mv}) and so further increase lung oedema.

Renal impairment is commonly associated with severe lung injury, further complicating fluid management. Critically ill patients frequently require large-volume infusions for nutritional purposes and haemofiltration or dialysis is of great benefit; pump-assisted haemofiltration is particularly beneficial to patients with poor cardiac performance [74], and in experimentally induced septic shock the volume of filtration has been positively correlated with outcome, possibly due to the removal of circulating 'toxins' of molecular weight below 8000 Da [75, 76].

Circulatory support

Lung injury influences both cardiac output and SVR, particularly when sepsis or multisystem organ failure are involved. Therapeutic endeavours to restrict fluid input, a raised PVR, high intrathoracic pressures consequent upon mechanical ventilation and fluid restriction, can all adversely influence cardiac performance. Systemic vascular resistance is lowered in sepsis by vasodilatation and a loss of peripheral microvascular control. Invasive monitoring permits the measurement of cardiac output, PVR and the calculation of SVR, all of which are necessary if the effects of supportive therapy are to be effectively monitored. Lowering PVR using prostacyclin or adenosine [77] is said to be of benefit in sepsis and ARDS [39], but may not increase DO_2 [78] unless inotropes such as dopamine or dobutamine are employed. Treatment directed against an inappropriately low SVR and low organ perfusion pressures may involve the use of a pressor agent such as noradrenaline.

Nutrition

The incidence of malnutrition in patients with acute respiratory failure is high and may adversely effect outcome. Furthermore, weaning from mechanical ventilation becomes difficult in malnourished patients with weak respiratory muscles [79, 80]. Cell-mediated immunity is depressed [81], as is the production of surfactant [82]. Low levels of vitamin E are associated with an increased risk of free radical mediated tissue damage [83]. Feeding supplements can be administered enterally or intravenously: enteral feeding may reduce the incidence of nosocomial infection even when used in low volumes, because it provides a supply of essential nutrients to the gut mucosa, which may prevent translocation of bacteria from the gut into the portal circulation [84]. However, enteral feeding places a further stress on fluid restriction and, if carbohydrates are used, is associated with a higher production of CO_2, with an increase in ventilation requirements. Lipid metabolism produces less CO_2 than carbohydrate and a change from standard composition feeds to a high-fat feed can lead to a 17% reduction in the respiratory quotient in ventilated patients [85]. However, lipid may induce prostacyclin production by the pulmonary vascular endothelium, leading to increased $\dot{V}/\dot{Q}$ mismatch [86, 87].

Bacteriology

There is no evidence that prophylactic antimicrobial therapy in ARDS improves survival. Extrapulmonary sources of infection may induce lung injury and the incidence of ARDS in association with the sepsis syndrome is 50–60% [88]. Immediate instigation of antimicrobial therapy is appropriate in such cases because multisystem organ failure commonly ensues [89]. The precipitating organism cannot always be identified, although all the signs of sepsis are present. Patients with prolonged (over 24 h) respiratory support have an increased incidence of pulmonary infection [90]. The patient with lung injury is therefore at increased risk of pneumonia associated with general debilitation and also by virtue of being ventilated [91]. The continual microaspiration of oropharyngeal secretions is thought by some to lead to nosocomial pneumonia in intubated patients [92], and prevention of colonization from the gastrointestinal tract has been intensively studied. Ventilated trauma patients given systemic antibiotics combined with selective gut decontamination showed a decrease in the incidence of pneumonias seen during ventilation [93]. A more recent analysis of many studies of selective gut decontamination found that the overall incidence of nosocomial infection was decreased, but with no influence on overall mortality [94]. The practice of using H_2-receptor blockers to prevent stress ulceration is associated with gastric colonization and an increased risk of nosocomial pneumonia. Sucraflate maintains gastric pH, decreasing the risk of gastric colonization, and has been shown to reduce the incidence of nosocomial pneumonia in patients in intensive care units [95].

Pharmacological interventions

Steroid therapy was advocated for patients at risk from ARDS and for those detected early in the course of the disease in the past, on the basis of favourable reports from non-randomized trials. A prospective study by Schumer also suggested that steroids reduce the mortality rate in septic shock from 38.4% to 10.5% [96]. However, two large randomized prospective studies have not shown any benefit from corticosteroid therapy and suggest that mortality in patients with sepsis may even be increased [97, 98]. Steroids have recently been used in patients recovering from ARDS but with concomitant signs of sepsis: if, following extensive investigation, no source for the sepsis was found steroids were given with some success. These results suggest that further trials are needed for steroids in the late phase of ARDS [99].

Speculation on the role of various inflammatory mediators has led to the development of therapies directed specifically against these processes. The use of an antibody directed against TNF in induced sepsis has had good results in animal studies [100]. Pentoxyfylline, a methylxanthine derivative, reduces the adherence of neutrophils to endothelium and also interferes with the production of reactive oxygen species. The drug has been shown to reduce mortality in experimentally induced shock [101, 102].

ARDS is a frequent complication of sepsis. A human monoclonal IgM antibody, HA-lA, directed against Gram-negative endotoxin has been shown to reduce mortality in patients with ARDS [103]. In early ARDS or those at high risk, protection against free radical mediated injury using *N*-acetylcysteine has been shown to reduce injury. The liver frees the cysteine for incorporation into glutathione, a powerful scavenger of reactive oxygen species. A multicentre trial is now under way [104].

Few directed pharmacological interventions are in general use for established ARDS. Prostaglandin (PG) E_1 and PGE_2, by preventing platelet adherence, reducing pulmonary hypertension, decreasing lymphokine production, decreasing oxygen radical generation by macrophages and inducing T-lymphocyte suppressor function, are thought to be of therapeutic benefit. An increased 30-day survival in patients with ARDS treated with PGE_1 has been demonstrated, although most of those treated were from a surgical intensive care unit, with little or no documentation of PAOP. A subsequent multicentre trial failed to show any benefit from prostaglandin therapy [105].

The increased free radical activity associated with ARDS reduces the concentration of surfactant in the alveoli. Surfactant production by type II pneumocytes is further influenced by hypoxia, hyperoxia and infection. In animal studies of induced ARDS surfactant replacement has been shown to reduce the shear forces in the damaged lung and so ameliorate the injury [106] and preliminary clinical studies have been encouraging [107].

The wide range of pathways leading to lung injury suggests that no one therapeutic intervention will prevent pulmonary damage. A policy of multiple therapies aimed at overcoming this biological redundancy, through preventing the activation of inflammatory cells and inhibiting the substances they release, may therefore prove to be the most effective approach.

Conclusions

The mortality from ARDS remains at 50–60%, despite considerable advances in our understanding of its pathophysiology. Therapies remain almost entirely supportive. The most promising approach probably lies in developing interventions directed at the level of endothelial cell/inflammatory cell interaction.

References

1. Ashbaugh DG, Bigelow DB, Petty,TL, Levine BE. Acute respiratory distress in adults. *Lancet* 1967; **ii:** 319–323.
2. Fowler AA, Hamman RF, Good JT *et al.* Adult respiratory distress syndrome: risk with common predictors. *Ann Intern Med* 1983; **98:** 593–597.
3. Murray JF. An expanded definition of ARDS. *Am Rev Respir Dis* 1988; **138:** 720–723.
4. Kreutzfelder E, Joka T, Kienecke H *et al.* Adult respiratory distress syndrome as a specific manifestation of a general permeability defect in trauma patients. *Am Rev Respir Dis* 1988; **137:** 95–99.
5. Liu SF, Crawley DG, Barnes PJ, Evans TW. Endothelium-derived relaxant factor modulates hypoxic pulmonary vasoconstriction in isolated blood–perfused rat lungs. *Am Rev Respir Dis* 1991; **143:** 32–37.
6. Vallance P, Collier J, Moncada S. Effects of endothelially derived nitric oxide on peripheral arterial tone in man. *Lancet* 1989; **ii:** 997–1000.
7. Montgomery B, Stager MA, Carrico CJ, Hudson LD. Causes of mortality in patients with the adult respiratory distress syndrome. *Am Rev Respir Dis* 1985; **132:** 485–489.
8. Lung Program, National Heart and Lung Institute. *Respiratory Diseases: task force on problems, research approaches, needs, Washington, D.C.* Government printing office, 1972; 17. DHEW publication number NIH 73–432.
9. Webster NR, Cohen AT, Nunn JF. Adult respiratory distress syndrome – how many cases in the UK? *Anaesthesia* 1988; **43:** 923–926.
10. Villar J, Slutsky AS. Incidence of the adult respiratory distress syndrome. *Am Rev Respir Dis* 1989; **140:** 814–816.

11. Messent M,Keogh BF, Morgan CJ, Evans TW. Incidence outcome and prediction of ARDS following cardiopulmonary bypass. *Anaesthesia* 1992; **47:** 267–268.
12. Fein AM, Lippman M, Holtzman H, Elraz A, Goldberg SK. The risk factors, incidence and prognosis of ARDS following septicaemia. *Chest* 1983; **83:** 40–42.
13. Kaplan RL, Sahn SA, Petty TL. Incidence and outcome of the respiratory distress syndrome in Gram–negative sepsis. *Arch Intern Med* 1979; **139:** 867–869.
14. Rocker GM, Pearson D, Wiseman MS, Shale DJ. Diagnostic criteria for adult respiratory distress syndrome: time for reappraisal. *Lancet* 1989; **i:** 120–123.
15. Fowler AA, Haman RF, Zerbe GO, Benson KN, Hyers TM. Adult respiratory distress syndrome: prognosis after onset. *Am Rev Respir Dis* 1985; **132:** 472–478.
16. Zapol WM, Trelstad RL, Coffey JW *et al.* Pulmonary fibrosis in severe acute respiratory failure. *Am Rev Respir Dis* 1979; **119:** 547–554.
17. Peters JI, Belol RC,Prihoda TJ *et al.* Clinical determinants of abnormalities in pulmonary function in survivors of the adult respiratory distress syndrome. *Am Rev Respir Dis* 1989; **139:** 1163–1168.
18. Staub NC. State of the art: pathogenesis of pulmonary oedema. *Am Rev Respir Dis* 1974; **109:** 358.
19. Heffner JE, Sahn SS, Repine JE. The role of platelets in the adult respiratory distress syndrome. *Am Rev Respir Dis* 1987; **135:** 482–492.
20. Tate RM, Repine JE. Neutrophils and the adult respiratory distress syndrome. *Am Rev Respir Dis* 1984; **130:** 552.
21. Shalaby MR, Aggarwal BB, Rinderknect T, Svedersky LP, Finkle BS, Palladino MA. Activation of human polymorphonuclear neutrophil functions by interferon gamma and tumour necrosis factor. *J Immunol* 1985; **135:** 2069–2073.
22. Hammerschmidt DE, Weaver LJ, Hudson LD *et al.* Association of complement activation and elevated plasma C5a with adult respiratory distress syndrome. *Lancet* 1980; **i:** 947–949.
23. Deuel TF, Huang JS. Platelet–derived growth factor: structure, function and roles in normal and transformed cells. *J Clin Invest* 1982; **69:** 1046–1049.
24. Stephens KE, Ishikaza A, Larrick JW, Raffin TA. Tumour necrosis factor causes increased pulmonary permeability and oedema. *Am Rev Respir Dis* 1988; **137:** 1364–1370.
25. Millar AB, Singer M, Meager A *et al.* Tumor necrosis factor in bronchopulmonary secretions of patients with adult respiratory distress syndrome. *Lancet* 1989; **ii:** 712–713.
26. Lui SF, Dewar A, Barnes PJ, Evans TW. Effects of tumor necrosis factor on hypoxic pulmonary vasoconstriction in isolated perfused rat lungs. *J Appl Physiol* 1992; **72:** 1044–1049.
27. Carvalho ACA. Blood alterations in ARDS. In: *Acute Respiratory Failure.* Zapol WM, Falke KJ eds. New York: Marcel Dekker, 1985; 303–306.
28. Evans TW, Rogers DF, Belvisi M, Chung KF, Barnes PJ. Involvement of platelet activating factor in endotoxin-induced microvascular leak in guinea-pig airway. *Eur Respir J* 1990; 3: 299–303.
29. Harrison NK, Laurent GJ, Evans TW. A method for measuring type III collagen synthesis by the human lung: effect of cardioplmonary bypass. *Int Care Med* 1993; in press.
30. Evans TW, McAnulty R, Rogers DF, Chung KF, Barnes PJ, Laurent GL. Bleomycin–induced lung injury in the rat: effects of the platelet–activating factor PAF receptor antagonist BN 52021 and platelet depletion. *Environ Hlth Perspect* 1990; **85:** 65–69.
31. Evans TW, Rogers DF, Aursudkij B, Chung KF, Barnes PJ. Regional and time-dependent effects of inflammatory mediators on airway microvascular permeability in the guinea-pig. *Clin Sci* 1989; **76:** 479–485.
32. Brigham KL. Oxidant stress and the adult respiratory distress syndrome. *Eur Respir J* 1990; **3** (Suppl.11): 482–484.
33. Cochrane C, Spragg R, Revack S, Cohen Z, McGuire W. The presence of neutrophil elastase and the evidence of oxidation activity in bronchoalveolar lavage fluid of patients with the adult respiratory distress syndrome. *Am Rev Respir Dis* 1983; **127:** S25–S27.
34. Brigham KL, Meyrick BO, Berry LC, Repine JE. Antioxidants protect cultured bovine lung endothelial cells from injury by endotoxin. *J Appl Physiol* 1987; **632:** 840–850.
35. Shiki Y, Meyrick BO, Brigham KL, Burr IM. Endotoxin increases superoxide dismutase in cultured bovine pulmonary endothelial cells. *Am J Physiol* 1987; **252:** C436–C440.
36. Reilly JM, Cunnion RE, Burch–Whitman C *et al.* A circulating myocardial depressant substance is associated with cardiac dysfunction and peripheral hypoperfusion in patients with septic shock. *Chest* 1989; **95:** 1072–1080.
37. Cunnion RE, Parrillo JE. Myocardial dysfunction in sepsis. *Chest* 1989; **95:** 941–944.
38. Daneck ST, Lynch JP, Weg JG *et al.* The dependance of oxygen uptake on oxygen delivery in the adult respiratory distress syndrome. *Am Rev Respir Dis* 1980; **122:** 387–395.
39. Bhari D, Smithies M, Gimson A *et al.* The effects of vasodilation with prostacyclin on oxygen delivery and uptake in critically ill patients. *N Engl J Med* 1987; **317:** 397–403.

40. Ronco JJ, Phang TP, Walley KR *et al.* Oxygen consumption is independent of changes in oxygen delivery in severe adult respiratory distress syndrome.*Am Rev Respir Dis* 1991; **143:** 1267–1273
41. Gattinoni L, Presenti A, Bagliari S. Inflammatory pulmonary oedema and positive end expiratory pressure: correlation between imaging and physiological studies. *J Thorac Imaging* 1988; 3: 59–64.
42. Teboul JL, Zapol WM, Brun–Bussion C *et al.* A comparison of pulmonary artery occlusion pressure and left ventricular end diastolic pressure during mechanical ventilation with PEEP in patients with severe ARDS. *Anaesthesiology* 1989; **70:** 261–266.
43. Rocker GM, Pearson D, Stephens M, Shale DJ. An assessment of a double–isotope method for the detection of transferrin accumulation in the lungs of patients with widespread pulmonary infiltrates. *Clin Sci* 1988; 75: 47–52.
44. Hunter DN, Morgan CJ, Evans TW. The use of radionuclide techniques in the assessment of alveolar-capillary membrane permeability on the intensive care unit. *Int Care Med* 1990; **16:** 363–371.
45. Macnaughton PD, Braude S, Keogh BF *et al.* Serial measurement of pulmonary physiology in ARDS. *Thorax* 1991; **46:** 754P.
46. Downs JB, Stock MC. Airway pressure-release ventilation: a new concept in ventilatory support. *Crit Care Med* 1987; **15:** 459–461.
47. Clark JM, Lambertsen CJ. Pulmonary oxygen toxicity: a review. *Pharmacol Rev* 1971; **23:** 37–133.
48. Ralph DD, Roverston HT, Weaver JL *et al.* Distribution of ventilation and perfusion during positive end expiratory pressure in adult respiratory distress syndrome. *Am Rev Respir Dis* 1985; **131:** 54–60.
49. Pepe PE, Hudson LD, Carrico CJ. Early application of positive end expiratory pressure in patients at risk for the adult respiratory distress syndrome. *N Engl J Med* 1984; **311:** 281–290.
50. Haake R, Schlichti R, Ulstad DR. Barotrauma: pathophysiology, risk factors and prevention. *Chest* 1987; **91:** 608–613.
51. Petersen GW, Baier H. Incidence of pulmonary barotrauma in a medical ICU. *Crit Care Med* 1983; **11:** 67–69.
52. Cole AGH, Weller SF, Sykes MK. Inverse ratio ventilation compared with PEEP in adult respiratory failure. *Int Care Med* 1984; **10:** 227–232.
53. Tharratt RS, Allen RP, Albertson TE . Pressure controlled inverse ratio ventilation in severe adult respiratory failure. *Chest* 1988; **94:** 755–762.
54. Lain DC, DiBenedetto R, Morris SL *et al.* Pressure controlled inverse ratio ventilation as a method to reduce peak inspiratory pressure and provide adequate ventilation and oxygenation. *Chest* 1989; **95:** 1081–1088.
55. Mathay MA. New modes of mechanical ventilation in ARDS: how should they be evaluated? *Chest* 1989; **95:** 1175–1176.
56. Hickling KG, Henderson S, Jackson R. Low mortality associated with low volume pressure limited ventilation with permissive hypercapnia in severe adult respiratory distress syndrome. *Int Care Med* 1990; **16:** 372–377.
57. Baudouin S, Barnes PJ, Evans TW. The effect of L–NMMA on the response of the rat pulmonary circulation to hypoxia with hypercapnia. *Eur Respir J* 1991; **4** (Suppl. 14): 337s.
58. Carlon GC, Howland SW, Ray C *et al.* High frequency jet ventilation. A prospective randomised evaluation. *Chest* 1983; **84:** 551–559.
59. Keogh BF, Heard S, Calkins J *et al.* Ultra high frequency ventilation in severe ARDS: preliminary results from multicentre study. *Eur Respir J* 1991; **4** (Suppl 14): 176.
60. Woodring JH. Pulmonary interstitial emphysema in the adult respiratory distress syndrome. *Crit Care Med* 1985; **13:** 786–791.
61. Lachmann B, Danzmann E, Heandly B, Jonsson B. Ventilator setting and gas exchange in respiratory distress syndrome. In: *Applied Physiology in Clinical Respiratory Care.* Prakash O. ed. The Hague: Martinus Nijhoff, 1982; 141–176.
62. Keogh BF, Evans TW. Extracorporeal membrane oxygenation: a breath of fresh air or yesterday's therapy? *Thorax* 1991; **46:** 692–694.
63. Zapol WM, Snider MT, Hill JD *et al.* Extra corporeal membrane oxygenation in severe acute respiratory failure. A randomised prospective study. *JAMA* 1979; **242:** 2193–2196.
64. Hill JD, O'Brien TG, Muray JT. Prolonged extra corporeal oxygenation for acute post traumatic respiratory failure shock lung syndrome. *N Engl J Med* 1972; **286:** 629–634.
65. Iatridis A. Review of ECMO in adults – North American experience. *Perfusion* 1988; **3:** 37–40.
66. Gattinoni L. Extracorporeal respiratory support for acute respiratory failure. *Curr Op Anaesth* 1991; **4:** 4261–265.
67. Gattinoni L, Presenti A, Mascheroni D *et al.* Low fequency positive-pressure ventilation with extracorporeal CO_2 removal in severe acute respiratory failure. *JAMA* 1986; **256:** 881–886.
68. Muller E, Knoch E, Holterman M *et al.* Extracorporeal CO_2 removal in severe ARDS. Report of 100 cases. *Am Rev Respir Dis* 1991; **143:** A249.

69. Rossiant R, Slama K, Pappert D *et al.* Extra-corporeal lung assist with heparin coated systems. *Am Rev Respir Dis* 1991; **143:** A263.
70. Mudalier MY, Hunter DN, Morgan CJ, Evans TW. Extracorporeal gas exchange for respiratory failure. *Hosp Update* 1991; **17:** 410–415.
71. Tsang V, Evans TW, Morgan CJ, Yacoub M. Heart–lung transplantation for the adult respiratory distress syndrome. *Crit Care Med* 1991; **19:** 286–287.
72. Kallis P, Al-Saady NM, Bennet D, Treasure T. Clinical use of intravascular oxygenation. *Lancet* 1991; **337:** 549.
73. Sibbald WJ, Short AIK, Warshawski FJ *et al.* Thermal dye measurements of extravascular lung water in critically ill patients – intravascular Starling forces and extravascular lung water in the adult respiratory distress syndrome. *Chest* 1985; **87:** 585–592.
74. Morgan JM, Morgan C, Evans TW. Clinical experience of pump assisted arteriovenous haemofiltration in the management of patients in oliguric renal failure following cardiothoracic surgery. *Int J Cardiol* 1989; **23:** 365–371.
75. Gotloib L, Brazilay E, Shustack A *et al.* Haemofiltration in septic ARDS, the artificial kidney as an artificial endocrine lung. *Resuscitation* 1986; **13:** 123.
76. Groeneveld ABJ. Septic shock and multiple organ failure: treatment with haemofiltration. *Int Care Med* 1990; **16:** 489–490.
77. Morgan JM, McCormack DG, Griffiths MJD *et al.* Adenosine as a vasodilator in primary pulmonary hypertension. *Circulation* 1991; **84:** 1145–1149.
78. Melot C, Lejune P, Leeman M, Moraine JJ, Naeige R. Prostaglandin E_1 in the adult respiratory distress syndrome. *Am Rev Respir Dis* 1989; **139:** 106–110.
79. Arora KS, Rochester D. Respiratory muscle strength and maximal voluntary ventilation in undernourished patients. *Am Rev Respir Dis* 1982; **126:** 5–8.
80. Bassili HR, Dietel M. Effect of nutritional support on weaning patients from ventilators. *JPEN* 1981; **5:** 161–163.
81. Hunter AMB, Carey MA, Larsh HW. The nutritional status of patients with chronic obstructive pulmonary disease. *Am Rev Respir Dis* 1981; **124:** 376–381.
82. Gross I. Nutritional and hormonal influences on lung phospolipid metabolism. *Fed Proc* 1977; **36:** 2665–2669.
83. Richard C, Lemonnier F, Thibault M *et al.* Vitamin E deficiency and lipoperoxidation during adult respiratory distress syndrome. *Crit Care Med* 1990; **18:** 4–9.
84. Moore FA, Moore EE, Jones TN *et al.* TEN versus TPN following major abdominal trauma: reduced septic mortality. *J Trauma* 1989; **29:** 916–923.
85. Lathrop JC, Bommarito A, Letson JA *et al.* The effects of high fat enteral feeding on patients requiring mechanical ventilation. *Pharm Pract News* 1986; **Sept.:** 32.
86. Skeie B, Askanazi J, Rothkopf MM *et al.* Intravenous fat emulsions and lung function: A review. *Crit Care Med* 1989; **16:** 183–194.
87. Baudouin SV, Barnes PJ, Evans TW. The effect of lipid on pulmonary vasoconstriction in the rat. *Thorax* 1993; abstract, in press.
88. Pepe PE, Potkin RT, Reus DH *et al.* Clinical predictors of the adult respiratory distress syndrome. *Am J Surg* 1982; **144:** 124–130.
89. Bell RC, Coalson JJ, Smith JD *et al.* Multiple system organ failure and the adult respiratory distress syndrome. *Ann Intern Med* 1983; **99:** 293–298.
90. Langer M, Mosconi P, Cigada M *et al.* Long term respiratory support and risk of pnuemonia in critically ill patients. *Am Rev Respir Dis* 1989; **140:** 302–305.
91. LaForce FM. Hospital aquired Gram–negative rod pnuemonias: An overview. *Am J Med* 1981; **70:** 664–669.
92. Stoutenbeck CP, Van Seane HK, Miranda DR *et al.* The effect of oropharangael decomtamination using topical non-absorbable antibiotics on the incidence of nosocomial respiratory tract infection in multiple trauma patients. *J Trauma* 1987; **27:** 375–362.
93. Vandenbrouke–Grauls CMJE, Vandenbrouke JP. Effect of selective decontamination of the digestive tract on respiratory tract infections and mortality in the intensive care unit. *Lancet* 1991; **338:** 859–862.
94. Driks MR, Craven DE, Celli BR *et al.* Nosocomial pnuemonia in intubated patients given sucraflate with antacids or histamine type 2 blockers.The role of gastric colonisation. *N Engl J Med* 1987; **317:** 1376–1382.
95. Schumer W. Steroids in the treatment of clinical septic shock. *Ann Surg* 1976; **184:** 333–341.
96. Bernard GR, Luce JM, Sprung CL *et al.* High–dose corticosteroids in patients with the adult respiratory distress syndrome. *N Engl J Med* 1987; **317:** 1565–1570.
97. Bone RC, Fisher CJ, Clemmer TP *et al.* A controlled clinical trial of high dose methylprednisolone in the treatment of severe sepsis and septic shock. *N Engl J Med* 1987; **317:** 653–658.

98. Meduri GU, Belenchia JM, Estes RJ *et al.* Fibroproliferative phase of ARDS: Clinical findings and the effects of corticosteriods. *Chest* 1991; **100:** 943–953.
99. Beutler B, Milsark IW, Cerami AC *et al.* Passive immunisation against cachectin/tumour necrosis factor protects mice from the lethal effects of endotoxin. *Science* 1985; **229:** 869–871.
100. Welsh CH, Lien D, Worthen GS, Weil JV. Pentoxifylline decreases endotoxin–induced pulmonary neutrophil sequestration and extravascular protein accumulation in the dog. *Am Rev Respir Dis* 1989; **138:** 1106–1114.
101. Coccia MT, Waxman K, Soliman H *et al.* Pentoxifylline improves survival following haemorrhagic shock. *Crit Care Med* 1989; **17:** 36–38.
102. Zeigler EJ, Fisher CJ, Sprung CL *et al.* Treatment of Gram negative bacteraemia and septic shock with HA-lA human monoclonal antibody against endotoxin. *N Engl J Med* 1991; **324:** 429–436.
103. Van Asbeck BS, Hoidal J, Vercellotti GM *et al.* Protection against lethal hyperoxia by tracheal insufflation of erythrocytes: role of red cell glutathione. *Science* 1985; **227:** 756–759.
104. Holdcroft JW, Vassar MJ, Weber CJ. Prostaglandin E_1 and survival in patients with adult respiratory distress syndrome. *Ann Surg* 1986; **203:** 371–378.
105. Bone RC, Slotman G, Muander R *et al.* Randomized doubleblind, multicentre study of prostaglandin E_1 in patients with the adult respiratory distress syndrome. *Chest* 1989; **96:** 114–119.
106. Lachman B. Animal models and clinical pilot studies of surfactant replacement in adult respiratory distress syndrome. *Eur Respir J* 1989; **2** (Suppl. 3): 98–103.
107. Haslam PL, Hughes DA, Dewar A, Braude S, Yacoub M, Evans TW. Alerations in BAL cells and phospholipid profiles associated with corticosteroid response in adult respiratory distress syndrome. *Eur Respir J* 1991; **4** (Suppl. 14): 175s.

10

Mechanisms for the pathogenesis of pulmonary fibrosis

N.K. Harrison and G.J. Laurent

Introduction

Pulmonary fibrosis: an expanded definition

The diagnosis of pulmonary fibrosis is usually applied to patients with interstitial lung disease who show reticular or reticulonodular shadowing on a chest radiograph and have evidence of small lungs, together with diminished carbon monoxide diffusing capacity on lung function tests. The patient is usually breathless, although in the early stages of disease all these parameters may be normal. The pattern and distribution of shadowing on chest radiograph (Figure 10.1 a) and thoracic computed tomography (CT) scan may give a clue to the underlying condition, but the widespread reticulonodular shadowing of advanced pulmonary fibrosis is non-specific (Figure 10.1 b).

A biochemical definition of pulmonary fibrosis is more problematical [1] but put most simply it is increased deposition of collagen and other extracellular matrix proteins in the lung. In general, this increase in collagen deposition is a consequence of lung injury and subsequent inflammation which lead to activation of lung fibroblasts – events analogous to processes which occur during wound healing [2]. The precise mechanisms of fibroblast activation are complex and probably vary in different clinical conditions.

By applying the biochemical definition it is apparent that, in addition to interstitial lung diseases, a wide range of common pulmonary conditions involve a 'fibrotic' process. These include subepithelial fibrosis of the airways in asthmatics, pulmonary vascular remodelling in patients with primary and secondary pulmonary hypertension, bronchopulmonary dysplasia in pre-term infants with respiratory distress syndrome and pulmonary fibrosis in patients who survive adult respiratory distress syndrome. Although the interrelationships between lung injury, inflammatory mediators and fibroblast activation are complex and probably vary in these different clinical conditions, it is likely that they also have some elements in common.

The aim of this chapter is to describe the important role played by extracellular matrix proteins in maintaining normal lung structure and to elucidate the processes which activate lung fibroblasts resulting in enhanced collagen deposition, distortion of lung architecture and loss of lung function.

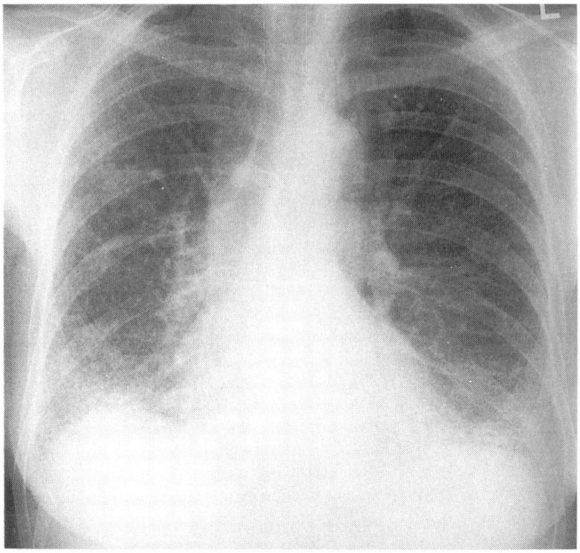

a

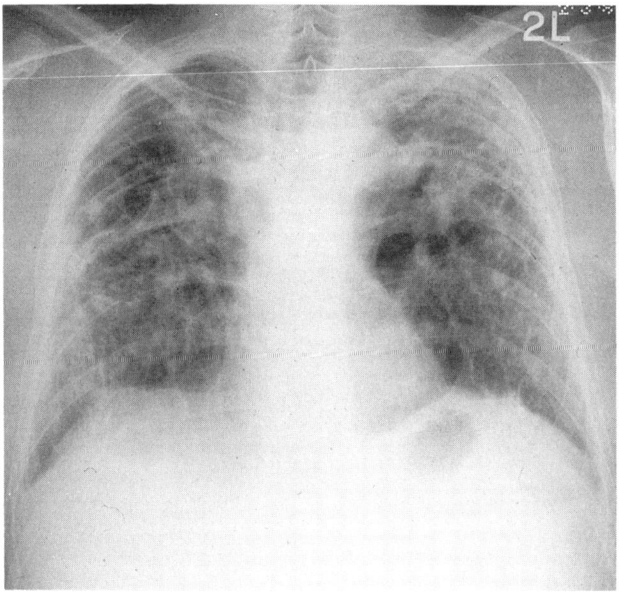

b

Figure 10.1 (a) Chest rediograph from a patient with cryptogenic fibrosing alveolitis showing characteristic reticular shadowing in the lower zones; (b) chest radiograph showing extensive reticulonodular shadowing characteristic of end-stage pulmonary fibrosis. This patient has extrinsic allergic alveolitis

Collagens, extracellular matrix and the structure of normal lung

Collagens are the most abundant proteins in the lung, comprising 15–20% of its dry weight and 60% of its extracellular matrix. A continuous network of interstitial collagen fibres (types I and III) courses distally from the trachea providing a structural framework for the smaller airways and alveolar units. They form a three-dimensional meshwork, within which are embedded interstitial cells and other matrix proteins of the lung (Figure 10.2). The trachea and larger bronchi are strengthened by a series of incomplete cartilaginous rings made up of type II collagen. With repeated subdivision of the smaller bronchi the supporting cartilage becomes more sparse and eventually disappears at the level of the respiratory bronchioles. The pulmonary arteries and arterioles, which transport deoxygenated blood to the alveolar units, also form an integral part of lung structure. They are located adjacent to airways and run distally with the bronchi to the bronchioles beyond which they form a capillary network enmeshing the alveolar air sacs. Pulmonary endothelial and epithelial cells produce type IV collagen, laminin, type V collagen and other components of basement membrane which forms a substratum to which they are attached (Figure 10.2).

Although collagens are the major extracellular proteins in the lung, other macromolecules form an important part of lung structure. Elastins cross-link to each other to form a highly elastic three-dimensional network constituting 30% of lung matrix [3]. They are distributed as fibres in the walls of the airways, alveoli and blood vessels

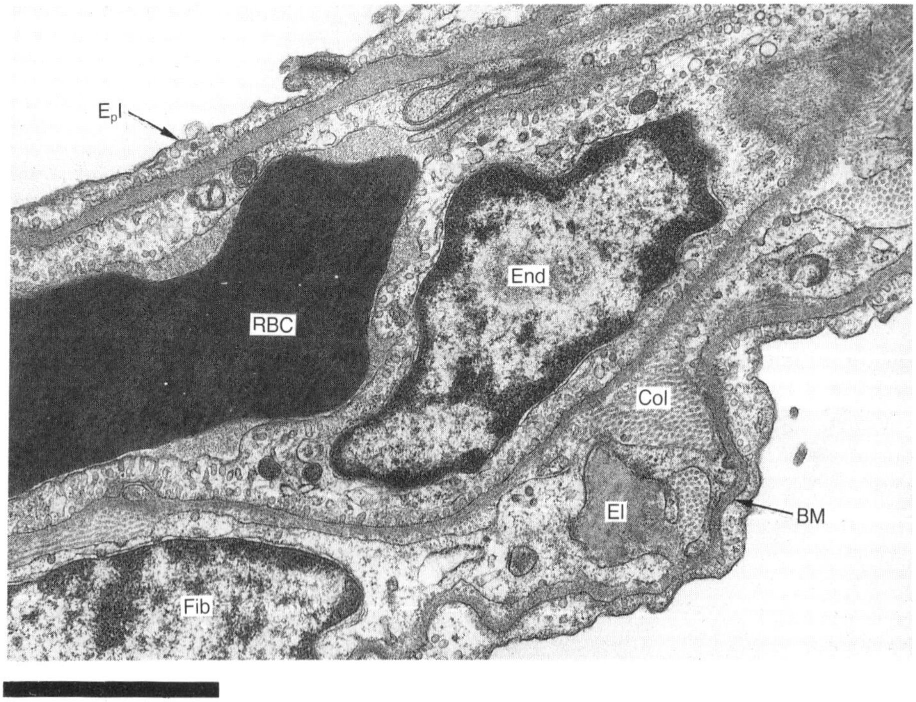

Figure 10.2 Electron micrograph of the normal human alveolar wall. EpI, Type I epithelial cell; End, endothelial cell; RBC, red blood cell within a capillary; Fib, fibroblast; BM, basement membrane; Col, collagen; El, elastin. Stain: uranyl acetate and lead citrate. Bar = 2 μm. (Courtesy of Ann Dewar)

in close association with collagens (Figure 10.2). Elastins convey upon the lungs an ability to stretch and undergo elastic recoil, although at the level of the alveoli this is subsidiary to surface tension forces.

Proteoglycans are a group of structurally diverse, highly charged molecules with molecular weights of up to several millions. They have a protein core to which sulphated carbohydrate side chains (glycosaminoglycans) attach and are found on most cell surfaces as well as being present in the extracellular matrix. Proteoglycans avidly bind cations and water, thereby regulating the viscoelastic properties of the lung [4]. They also influence cell–cell and cell–matrix interactions in the lungs and function as adhesive molecules which can bind collagens, laminin, fibronectin and various growth factors; properties which are thought to be critical in the regulation of lung growth and development.

A related glycosaminoglycan is hyaluronan which contains the disaccharide-repeating unit, *N*-acetylglucosamine-glucuronic acid. It does not contain a protein core, but it has strong water-retaining properties and can aggregate proteoglycan molecules to form a network in the pericellular domain of many nucleated cells [5]. It thus has a profound influence on interstitial fluid balance and solute movement in the lung. Hyaluronan cannot usually be detected in normal human lung epithelial lining fluid but can be recovered in high concentration from bronchoalveolar lavage fluid of patients with interstitial lung diseases and adult respiratory distress syndrome [6]. Concentrations of hyaluronan are closely related to lung water content and increased levels have been observed in the early stages of bleomycin-induced lung injury in rats, suggesting that it may play a role in the development of alveolar oedema [7].

Two other important extracellular matrix components are fibronectin and laminin. Fibronectin, a 440 kDa dimeric glycoprotein functions primarily as an adhesive molecule. It is secreted by several cells, including lung fibroblasts and possesses binding sites for a variety of cell types and for collagens, elastin, proteoglycans and fibrinogen. Fibronectin exerts important influences on the morphology and differentiation of normal lung [8] and, in keeping with this role, has been shown to act as both a chemoattractant and a growth factor for lung fibroblasts [9, 10].

Laminin, also a glycoprotein, has a unique cross-shaped structure with one long and three short arms. It has binding sites for type IV collagen and proteoglycans and is a ubiquitous component of all basement membranes [11].

In summary, lung collagens form a three-dimensional meshwork into which both interstitial cells and other extracellular proteins are embedded. Together, these elements maintain lung structure and function. In addition, as part of the lungs' capacity to respond to injury, they have evolved intricate defence systems such as antioxidant molecules in the epithelial lining fluid and rapidly responding inflammatory and immune networks. When these systems are overcome or chronically challenged, lung fibroblasts become activated, upregulate procollagen production and deposit collagen fibrils as organized fibrotic tissue. Equally important is the termination of this fibrotic response when lung injury ceases.

These events are facilitated by the maintenance of a dynamic equilibrium between collagen synthesis and degradation in lung fibroblasts, even in mature animals [12, 13]. In order to understand the associations between inflammatory and immune responses that follow lung injury and the repair processes that result in pulmonary fibrosis, a knowledge of the biochemical mechanisms that regulate this equilibrium is essential.

Theories of the pathogenesis of pulmonary fibrosis

There are several potential mechanisms for the activation of fibroblasts and increased collagen deposition at specific sites in the lung: first, an increase in fibroblast number resulting from fibroblast proliferation, recruitment of fibroblasts from undifferentiated stem cells or by chemoattraction of cells from adjacent areas; second, an increased collagen biosynthesis by individual lung fibroblasts, which could occur at numerous sites in the collagen biosynthetic pathway; third, diminished collagen degradation, either through a reduction in the rate at which newly synthesized procollagens are degraded or by reduced enzymatic breakdown of collagens in the extracellular matrix. Evidence relating to each of these mechanisms and other possible influences on lung fibroblasts will be examined in the following sections.

Fibroblast proliferation

Evidence that fibroblast proliferation is an important mechanism in the pathogenesis of diseases such as fibrosing alveolitis is based on two lines of evidence. First, morphological studies have demonstrated that fibroblast numbers are increased in both human disease (for review see [14]) and in animal models of pulmonary fibrosis [15]. Secondly, alveolar macrophages from patients with pulmonary fibrosis spontaneously release a variety of fibroblast mitogens when cultured *in vitro*.

Current theories of cell division propose that two different kinds of signal, referred to as competence and progression factors acting at different stages of the cell cycle, are required for mitosis to occur ([16], see Figure 10.3). Mitogens of both classes are released by macrophages. These include the competence factors fibronectin and platelet-derived growth factor and the progression factor insulin-like growth factor 1 [17–19].

The importance of fibronectin as an adhesive molecule in the extracellular matrix was discussed earlier in this chapter. However, it can also act as a chemoattractant for fibroblasts and as a competence factor inducing cells in the G_0 phase of the cell cycle to enter G_1 (Figure 10.3). Macrophages are known to infiltrate the lungs of patients with pulmonary fibrosis (Figure 10.4) and spontaneously secrete enhanced amounts of fibronectin, compared with macrophages derived from healthy lungs [9, 19]. Consequently, it has been proposed that macrophage-derived fibronectin plays a role in the pathogenesis of fibrosing lung disease. However, the relevance of these observations is uncertain because preparations of fibronectin derived from macrophage-conditioned media may contain growth-factor contaminants [20]. A further consideration is that fibronectin in the lung may derive from other sources. For example, lung fibroblasts are themselves capable of secreting considerable quantities of fibronectin when cultured *in vitro* [21]. Also fibronectin is present in the circulation [22], and significant concentrations could enter the lung interstitium following endothelial cell injury.

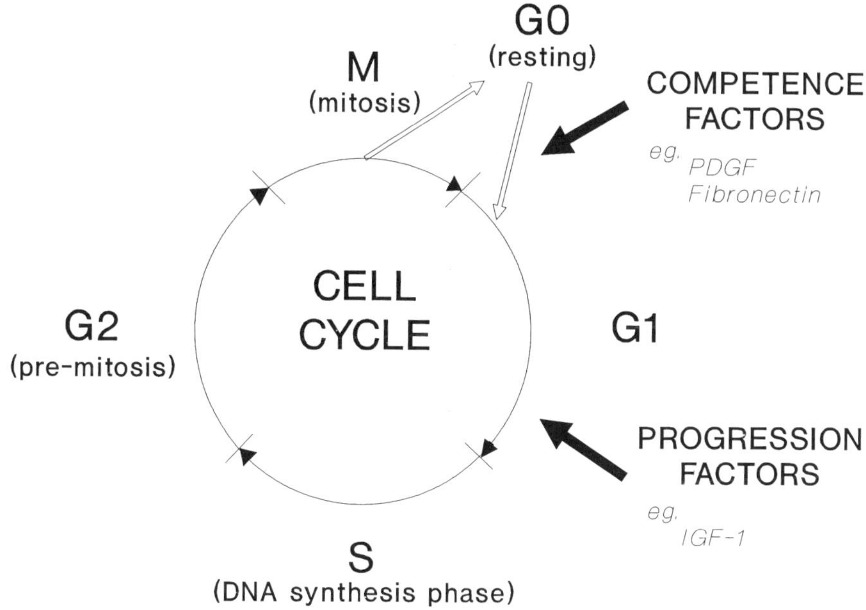

Figure 10.3 The cell cycle

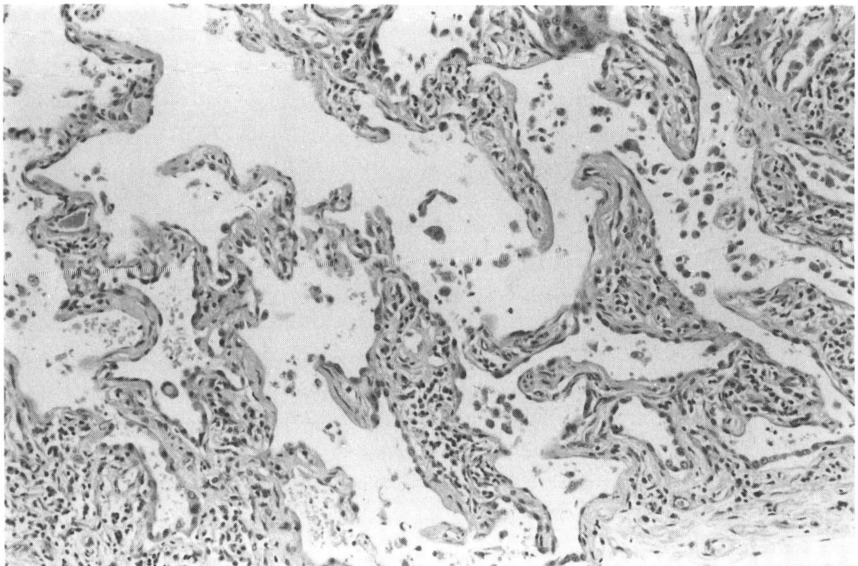

Figure 10.4 Fibrosing alveolitis: inflammatory changes consist of macrophage accumulation in the alveolar spaces and lymphocytes and plasma cell infiltration of the alveolar walls, which are thickened by excess collagen deposition and contain increased numbers of fibroblasts. Stain: haematoxylin and eosin, original magnification ×180. (Courtesy of Professor Bryan Corrin)

Platelet-derived growth factor (PDGF) is a 32 kDa heterodimeric peptide which can exist as different isoforms (designated AA, AB and BB). It acts as a competence factor for fibroblast proliferation and is a potent chemoattractant for mesenchymal cells *in vitro* [23]. It was originally isolated from platelets [24] but is now recognized to be produced by several cell types, including macrophages. Alveolar macrophages from patients with fibrosing alveolitis spontaneously release PDGF and express mRNA for PDGF when cultured *in vitro* [18]. Similar findings have been reported for macrophages from asbestos-exposed rats [25], but these experiments also indicated PDGF is associated with α_2-macroglobulin and other less well-characterized binding proteins – raising questions about its bioavailability both *in vitro* and *in vivo*.

A recent study of lung tissue from patients with fibrosing alveolitis indicated that tissue macrophages produced PDGF-like molecules and expressed mRNA transcripts of PDGF genes [26]. However, other investigators employing similar techniques found that macrophages produced relatively little PDGF by comparison with type II alveolar epithelial cells that demonstrated strong expression of PDGF mRNA and marked staining for PDGF-like proteins, suggesting that regenerating alveolar epithelium may be an important source of this mediator [27].

Insulin-like growth factor 1 (IGF-1, also called somatomedin C) is a 70-amino acid peptide with a molecular weight of 7.6 kDa. IGF-1 acts as a potent progression factor for fibroblasts, stimulating competence-primed cells to complete G_1 and progress to S phase (DNA synthesis phase) of the cell cycle (see Figure 10.3). It is also capable of stimulating collagen production by human lung fibroblasts [28]. Alveolar macrophages from patients with cryptogenic fibrosing alveolitis and asbestosis have been shown spontaneously to release a progression-type growth factor for human lung fibroblasts [17]. A component of this has since been purified and characterized as a 25 kDa molecule with IGF-1-like activity [19]. Similar to fibronectin, IGF-1 occurs in high concentrations in the blood where it is bound to large carrier proteins. This circulating IGF-1 is thought to be synthesized mainly in the liver [29]. Furthermore, IGF-1-like molecules are synthesized *in vitro* by a number of other cell lines including fetal lung fibroblasts [30, 31]. Attempts to quantify production rates of IGF-1-like molecules by macrophages in cell culture have met with difficulties because of the presence of binding proteins [31], but the amount produced by alveolar macrophages is probably small compared with other potential sources.

The ease by which alveolar macrophages can be obtained using the technique of bronchoalveolar lavage may have led to an exaggerated view of its importance in the pathogenesis of pulmonary fibrosis. It is also uncertain whether growth factors produced by alveolar macrophages would be available at sufficiently high concentrations to activate interstitial lung fibroblasts, although it has been argued that injury to the alveolar epithelium, by oxidants released from macrophages or neutrophils in the alveolar space, may render it more permeable to growth factors [32].

Sources of fibroblast growth factors other than the alveolar macrophage must be also considered. It is known that lymphocytes produce mediators which stimulate fibroblast proliferation and collagen biosynthesis [33, 34], although many of these mediators have not been fully characterized. Furthermore, infiltration of the lung interstitium by lymphocytes is a characteristic feature of many lung diseases associated with fibrosis (Figure 10.4). It is difficult to extract lymphocytes from the lung interstitium in sufficient numbers to study their behaviour *in vitro* and few workers have attempted such studies. However, recent experiments by Selman and coworkers showed that T lymphocytes from the lungs of patients with cryptogenic fibrosing alveolitis and extrinsic allergic alveolitis released a mediator which inhibited fibroblast proliferation [35]. By contrast, circulating T lymphocytes from the same patients and from controls released a mediator which caused a modest stimulation of fibroblast proliferation, confirming a similar observation from an earlier study [36]. These findings indicate that there are differences in behaviour between lung and blood lymphocytes, and illustrate the danger of drawing generalized conclusions about lung lymphocytes from studies of cells derived from the circulation.

Attempts to isolate mediators from purified preparations of individual cell types cultured *in vitro* may also give a misleading impression of their importance as activators of lung fibroblasts *in vivo*. An alternative approach was taken by Cantin and coworkers, who sampled lung epithelial lining fluid from patients with interstitial lung disease by the technique of bronchoalveolar lavage and determined the overall effect of lavage concentrates on human lung fibroblasts [37]. This approach may allow the overall effects of mediators present *in vivo* to be determined, but it does not identify their source. They found that lavage fluid from patients with cryptogenic fibrosing alveolitis stimulated fibroblast thymidine-uptake significantly more than did controls, suggesting it contained fibroblast growth factors. Furthermore, this stimulatory activity correlated with indices of lung collagen production *in vivo*.

Alternative hypotheses have been proposed to explain the increased lung fibroblast numbers in patients with pulmonary fibrosis. Jordana and colleagues demonstrated that fibroblasts derived from fibrotic lung tissue proliferate significantly faster than controls when cultured *in vitro* [38]. They observed a marked heterogeneity in the proliferative characteristics of lung fibroblasts, with certain clonally derived cell lines exhibiting a 'fast-replicating' phenotype and proposed that the conditions of injury and repair prevailing in the lower respiratory tract might select out fast-replicating fibroblast clones. In a similar study, Raghu and coworkers found variability in the rate of fibroblast proliferation [39]. Fibroblasts derived from lung biopsies which showed histological evidence of early disease had greater proliferative potential than those from areas with more established fibrosis.

In summary, lung fibroblast numbers appear to be increased in patients with pulmonary fibrosis and alveolar macrophages from such patients release mediators which stimulate fibroblast proliferation. However, it is uncertain whether the concentration of these macrophage products at the site where they are released enables them to exert important influences on fibroblasts in the lung interstitium. The potential role of other cells (such as interstitial lymphocytes, mast cells or alveolar type II epithelial cells) in the production of mediators which might regulate fibroblast proliferation is largely unknown. Furthermore, a relationship between fibroblast numbers and lung collagen production has never been demonstrated in human disease or animal models, and therefore it seems likely that mediators which stimulate fibroblast collagen production are also important.

Collagen production by lung fibroblasts

Regulation of collagen production by lung fibroblasts may occur at the level of procollagen gene transcription, translation of procollagen mRNA, or sites of post-translational modifications to procollagen molecules. The coordinated production of the various collagen types is complex. There are now known to be over 25 different procollagen genes located on several different chromosomes. However, the elements that regulate transcription of the interstitial procollagens types I, II, III and V, which comprise over 95% of all lung collagen, are thought to be generally similar.

Transcription and translation of procollagen genes

The mechanisms of transcription and translation of the procollagen type I(α_1) gene are outlined in Figure 10.5. DNA transcription by an RNA polymerase produces its complementary sequence which undergoes further processing within the nucleus during which some sequences (introns) are excised and those remaining (exons) are respliced. The product is a 6 kb mRNA which leaves the nucleus to be translated on membrane-bound polysomes. The resultant polypeptide chain then undergoes extensive post-translational modifications catalysed by a series of hydroxylating and glycosylating enzymes (for review see [40]).

The hydroxylation of proline is vital for the ultimate tertiary structure and function of the collagen molecule and is therefore a potentially vulnerable point in the collagen

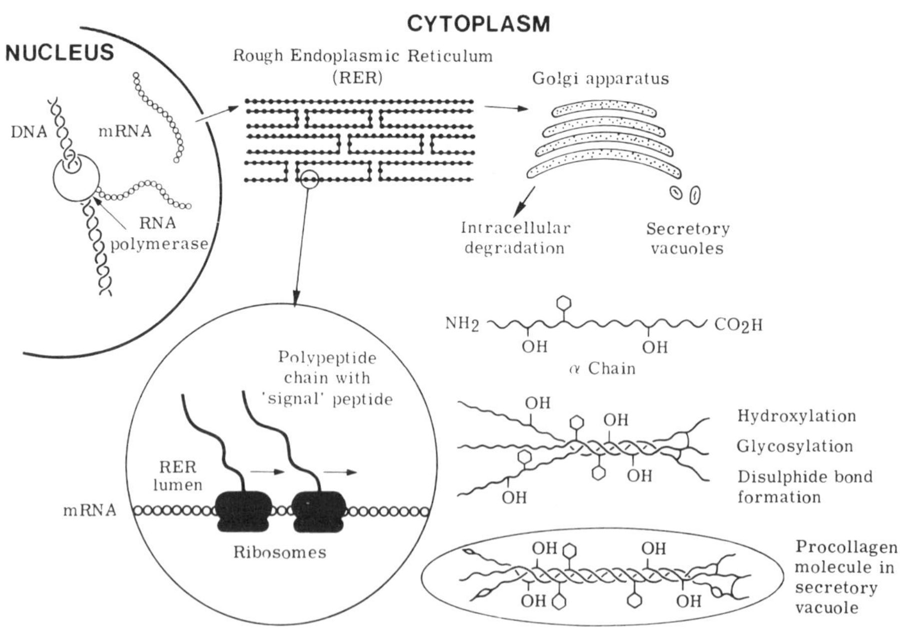

Figure 10.5 Biochemical pathways for the transcription and translation of procollagen genes. Reprinted from [40], with permission

biosynthetic pathway, which could be open to therapeutic manipulation. For example, the use of proline analogues that result in under-hydroxylation of α chains has been shown to reduce the stability of procollagen, make it more susceptible to intracellular degradation and delay secretion [41]. Furthermore, the anthracyclines doxorubicin and daunorubicin, potent irreversible inactivators of prolyl hydroxylase [42], have been shown to impair wound healing in experimental animals [43].

Procollagen secretion

As procollagen molecules are secreted from cells, peptides are cleaved by proteases which are specific for either the N- or the C-terminal ends, but not specific for each collagen type. A number of biological functions have been ascribed to these so-called procollagen peptides. Before secretion they are thought to prevent premature fibril formation [44], but after secretion they may direct fibril assembly, and it has been demonstrated that cleavage of the C-terminal propeptide is the rate-controlling step for assembly of type I fibrils *in vitro* [45]. Furthermore, the N-terminal propeptides of collagen types I and III exert a negative feedback on collagen synthesis by fibroblasts cultured *in vitro* [46].

Procollagen peptides have recently assumed clinical importance as potential markers of collagen production *in vivo*. Several features make them useful for this purpose: they are thought to be released in stoichiometric amounts when collagens are secreted from cells, they are immunologically distinct for each collagen type; their high carbohydrate content renders them antigenic. Consequently, radioimmunoassays to detect procollagen peptides in biological fluids have been developed and several are commercially available, the most widely used of which measure the N-terminal propeptide of type III collagen. Elevated levels of type III procollagen N-terminal peptides have been detected in serum of patients with a variety of fibroproliferative disorders [47] and these assays have also been applied to bronchoalveolar lavage fluid from patients with pulmonary fibrosis [48–50].

Two research areas have been particularly important in improving our understanding of the regulation of lung collagen production: the development of molecular biological techniques that permit the investigation of elements which regulate collagen gene expression, and the discovery and characterization of polypeptide mediators with potent effects on the mesenchymal cells which produce collagen.

One such mediator is transforming growth factor-beta (TGFβ) a 25 kDa dimeric peptide composed of two identical disulphide-bonded subunits which occurs in at least five different isoforms. TGFβ was originally purified from human platelets, human placenta and bovine kidney, but is widely distributed throughout the animal kingdom, being totally conserved in human, bovine and porcine species [51]. TGFβ_1 has potent stimulatory effects on the synthesis of procollagen and fibronectin by lung fibroblast cell lines [52] and this is associated with an increase in steady-state levels of mRNA for these proteins [53]. It also has the potential to inhibit collagenase secretion by fibroblasts [54].

Several recent studies have demonstrated both that TGFβ_1 is present at sites of extracellular matrix gene expression in human pulmonary fibrosis [55, 56] and that fibroblast cell lines derived from lungs of patients with pulmonary fibrosis respond to TGFβ_1 by upregulating procollagen gene expression [57] and by reducing rates at which newly synthesized procollagen is degraded [58].

In addition to TGFβ, a variety of mediators released by activated resident or inflammatory cells could influence collagen gene expression in the lungs following injury. However, their interactions are complex and some observations appear contradictory. For example, interleukin-l (IL-1) increases type I procollagen mRNA levels [59], yet in combination with tumour necrosis factor, levels are reduced [60]. Interferon gamma reduces steady-state type I procollagen mRNA levels [61], but does not appear to affect type I collagen transcription [62]. Cytokines and other agents which have the potential to modulate collagen gene expression are summarized in Table 10.1. Continued investigation of the mechanisms of action of these agents is important and it is hoped that such studies will lead to the development of agents with the potential to block lung collagen production at the molecular level.

Table 10.1 Agents that alter procollagen gene expression

	Agent	Reference
Increase		
	TGFβ	57
	IGF-1	28
	IL-1	59
	TNF-α (serum absent)	109
	Bleomycin	117
Decrease		
	Prostaglandin E_2	118
	Corticosteroids	119
	Interferon gamma	62
	TNF-α (serum present)	120

Collagen degradation

Reduced collagen degradation may also lead to increased lung collagen content. Regulation of this can occur at intracellular and extracellular sites.

Intracellular mechanisms

Over the last 30 years two independent lines of evidence have suggested the existence of pathways which rapidly degrade newly synthesized procollagens *in vivo*: first, experiments by Jackson and Bentley [63] and by Nimni and coworkers [64] indicated that procollagen turnover is most rapid for collagens soluble in solutions of low ionic strength (i.e. those most recently synthesized); secondly, experiments by Barnes and coworkers demonstrated the rapid appearance of radiolabelled hydroxyproline after the injection of radiolabelled proline into guinea-pigs [65]. As hydroxylation of proline occurs as a post-translational event during procollagen synthesis, this observation suggested the radiolabelled hydroxyproline was derived from the degradation of a larger substrate molecule. The precise nature of this substrate and the site at which degradation occurs was investigated by Bienkowski and coworkers, who examined the kinetics of uptake of radiolabelled proline into protein and the appearance of radiolabelled hydroxyproline, either as the free amino acid or as low molecular weight peptides [66]. They concluded that the substrate was most likely to be procollagen and that degradation occurred intracellularly.

Two sites have been proposed for the intracellular degradation of procollagen. Studies *in vitro* have indicated that under conditions of optimal hydroxylation of proline, rates of procollagen degradation are of the order of 15 ± 5%, a level described as 'basal degradation' [67]. This process is not blocked by agents such as chloroquine, which inhibits lysosomal enzymes, or by colchicine, which disrupts microtubules and inhibits transport of secretory proteins beyond the Golgi [68], suggesting that intracellular proteases located in the endoplasmic reticulum or Golgi apparatus may be responsible.

Rates of intracellular degradation of procollagen increase in response to agents which inhibit hydroxylation of proline [69]. This enhanced degradation can be blocked by inhibitors of lysosomal proteases and by colchicine. It can also be increased by prostaglandin E_2 and epidermal growth factor [70], and thus represents a potential site at which procollagen production may be regulated.

Extracellular mechanisms

The extracellular degradation of collagen is thought to result largely from the action of neutral proteases. Fibroblasts actively produce collagenase, gelatinase and stromelysin, enzymes which can cleave collagen or its breakdown products [71]. However, leucocytes also produce collagenases which may contribute to remodelling of lung extracellular matrix in disease states.

Neutrophil collagenase, a metalloproteinase found pre-formed in neutrophil specific granules, is one such protease. It is produced in a latent form and activated extracellularly. It cleaves collagens type I, II and III but has greatest activity against type I [72]. Neutrophils also possess a gelatinase capable of degrading collagen [73]. Macrophages secrete both collagenase and stromelysin, with identical properties to those produced by fibroblasts [74, 75]. They also produce a gelatinase immunologically identical to neutrophil gelatinase [76].

In the circulation, collagenases are inhibited by α_2-macroglobulin and β_1-anticollagenase, and in tissues by the tissue inhibitor of metalloproteinases. The latter is produced by fibroblasts [77] and represents another site at which collagen deposition could be regulated.

The relevance of changes in the rates of collagen degradation to the pathogenesis of pulmonary fibrosis has received relatively little attention. There is evidence that a reduction in the degradation of newly synthesized collagen contributes to the development of bleomycin-induced pulmonary fibrosis in rabbits [78]. There is also evidence that the increase in procollagen production induced by $TGF\beta_1$ in rat fetal fibroblasts is associated with a reduction in the rate at which newly synthesized procollagen is degraded [79].

Extracellular degradation of collagen molecules or fibrils will be influenced by the relative levels of collagenase and collagenase inhibitors in the lungs. Little is known about these in the context of pulmonary fibrosis, but one recent *in vitro* study, which examined rates of collagen metabolism in fibrotic human lung tissue, demonstrated that enhanced lung collagen concentrations were associated with normal rates of collagen production but reduced levels of collagenolytic activity [80]. This suggests that, in established pulmonary fibrosis, progression of disease may be related to impaired extracellular degradation of collagen, but such results may not be relevant to early pathogenesis. Furthermore, they are at odds with the observation that bronchoalveolar lavage fluid from patients with fibrosing alveolitis had an enhanced ability to degrade exogenous type I collagen substrate [81]. However, the technique of bronchoalveolar lavage samples the lung epithelial lining fluid and this may not reflect enzymatic processes occurring in the lung interstitium.

The role of epithelial and endothelial barriers

Agents that injure pulmonary endothelial or epithelial cells are known to result in pulmonary fibrosis. Such agents may preferentially injure endothelial cells (e.g. hyperbaric oxygen and ionizing radiation), whereas others (e.g. bleomycin and paraquat) are more injurious to type I epithelial cells [82]. These observations demonstrate that the route by which such agents reach the lung does not necessarily govern the site of injury. In asbestosis, which clearly results from inhalation of asbestos fibres, ultrastructural studies demonstrate injury to alveolar epithelium, but asbestos fibres can be observed in pulmonary endothelial cells [83]. In other conditions such as fibrosing alveolitis where the nature of the injurious agent(s) remains uncertain, there is ultrastructural evidence of both epithelial (Figure 10.6) and endothelial cell (Figure 10.7) injury from the earliest stages of disease [84, 85].

Evidence from animal experiments indicates that epithelial cells may play an important role in the regulation of collagen deposition. For example, if a tracheal ring with denuded epithelium is grafted into a mouse, the lumen gradually becomes obliterated by connective tissue but re-epithelialization prevents this process [86]. There is evidence that epithelial cell loss occurs in pulmonary fibrosis in humans. Electron microscopy of lung tissue in the early stages of fibrosing alveolitis and systemic sclerosis has demonstrated extensive areas of bare epithelial basement membrane ([84, 85] and Figure 10.6). Based on these observations, it has been suggested that epithelial cells normally release inhibitory mediators such as PGE_2 (which inhibits fibroblast proliferation and collagen production) and that denuding the alveolar epithelium might therefore result in a shift towards fibroblast activation [84]. Evidence that regenerating epithelial cells might also produce PDGF-like molecules with the capacity to stimulate fibroblast proliferation has been presented above [27], and might be a further mechanism by which epithelial injury contributes to interstitial fibrosis. This hypothesis may also be relevant to subepithelial fibrosis in asthmatic patients in whom bronchial epithelial cell loss is a characteristic feature.

It is increasingly recognized that the endothelial cell produces mediators which may interact with mesenchymal cells and connective tissue beneath its basement membrane. These include heparin-binding growth factors, PDGF, TGFβ [87] and endothelins which, in addition to regulating vasomotor tone, may have important effects on mesenchymal cell proliferation and chemotaxis. Therefore, endothelial injury and/or regeneration could lead to an imbalance of mediators derived from

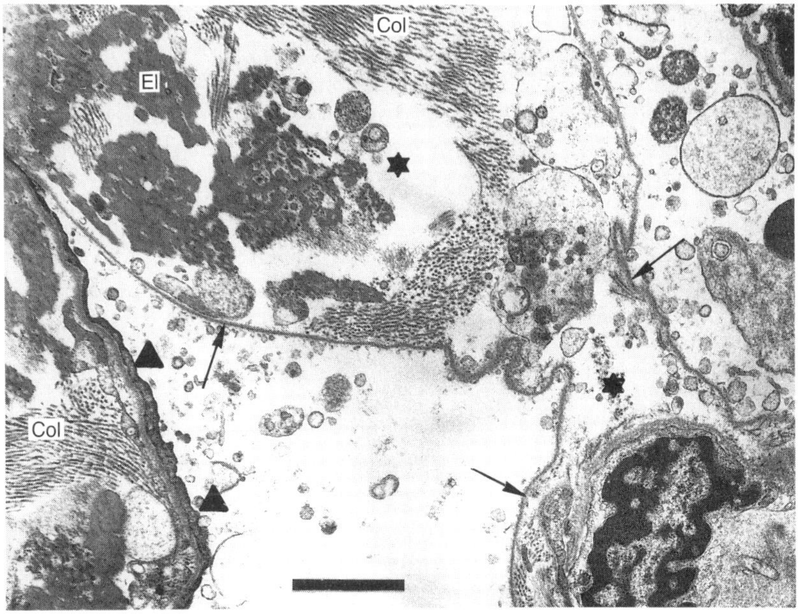

Figure 10.6 Electron micrograph of the human lung in the early stages of fibrosing alveolitis, showing interstitial oedema (stars). Extensive epithelial cell loss has led to denudation of the basement membrane (arrows). Residual alveolar epithelium is pyknotic (arrowheads). Col, Collagen; El, elastin. Stain: uranyl acetate and lead citrate. Bar = 2 μm. (Courtesy of Ann Dewar)

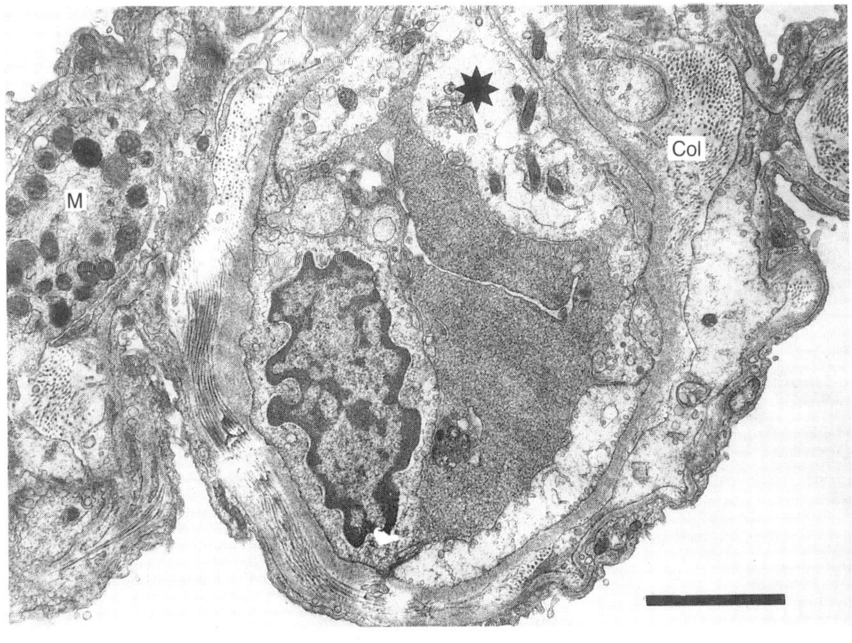

Figure 10.7 Endothelial injury in the early stages of fibrosing alveolitis. There is cytoplasmic endothelial swelling (star). A mast cell (M) can be seen in close contact with thin cytoplasmic processes of a fibroblast. Col, Collagen. Stain: uranyl acetate and lead citrate. Bar = 2 μm. (Courtesy of Ann Dewar)

endothelial cells and result in excessive collagen deposition by fibroblasts.

In summary, loss of or injury to epithelial and endothelial surfaces could affect the regulatory influences which these cells exert on fibroblasts and connective tissue beneath their basement membranes. For this reason, prevention of damage to these structures, or facilitation of their regeneration represents another potential site at which novel forms of therapy may be directed.

Increased vascular permeability

There is evidence from clinical studies and animal models that pulmonary vascular leakage of proteins occurs many days before lung fibrosis is detectable by biochemical or histological techniques [50, 88, 89]. Two independent lines of evidence suggest that increased pulmonary vascular permeability is associated with the development of pulmonary fibrosis: first, injured pulmonary capillary endothelial cells and interstitial oedema have been observed in ultrastructural studies of the lungs in patients with pulmonary fibrosis (Figures 10.5 and 10.6); secondly, clearance of radiolabelled, low-molecular-weight solutes from lungs to blood is increased in patients with pulmonary fibrosis [90, 91].

The association between increased pulmonary vascular permeability with pulmonary fibrosis raises the possibility that proteins derived from the circulation may activate lung fibroblasts. Fibrin deposits can be observed covering bare epithelial basement membrane in patients with cryptogenic fibrosing alveolitis and systemic sclerosis [84, 85], providing circumstantial evidence that thrombin has initiated the polymerization of fibrinogen molecules in the alveolar space with the consequent release of fibrinopeptides A and B together with other soluble products of clot formation. Thrombin has been reported to initiate fibroblast cell division [92], to stimulate human lung fibroblast proliferation *in vitro* [93] and to enhance lung fibroblast proliferation in bleomycin-induced pulmonary fibrosis in animals [94]. Fibrin can act as a matrix upon which fibroblasts may grow [95] and the soluble products of clot formation are known to act as chemoattractants for fibroblasts [96] and to stimulate human lung fibroblast proliferation [93]. Characterized growth factors for fibroblasts such as fibronectin, PDGF and IGF-1 are all present in blood and are known to be partly responsible for the stimulatory effects of serum on fibroblast proliferation and collagen production [97].

Taken together, these data provide compelling evidence that pulmonary vascular leakage of proteins may activate lung fibroblasts and initiate deposition of collagen in the lung interstitium. This hypothesis is supported by other clinical observations. Lung diseases associated with profound but transient pulmonary vascular leakage (such as the adult respiratory distress syndrome) also frequently progress to pulmonary fibrosis [98]. Similarly, conditions characterized by chronic interstitial oedema (such as mitral stenosis and pulmonary veno-occlusive disease) may also result in pulmonary fibrosis [99].

Mast cells

Several lines of evidence suggest that lung mast cells may be involved in the pathogenesis of pulmonary fibrosis. Increased numbers of mast cells have been observed in the lungs of patients with pulmonary fibrosis (Figure 10.7), and elevated levels of histamine have been observed in bronchoalveolar lavage fluid from patients with cryptogenic fibrosing alveolitis [100]. It is also known that alveolar macrophages can release a factor causing human lung mast cells to release histamine [101] and histamine can, under certain circumstances, stimulate fibroblast proliferation [102]. Mast cells also release heparin, which binds to endothelial cells and stimulates release of growth factors, which in turn can stimulate fibroblast proliferation [103]. Degranulated mast cells have also been identified in other fibrotic conditions such as scleroderma [104], supporting the hypothesis that mast cells represent a link between activated endothelial cells, macrophages and fibroblasts in the skin of patients with this condition. Taken together, these findings indicate that mast cells in the lung have the potential to stimulate collagen deposition. Such a mechanism may be relevant to the development of subepithelial fibrosis in asthma, a condition in which the presence of degranulated mast cells has long been recognized.

The fibroblast as an effector cell

Lung fibroblasts are not simply target cells which respond to inflammatory mediators in their environment: they are increasingly recognized as effector cells in their own right (for a review, see [105]). Their ability to produce fibronectin and an IGF-1-like molecule was discussed earlier in this chapter. They also secrete prostaglandin E_2, which has potent paracrine and autocrine effects, inhibiting fibroblast proliferation and collagen synthesis [106]. There is also evidence that fibroblasts can amplify the production of mediators produced by other cells. Activated alveolar macrophages produce large quantities of tumour necrosis factor [107] but only limited amounts of IL-1 [108]. However, lung fibroblasts are capable of secreting IL-1 in response to the synergistic actions of IL-1 and tumour necrosis factor [109]. Thus, the production of IL-1 by fibroblasts may represent an amplification mechanism for this inflammatory mediator which can stimulate fibroblast collagen production [59, 110].

Fibroblasts produce interleukin-6 (IL-6, also called interleukin beta 2), which stimulates lymphocyte proliferation and induces release of acute-phase proteins from the liver [111]. It is therefore possible that IL-6 secreted by lung fibroblasts stimulates lymphocyte proliferation in the lung and is responsible, at least in part, for the systemic symptoms of which patients with interstitial lung disease frequently complain, particularly in the early stages.

Human lung fibroblasts have been shown spontaneously to release granulocyte/macrophage colony-stimulating factor (GM-CSF), which enhances *in vitro* survival of eosinophils [112]. Fibroblasts can also interact, via specific cell-surface moieties, with eosinophils, and are activated to proliferate by eosinophil products [113]. These results suggest that fibroblasts, as well as being influenced by inflammatory cell products, can modulate the inflammatory cell population which infiltrates the lung.

Preliminary studies indicate that rat lung fibroblasts are capable of producing both PDGF [114] and TGFβ analogues [115], although these observations have not yet been confirmed in human lung fibroblast cell lines. However, taken with the recent observation using immunohistochemical techniques that human skin fibroblasts may stain positively for TGFβ_1 and TGFβ_2 [116], these data indicate that, under some circumstances, fibroblasts produce the very mediators to which they have traditionally been considered responders.

In summary, there is strong evidence that fibroblasts can exert powerful influences on their environment. In addition to producing collagens, collagenases and collagenase inhibitors, they produce mediators which regulate the synthesis and secretion of these proteins by autocrine and paracrine effects. They may also regulate inflammatory cell accumulation in the microenvironment of the lung interstitium and have the ability to amplify mediators produced by these cells. Finally, through the release of IL-6 they may induce the production of acute-phase proteins by the liver and this may be the cause of the systemic symptoms often noted in patients with conditions such as cryptogenic fibrosing alveolitis, particularly in its early stages.

Summary

The various mechanisms by which fibroblasts are activated may seem remote to the clinician confronted by a patient with pulmonary fibrosis. However, excess collagen deposition is a feature of many common pulmonary diseases and is just as relevant to 'steroid-resistant' asthmatics with 'fixed' airways obstruction or patients with pulmonary hypertension, as it is to those with fibrosing alveolitis or asbestosis. Given the current paucity of treatment for all these conditions there is a clear need to increase our understanding of the ways by which connective tissue deposition is regulated in the lungs, so that new therapies can be developed.

References

1. Murray JC, Laurent GJ. What is pulmonary fibrosis? *Thorax* 1988; **43:** 9–11.
2. Laurent GJ. Regulation of lung collagen production during wound healing. *Chest* 1991; **99:** 67S–69S.
3. Starcher BC. Elastin and the lung. *Thorax* 1986; **41:** 577–585.
4. Roberts CR. Lung proteoglycans in health and disease. In: Selman Lama M, Barrios R, eds. *Interstitial Pulmonary Diseases: Selected Topics*. Boca Raton: CRC Press, 1991; 99–376.
5. Laurent TC. Structure of hyaluronic acid. In: Balazs EA, ed. *Chemistry and Molecular Biology of the Intercellular Matrix*. New York: Academic Press, 1970; 703–732.
6. Hallgren R, Samuelsson T, Laurent TC, Modig J. Accumulation of hyaluron in the lung in adult respiratory distress syndrome. *Am Rev Respir Dis* 1989; **139:** 682–687.
7. Nettelbladt O, Bergh J, Schenholm M, Tengblad A, Hallgren R. Accumulation of hyaluronic acid in the alveolar interstitial tissue in bleomycin-induced alveolitis. *Am Rev Respir Dis* 1989; **139:** 759–762.
8. Ruoslahti E. Fibronectin and its receptor. *Ann Rev Biochem* 1988; **57:** 375–413.
9. Rennard SI, Hunninghake GW, Gadek JE, Fales Hr Crystal RG. Production of fibronectin by human alveolar macrophages: mechanism for recruitment of fibroblasts to sites of tissue injury in interstitial lung disease. *Proc Natl Acad Sci USA* 1981; **78:** 7147–7151.
10. Bitterman PB, Rennard SI, Adelberg S, Crystal RG. Role of fibronectin as a growth factor for fibroblasts. *J Cell Biol* 1983; **97:** 1925–932.
11. Laurie GW, Leblond CP, Martin GR. Light microscopic localization of type IV collagen, laminin, heparan sulphate proteoglycan and fibronectin in the basement membranes of a variety of rat organs. *Am J Anat* 1983; **167:** 71–78.
12. Laurent GJ. Rates of collagen synthesis in lung, skin and muscle obtained *in vivo* by a simplified method using [^{3}H] proline. *Biochem J* 1982; **206:** 535–544.
13. Mays PK, McAnulty RJ, Laurent GJ. Age-related changes in lung collagen metabolism: a role for degradation in regulating lung collagen production. *Am Rev Respir Dis* 1989; **140:** 410–416.

14. Bassett F, Soler P. Connective tissue in pulmonary alveolar damage and repair. *Bull Finjl Longafw* 1987; **12:** 68–72.
15. Adler KB, Callahan LM, Evans JN. Cellular alterations in the alveolar wall in bleomycin-induced pulmonary fibrosis in rats. *Am J Rev Respir Dis* 1986; **133:** 1043–1048.
16. McIntosh JR, Koonce MP. Mitosis. *Science* 1989; **249:** 622.
17. Bitterman PB, Rennard SI, Hunninghake GW, Crystal RG. Human alveolar macrophage growth factor for fibroblasts: regulation and partial characterisation. *J Clin Invest* 1982; **70:** 806–822.
18. Martinet Y, Rom WN, Grotendorst GR, Martin GR, Crystal RG. Exaggerated spontaneous release of platelet-derived growth factor by alveolar macrophages from patients with idiopathic pulmonary fibrosis. *N Engl J Med* 1987; **317:** 202–209.
19. Rom WN, Basset P, Fells GA, Nukiwa T, Trapnell BC, Crystal RG. Alveolar macrophages release an insulin-like growth factor 1-type molecule. *J Clin Invest* 1988; **82:** 1685–1693.
20. Fava RA, McClure DB. Fibronectin-associated transforming growth factor. *J Cell Physiol* 1987; **131:** 184–189.
21. Mann DM, McKeown-Longo PJ, Mills AJ. Binding of soluble fibronectin and its subsequent incorporation into the extracellular matrix by early and late passage human skin fibroblasts. *J Biol Chem* 1988; **263:** 2756–2760.
22. Hayashi M, Yamada KM. Differences in domain structures between plasma and cellular fibronectin. *J Biol Chem* 1981; **256:** 11292–11300.
23. Marinelli WA, Polunovsky VA, Harmon KR, Bitterman PB. Role of platelet-derived growth factor in pulmonary fibrosis. *Am J Respir Cell Mol Biol* 1991; **5:** 503–504.
24. Antoniades HN, Scher CD, Stiles CD. Purification of human platelet-derived growth factor. *Proc Natl Acad Sci USA* 1979; **76:** 1809–1813.
25. Bonner JC, Osornio-Vargas AR, Badgett A, Brody AR. Differential proliferation of rat lung fibroblasts induced by the platelet-derived growth factor-AA, -AB, and -BB isoforms secreted by rat alveolar macrophages. *Am J Respir Cell Mol Biol* 1991; **5:** 539–547.
26. Vignaud J-M, Allam M, Martinet N, Pech M, Plenat F, Martinet Y. Presence of platelet-derived growth factor in normal and fibrotic lung is specifically associated with interstitial macrophages, while both interstitial macrophages and alveolar epithelial cells express the *c-sis* proto-oncogene. *Am J Respir Cell Mol Biol* 1991; **5:** 531–538.
27. Antoniades HN, Bravo MA, Avila RE, Galanopoulos T, Selman Lama M. Platelet-derived growth factor in idiopathic pulmonary fibrosis. *J Clin Invest* 1990; **86:** 1055–1064.
28. Goldstein RH, Poliks CF, Pilch PF, Smith BD, Fine A. Stimulation of collagen formation by insulin and insulin-like growth factor I in cultures of human lung fibroblasts. *Endocrinology* 1989; **124:** 964–970.
29. Scott CD, Martin JL, Baxter RC. Production of insulin-like growth factor 1 and its binding protein by adult rat hepatocytes in primary culture. *Endocrinology* 1985; **116:** 1094–1105.
30. Atkinson PR, Weidman ER, Bhaumick B, Bala RM. Release of somatomedin-like activity by cultured WI-38 human fibroblasts. *Endocrinology* 1980; **106:** 2006–2012.
31. Stiles AD, Moats-Staats BM. Production and action of insulin-like growth factor 1/somatomedin C in primary cultures of fetal lung fibroblasts. *Am J Respir Cell Mol Biol* 1989; **1:** 21–26.
32. Rom WN, Travis WD, Brody AR. Cellular and molecular basis of the asbestos-related diseases. *Am Rev Respir Dis* 1991; **143:** 408–422.
33. Wahl SM, Gately CL. Modulation of fibroblast growth by a lymphokine of human T cell and continuous T cell line origin. *J Immunol* 1983; **130:** 1226–1230.
34. Postlethwaite AE, Smith GN, Mainardi CL, Seyer JM, Kang AH. Lymphocyte modulation of fibroblast function *in vitro*: stimulation and inhibition of collagen production by different effector molecules. *J Immunol* 1984; **132:** 2470–2477.
35. Selman M, Gonzalez G, Bravo M *et al*. Effect of lung T lymphocytes on fibroblasts in idiopathic pulmonary fibrosis and extrinsic allergic alveolitis. *Thorax* 1991: **45:** 451–455.
36. Cathcart MK, Edmur LI, Ahtiala-Stewart K, Ahmad M. Excessive helper T-cell function in patients with idiopathic pulmonary fibrosis: correlation with disease activity. *Clin Immunol Immunopathol* 1987; **43:** 382–394.
37. Cantin AM, Boileau R, Begin R. Increased procollagen III aminoterminal peptide-related antigens and fibroblast growth signals in the lungs of patients with idiopathic pulmonary fibrosis. *Am Rev Respir Dis* 1988; **137:** 572–578.
38. Jordana M, Schulman J, McSharry C *et al*. Heterogeneous proliferative characteristics of human adult lung fibroblast lines and clonally-derived fibroblasts from control and fibrotic human. *Am Rev Respir Dis* 1988; **138:** 579–584.
39. Raghu G, Chen Y, Rusch V, Rabinovitch PS. Differential proliferation of fibroblasts cultured from normal and fibrotic lungs. *Am Rev Respir Dis* 1988; **138:** 703–708.
40. Harrison NK. Laurent GJ. Lung collagen metabolism: the link between inflammation and pulmonary

fibrosis. In: Selman Lama M, Barrios R, eds. *Interstitial Pulmonary Diseases: Selected Topics*. Boca Raton: CRC Press, 1991; 47–75.

41. Uitto J, Prockop DJ. Incorporation of proline analogues into collagen polypeptides: effects on the production of extracellular procollagen and on the stability of the triple helical structure of the molecule. *Biochim Biophys Acta* 1974; **336:** 234–251.
42. Gunzler V, Hanauske-Abel HM, Myllyla AR, Kaska DD, Hanauske A, Kivirikko KI. Syncatalytic inactivation of prolyl 4-hydroxylase by anthracyclines. *Biochem J* 1988; **251:** 365–372.
43. Lawrence WT, Norton JA, Harvey AK, Gorschboth CM, Talbot CM, Grotendorst GR. Doxorubicin-induced impairment of wound healing in rats. *J Natl cancer Inst* 1986; **76:** 119–126.
44. Grant ME, Prockop DJ. The biosynthesis of collagen. *N Engl J Med* 1972; **286:** 194–199, 242–249, 291–300.
45. Miyahara M, Nijeha FK, Prockop DJ. Formation of collagen fibrils *in vitro* by cleavage of procollagens with procollagen proteinases. *J Biol Chem* 1982; **257:** 8442–8448.
46. Weistner M, Kreig T, Horlein D, Glanville RW, Fietzek P, Muller PK. Inhibitory effect of procollagen peptides on collagen biosynthesis in fibroblast cultures. *J Biol Chem* 1979; **254:** 7016–7023.
47. Risteli L, Risteli J. Radioimmunoassays for monitoring connective tissue metabolism. *Rheumatology* 1986; **10:** 216–245.
48. Low RB, Cutroneo KR, Davis GS, Giancola BS. Lavage type III procollagen N-terminal peptides in human pulmonary fibrosis and sarcoidosis. *Lab Invest* 1983; **48:** 755–759.
49. Bjermer L, Engstrom-Laurent A, Lundgren R, Rosenthall L, Hallgren R. Hyaluronate and type III procollagen peptide in bronchoalveolar lavage fluid as markers of disease activity in farmers lung. *BMJ* 1987; **295:** 803–806.
50. Harrison NK, McAnulty RJ, Haslam PL, Black CM, Laurent GJ. Evidence for protein oedema, neutrophil influx and enhanced collagen production in lungs of patients with systemic sclerosis. *Thorax* 1990; **45:** 606–610.
51. Derynk R, Jarrett JA, Chen EY *et al*. Human transforming growth factor-beta cDNA sequence and expression in tumour cell lines. *Nature* 1985; **318:** 66–69.
52. Fine A, Goldstein RH. The effect of transforming growth factor-β on cell proliferation and collagen formation by lung fibroblasts. *J Biol Chem* 1987; **262:** 6443–6446.
53. Ignotz RA, Massague J. Transforming growth factor–β stimulates expression of fibronectin and collagen and their incorporation into the extracellular matrix. *J Biol Chem* 1986; **261:** 4337–4345.
54. Overall CM, Wrana JL, Sodek J. Independent regulation of collagenase, 72kDa progelatinase and metalloproteinase inhibitor expression in human fibroblasts by transforming growth factor-beta. *J Biol Chem* 1989; **264:** 1860–1869.
55. Broekelmann TJ, Limper AH, Colby TV, McDonald JA. Transforming growth factor β_1 is present at sites of extracellular matrix gene expression in human pulmonary fibrosis. *Proc Natl Acad Sci USA* 1991; **88:** 6642–6646.
56. Khalil N, O'Connor RN, Unruh HW *et al*. Increased production and immunohistochemical localization of transforming growth factor-β in idiopathic pulmonary fibrosis. *Am J Respir Cell Mol Biol* 1991; **5:** 155–162.
57. Raghu G, Mastra S, Meyers D, Narayan AS. Collagen synthesis by normal and fibrotic lung fibroblasts and the effect of transforming growth factor–β. *Am Rev Respir Dis* 1989; **140:** 95–100.
58. Harrison NK, Argent AC, McAnulty RJ, Black CM, Corrin B, Laurent GJ. Collagen synthesis and degradation by systemic sclerosis lung fibroblasts: responses to TGF-β_1. *Chest* 1991; **99:** S71–72.
59. Goldring MB, Krane SM. Modulation by recombinant interleukin 1 of synthesis of types I and III collagens and associated procollagen mRNA levels in cultured human cells. *J Biol Chem* 1987; **262:** 16724–16729.
60. Elias JA, Freundlich B, Adams SL, Rosenbloom J. Regulation of human lung fibroblast collagen production by recombinant interleukin 1, tumour necrosis factor and interferon gamma. *Ann NY Acad Sci* 1990; **580:** 233–244.
61. Rosenbloom J, Feldman G, Freundlich B, Jimenez SA. Transcriptional control of human diploid fibroblast collagen synthesis by gamma-interferon. *Biochem Biophys Res Commun* 1984; **123:** 365–372.
62. Czaja MJ, Weiner FR, Eghbali M, Giambrone MA, Eghbali M, Zern MA. Differential effects of gamma interferon on collagen and fibronectin gene expression. *J Biol Chem* 1987; **262:** 3348–3351.
63. Jackson DS, Bentley JP. On the significance of the extractable collagens. *J Biophys Biochem Cytol* 1960; **7:** 37–42.
64. Nimni ME, De Guia E, Bavetta LA. Synthesis and turnover of collagen precursors in rabbit skin. *Biochem J* 1967; **102:** 143–147.
65. Barnes MJ, Constable BJ, Morton LF, Kodicek E. Studies *in vivo* on the biosynthesis of collagen and elastin in ascorbic acid-deficient guinea pigs. *Biochem J* 1970; **119:** 575–585.
66. Bienkowski RS, Baum BJ, Crystal RG. Fibroblasts degrade newly-synthesised collagen within the cells before it is secreted. *Nature* 1978; **276:** 413–416.

67. Bienkowski RS. Intracellular degradation of newly-synthesised collagen. *Collagen Rel Res* 1984; **4:** 399–412.
68. Berg RA, Schwartz ML, Crystal RG. Regulation of the production of secretory proteins: intracellular degradation of newly synthesized 'defective' collagen. *Proc Natl Acad Sci USA* 1980; **77:** 4746–4750.
69. Jimenez SA, Yankowski R. Secretion of unhydroxylated chick tendon procollagen. *Biochem Biophys Res Commun* 1975; **67:** 335–340.
70. Baum BJ, Moss J, Breul SD, Berg RA, Crystal RG. Effect of cyclic AMP on the intracellular degradation of newly synthesized collagen. *J Biol Chem* 1980; **255:** 2843–2847.
71. Sakamoto S, Sakamoto M. Degradative processes of connective tissue proteins with special emphasis on collagenolysis and bone resorption. *Mol Aspects Med* 1988; **10:** 299–428.
72. Hasty KA, Jeffrey JJ, Hibbs MS, Welgus HG. The collagen substrate specificty of human neutrophil collagenase. *J Biol Chem* 1987; **262:** 10048–10052.
73. Murphy G, Bretz U, Baggiolini M, Reynolds JJ. The latent collagenase and gelatinase of human polymorphonuclear leucocytes. *Biochem J* 1980; **192:** 517–525.
74. Welgus HG, Campbell EJ, Bar-Shavit Z, Senior RM, Teitelbaum SL. Human alveolar macrophages produce a fibroblast-like collagenase and collagenase inhibitor. *J Clin Invest* 1985; **76:** 219–224.
75. Frisch SM, Clark EJ, Werb Z. Coordinate regulation of stromelysin and collagenase genes as determined with cDNA probes. *Proc Natl Acad Sci* 1987; **84:** 2600–2604.
76. Hibbs MS, Mainardi CL, Kang AH. Type-specific collagen degradation by eosinophils. *Biochem J* 1982; **207:** 621–624.
77. Harris ED Welgus HG, Krane SM. Regulation of the mammalian collagenases. *Collagen Rel Res* 1984; **4:** 493–512.
78. Laurent GJ, McAnulty RJ. Protein metabolism during bleomycin-induced pulmonary fibrosis in rabbits. *Am Rev Respir Dis* 1983; **128:** 82–88.
79. McAnulty RJ, Campa JS, Cambrey AD, Laurent GJ. The effect of transforming growth factor β on rates of procollagen synthesis and degradation *in vitro*. *Biochim Biophys Acta* 1991; **1091:** 231–235.
80. Selman M, Montano M, Ramos C, Chapala R. Concentration, biosynthesis and degradation of collagen in idiopathic pulmonary fibrosis. *Thorax* 1986; **41:** 355–359.
81. Gadek JE, Kelman JA, Feells G *et al.* Collagenase in the lower respiratory tract of patients with idiopathic pulmonary fibrosis. *N Engl J Med* 1979; **301:** 737–742.
82. Crouch E. Pathobiology of pulmonary fibrosis. *Am J Physiol* 1990; **3:** L159–L184.
83. Garcia JGN, Gray LD, Dodson RF, Callahan KS. Asbestos-induced endothelial cell activation and injury. *Am Rev Respir Dis* 1988; **138:** 958–964.
84. Corrin B, Dewar A, Rodriguez-Rogin R, Turner-Warwick M. Fine structural changes in cryptogenic fibrosing alveolitis and asbestosis. *J Pathol* 1985; **147:** 107–119.
85. Harrison NK, Myers AR, Corrin B *et al.* Structural features of interstitial lung disease in systemic sclerosis. *Am Rev Respir Dis* 1991; **144:** 706–713.
86. Terzaghi M, Nettesheim P, Williams ML. Repopulation of denuded tracheal grafts with normal, preneoplastic and neoplastic epithelial cell populations. *Cancer Res* 1978; **38:** 4546–4553.
87. Kahaleh MB. Vascular disease in scleroderma. *Rheum Dis Clin North Am* 1990; **16:** 53–73.
88. Wangensteen D, Yankovich R, Hoidal J, Niewoehner D. Bleomycin induced changes in pulmonary microvascular albumin permeability and extravascular space. *Am Rev Respir Dis* 1983; **127:** 204–208.
89. Hay JG, Haslam PL, Staple LH, Laurent GJ. Role of iron and oxygen in bleomycin-induced pulmonary edema. *Adv Microcirc* 1987; **13:** 239–255.
90. Rinderknecht JL, Shapiro L, Krauthammer M *et al.* Accelerated clearance of small solutes from the lungs in interstitial lung disease. *Am Rev Respir Dis* 1980; **121:** 105–117.
91. Harrison NK, Glanville AR, Strickland B *et al.* Pulmonary involvement in systemic sclerosis: the detection of early changes by thin section CT scan, bronchoalveolar lavage and 99mTc-DTPA clearance. *Respir Med* 1989; **83:** 403–414.
92. Glen KC, Carney DH, Fenton JW II, Cunningham DD. Thrombin active site regions required for fibroblast receptor binding and initiation of cell division. *J Biol Chem* 1980; **25:** 6609–6616.
93. Gray AJ, Reeves JT, Harrison NK, Winlove P, Laurent GJ. Growth factors for human fibroblasts in the solute remaining after clot formation. *J Cell Sci* 1990; **96:** 271–274.
94. Tani K, Yasuoka S, Ogushi F *et al.* Thrombin enhances lung fibroblast proliferation in bleomycin-induced pulmonary fibrosis. *Am J Respir Cell Mol Biol* 1991; **5:** 34–40.
95. Brown LF, Dvorak AM, Dvorak HF. Leaky vessels, fibrin deposition and fibrosis: a sequence of events common to solid tumours and to many other types of disease. *Am Rev Respir Dis* 1989; **140:** 1104–1107.
96. Senior RM, Skogen WF, Griffin GL, Wilner GD. Effects of fibrinogen derivatives upon the inflammatory response. Studies with human fibrinogen peptide B. *J Clin Invest* 1986; **77:** 1014–1019.
97. Griffiths JB. Serum and growth factors in cell culture media – an introductory review. *Devel Biol Stand* 1987; **66:** 155–160.

98. Zapol WM, Trelstad RL, Coffey JW, Tsai I, Salvador RA. Pulmonary fibrosis in severe acute respiratory failure. *Am Rev Respir Dis* 1979; **119:** 547–554.
99. Heard BE, Steiner RE, Herdan A, Gleeson D. Oedema and fibrosis of the lungs in left ventricular failure. *Br J Radiol* 1968; **41:** 161–171.
100. Haslam PL, Cromwell O, Dewar A, Turner-Warwick M. Evidence of increased histamine levels in lung lavage fluids from patients with cryptogenic fibrosing alveolitis. *Clin Exp Immunol* 1981; **44:** 587–593.
101. Schulman ES, Liu MC, Proud D, MacGlashan DW, Lichenstein LM, Plant M. Human lung macrophages induce histamine release from basophils and mast cells. *Am Rev Respir Dis* 1985; **131:** 230–235.
102. Jordana M, Befus AD, Newhouse MT, Bienenstock J, Gauldie J. Effects of histamine on proliferation of human adult lung fibroblasts. *Thorax* 1988; **43:** 552–558.
103. Gajdusek C. Release of endothelial cell-derived growth factor (ECDGF) by heparin. *J Cell Physiol* 1984; **121:** 13–21.
104. Claman HN. On scleroderma: mast cells, endothelial cells and fibroblasts. *JAMA* 1989; **262:** 1206–1209.
105. Raghu G, Kavanagh T. The human lung fibroblast: a multifaceted target and effector cell. In: Selman Lama M, Barrios R eds. *Interstitial Pulmonary Diseases: Selected Topics.* Boca Raton: CRC Press, 1991; 1–34.
106. Goldstein RH, Polger P. The effect and interaction of bradykinin and prostaglandins on protein and collagen production by lung fibroblasts. *J Biol Chem* 1982; **257:** 8630–8633.
107. Martinet Y, Yamauchi K, Crystal RG. Differential expression of the tumour necrosis factor (cachectin) gene by blood and lung mononuclear phagocytes. *Am Rev Respir Dis* 1988; **138:** 659–665.
108. Wewers MD, Rennard SI, Hance AJ, Bitterman PB, Crystal RG. Normal human alveolar macrophages obtained by bronchoalveolar lavage have a limited capacity to release interleukin-1. *J Clin Invest* 1984; **74:** 2208–2218.
109. Elias JA, Reynolds MM, Kotloff RM, Kern JA. Fibroblast interleukin-1 beta synthesis: stimulation by recombinant interleukin-1 and tumour necrosis factor. *Proc Natl Acad Sci USA* 1989; **86:** 6171–6175.
110. Kahari V-M, Heino J, Vuorio E. Interleukin-1 increases collagen production and mRNA levels in cultured skin fibroblasts. *Biochim Biophys Acta* 1987; **929:** 142–147.
111. Gauldie J, Richards C, Harnish D, Lansdorp P, Baumann H. Interferon beta 2/B-cell stimulatory factor type 2 shares identity with monocyte-derived hepatocyte-stimulating factor and regulates the major acute phase protein response in liver cells. *Proc Natl Acad Sci USA* 1987; **84:** 7251–7255.
112. Vancheri C, Gauldie J, Bienenstock J *et al.* Human lung fibroblast-derived granulocyte-macrophage colony stimulating factor (GM-CSF) mediates eosinophil survival *in vitro*. *Am J Respir Cell Mol Biol* 1989; **1:** 289–295.
113. Shock A, Rabe KF, Chambers RC *et al.* Eosinophils adhere to and stimulate replication of human lung fibroblasts *in vitro*. *Clin Exp Immunol* 1991; **86:** 185–190 .
114. Fabisiak JP, Absher MP, Kelley J. Production of platelet-derived growth factor (PDGF)-like cytokines by rat lung fibroblasts *in vitro*. *Am Rev Respir Dis* 1990; **141:** A915.
115. Kelley J, Fabisiak JP, Absher M. Secretion of transforming growth factor-β (TGF-β) by lung fibroblasts. *Am Rev Respir Dis* 1990; **141:** A701.
116. Gruschwitz M, Muller PU, Sepp N, Hofer E, Fontana A, Wick G. Transcription and expression of transforming growth factor type beta in the skin of progressive systemic sclerosis: a mediator of fibrosis ? *J Invest Dermatol* 1990; **94:** 197–203.
117. Sterling KM, Harris MJ, Mitchell JJ, Cutroneo KR. Bleomycin treatment of chick fibroblasts causes an increase of polysomal type I procollagen mRNAs. *J Biol Chem* 1986; **258:** 14438–14444.
118. Varga J, Diaz-Perez A, Rosenbloom J, Jimenez SA. PGE_2 causes a coordinate decrease in the steady state levels of fibronectin and types I and III procollagen mRNAs in normal human dermal fibroblasts. *Biochem Biophys Res Commun* 1987; **263:** 5841–5845.
119. Cockayne D, Sterling KM, Shull S, Mintz KP, Illeyne S, Cutroneo KR. Glucocorticoids decrease the synthesis of type I procollagen mRNAs. *Biochemistry* 1986; **25:** 3202–3209.
120. Solis-Herruzzo JA, Brenner DA, Chojkier M. Tumour necrosis factor α inhibits collagen gene transcription and collagen synthesis in cultured human fibroblasts. *J Biol Chem* 1988; **263:** 5841–5845.

11

Cell biology of fibrosing lung disease

R.M. du Bois

Introduction

The body responds to tissue injury by a process of healing and repair. This involves the synthesis and secretion of extracellular matrix proteins, particularly collagen which is an appropriate and effective response to skin or bone injury.

Injury may occur in internal organs and is often the result of inflammatory processes. In these situations, the process of repair can produce functional derangement of the involved organ, particularly when the inflammatory process is persistent, resulting in progressive connective tissue deposition.

In the lung, a number of persistent inflammatory responses can produce severe tissue injury with fibrosis (honeycomb lung) at which stage the clinical, functional and pathological features are identical irrespective of the underlying pathogenetic mechanisms. It is the causative agent, the nature of the pathological (inflammatory) response, and the disease site which define the nature of the disease (Table 11.1). Good examples of this include histiocytosis X (which is characterized by the presence of an accumulation of Langerhans cells in bronchocentric areas of lung which may then become cystic with the development of stellate fibrosis); Wegener's granulomatosis (in which pulmonary vasculitis is characterized by the presence of neutrophils and granulomas within the pulmonary blood vessels); and fibrosing alveolitis (in which lung damage and interstitial fibrosis are accompanied by the presence of large numbers of inflammatory cells within both the interstitium and the alveolar air spaces). As fibrosing alveolitis (known as idiopathic pulmonary fibrosis in the USA) is by far the best studied example of fibrosing lung disease, the remainder of this chapter will be devoted to the cell biology of this condition.

Fibrosing alveolitis – general considerations

Scadding defined fibrosing alveolitis as a condition characterized by inflammation and fibrosis of the pulmonary interstitium and peripheral air spaces [1]. Fibrosing alveolitis may be mimicked by a number of disorders in which the appropriate clinical and histological features may be present, including occupational diseases such as asbestosis and hard metal disease, the fibrosing alveolitis associated with a

Table 11.1 Interstitial lung diseases – patterns of cell biology of the more common diseases

	Causative agent	*Predominant site of process*	*Predominant inflammatory cell(s)*
Fibrosing alveolitis	Not known	Acini	Lymphocyte, neutrophil, eosinophil
Extrinsic allergic alveolitis	Organic antigen	Bronchocentric	Lymphocyte
Sarcoidosis	Not known	Bronchovascular	Lymphocyte
Pulmonary eosinophilia	Drugs, helminths	Acini	Eosinophil
Wegener's granulomatosis	Not known	Blood vessels	Neutrophil*
Churg Strauss granulomatosis	Not known	Blood vessels	Eosinophil*
Histiocytosis X	Not known	Bronchocentric	Langerhans cell

*In addition to cells of the granuloma

wide range of rheumatological disorders (for example systemic sclerosis and rheumatoid arthritis), fibrosing lung diseases consequent upon treatment with drugs such as amiodarone or cytotoxic drugs, and the diseases produced by exposure to organic antigens such as the avian immunoglobulins which cause extrinsic allergic alveolitis [2–8]. When all known causes have been excluded, the remainder are referred to as cryptogenic fibrosing alveolitis (CFA), although it is likely that this still represents a heterogeneous population of patients with a variable history, differing rates of disease progression and, most likely, different trigger factors.

Epidemiology

The prevalence of fibrosing alveolitis is unknown but is thought to be roughly 5 per 100 000 of the population [9]. Deaths from fibrosing alveolitis are increasing and approximately 1200-1400 people die each year from the condition [10]. As a group, response to treatment remains poor, with only 20% of patients responding to corticosteroids and a similar number to corticosteroids and cyclophosphamide combination therapy [11, 12]. Median survival in most series is less than 5 years [13, 14]. Factors which predict a better outcome at presentation are a young age, less dyspnoea, less severely involved lungs (assessed by radiography and lung function studies including arterial blood oxygen partial pressures), a more cellular open lung biopsy and an increased number of lymphocytes in lung lavage returns [13–16].

A typical patient will present in their fifth to sixth decades of life, will be breathless on exertion with finger clubbing and fine inspiratory crackles at both bases. Chest radiography will show small lungs with a reticulonodular pattern at the bases and pulmonary physiological assessment will confirm the presence of a restrictive pulmonary defect. $Pa\text{O}_2$ and $Pa\text{CO}_2$ will be low. Blood tests are unhelpful unless there is diagnostic doubt, when avian or other precipitins may disclose an unsuspected extrinsic allergic alveolitis. Autoantibodies, although present in roughly one-third of all patients with fibrosing alveolitis may indicate the presence of an underlying rheumatological condition if present in high titre.

Aetiology

The aetiology of fibrosing alveolitis is unknown. Viral infections have been implicated but never proven. In one series of 13 patients with fibrosing alveolitis, antibodies to Epstein–Barr virus (10 patients) and IgA against viral–capsid antigen (13 patients) were found [17]. Studies of lung material obtained from patients with cryptogenic organizing pneumonitis, an entity distinct from, but often confused with, fibrosing alveolitis, have shown the presence of adenovirus DNA following amplification of DNA fragments using the polymerase chain reaction [18].

The significance of these observations is not known but it is possible that, in certain individuals, viral infection is the triggering mechanism for the subsequent progressive inflammation. Occupational or environmental triggers may be of relevance but the appropriate epidemiological studies have not yet been performed. However, a pilot study reported recently has suggested that exposure to metal dusts and wood fires may have a causative role [19].

Immunogenetics

A number of observations support the hypothesis that inherited immunogenetic factors are involved in the pathogenesis of fibrosing alveolitis. Bitterman *et al.* studied 17 individuals from three families in whom more than one member had fibrosing alveolitis [20]. Of these (in whom there was no clinical evidence of lung disease), eight were found to have inflammation within the lower respiratory tract defined by increased numbers of neutrophils, spontaneous production of alveolar macrophage derived neutrophil chemotactic and growth factors or positive gallium scans. These data support the contention that inflammation precedes lung damage and fibrosis. In all eight individuals with abnormalities in the lung, evidence of inflammation was present before fibrosis or damage had become apparent.

In inherited disorders such as neurofibromatosis and the Hermansky–Pudlak syndrome (a condition characterized by oculocutaneous albinism and abnormal platelets), there is a higher prevalence of fibrosing alveolitis, which suggests an inherited predisposition for these patients to develop lung fibrosis [21].

Numerous studies of HLA status have been inconclusive, but studies of gene linkage disequilibrium using α_1-antitrypsin phenotype and immunoglobulin polymorphisms have suggested that at least in the families studied, genetic foci on chromosome 14 may be involved in the pathogenesis of fibrosing alveolitis [22–25].

One reason why HLA studies may have been so disappointing is that they were not sufficiently selective or comprehensive. In some studies not all HLA loci were examined and in others the disease pattern of the patient population was almost certainly heterogeneous. It is unlikely that clear immunogenetic factors will be identified unless patients with early disease are studied. Once end-stage changes have occurred it is not possible to differentiate distinct pathogenetic processes in the surviving population [26].

A recent analysis of patients with pulmonary fibrosis in the context of systemic sclerosis has identified the association of a particular class II major histocompatibility complex haplotype (DR3/DRw 52a) with pulmonary fibrosis, whereas only two of 33 individuals with this haplotype had no evidence of fibrosis [27]. This difference was highly significant in both the limited and diffuse forms of scleroderma and no such class II association was observed in a control group of patients with fibrosing alveolitis in whom there was no unifying feature such as a specific collagen vascular disease.

Pathology

In typical cases, histological examination of biopsy material demonstrates the presence of fibrosis within the alveolar walls and variable numbers of inflammatory cells within both the interstitium and the air spaces [28–31]. Within the air spaces, mononuclear phagocytes are seen (particularly in more cellular samples) and in the interstitium, mononuclear phagocytes, lymphocytes and plasma cells are present in increased numbers. Eosinophils and neutrophils are relatively sparse. In more advanced disease, the most prominent histological appearance is severe interstitial fibrosis. The relative degrees of cellularity and fibrosis differ widely, not only between patients but also between biopsies from the same patient and, strikingly, in different regions of the same biopsy. This emphasizes that the pathological process does not involve the whole lung all at once but that different regions of the lung become involved in the disease process at different times. This is particularly emphasized by studies using electron microscopy of lung which appears normal on light microscopy [32, 33]. At this earliest stage of disease both epithelial and endothelial cells exhibit evidence of injury. In the endothelium, cell swelling, electrolucence and occasionally pyknosis is observed. The epithelial cells are also damaged, with patchy swelling and loss exposing basement membranes. Interstitial oedema is common. The degree of damage is similar in both cell types. Thickening, and in some areas loss, of basement membrane is apparent. Predominantly alveolar capillary basement membrane thickening was reported in one study [32]. It has been suggested that the disruption of basement membrane prevents normal epithelial repair after injury [34].

Associated with these areas of injury are regions in which type II epithelial cell proliferation is occurring. This is an attempt to 'repair' the defect and results in the alveolus becoming lined by a more cuboidal epithelium. This anatomical observation is reflected in a change in profile of lipids within the lower respiratory tract in CFA [35]. Pulmonary surfactant is a product of type II epithelial cells and changes in surfactant phospholipid composition have been described in disorders characterized by lung injury such as the adult respiratory distress syndrome (ARDS). One component, phosphatidylglycerol (PG) may be particularly important in CFA: in one study PG concentration was reduced compared with control subjects, restoration of normal values being associated with improvement in pulmonary function and radiographic indices [36]. This reduction in PG has been confirmed by other workers, but in these series a more normal initial phospholipid profile was predictive of a better outcome [37]. It is not clear whether these changes are any more than indices of derangement of type II cells but in the context that normal surfactant has immunosuppressive properties, any change may produce a more favourable milieu for local immune responses.

Pathogenesis

The current paradigm of the pathogenesis of fibrosing alveolitis is depicted in Figure 11.1. Concepts of fibrosis and fibrogenesis are considered elsewhere in this book, but the body of evidence would suggest that fibrosis within the lung in CFA is a response to injury provoked by chronic and persistent inflammation. Cellular inflammatory mechanisms are central to disease initiation and amplification and result from a highly complex network of cell–cell and cell–matrix protein interactions.

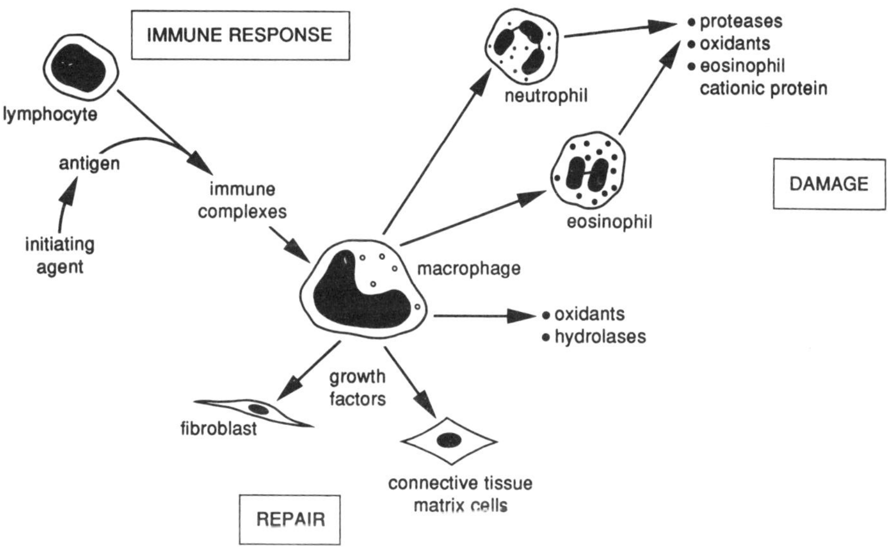

Figure 11.1 Pathogenetic mechanisms in fibrosing alveolitis

Three distinct but interrelated processes can be considered as causative factors in producing lung damage:

1. initiating factors;
2. immune mechanisms;
3. inflammatory mechanisms.

Initiating factors

It is likely that the first event in the pathogenesis of fibrosing alveolitis involves tissue injury: this is supported by animal studies using stimuli such as bleomycin [38-40]. Early injury is followed by an influx of acute then chronic inflammatory cells and subsequent fibrosis. The earliest evidence of human lung abnormalities observed in ARDS, a condition which may result in diffuse interstitial fibrosis in survivors, is damage to endothelial cells in association with damaged basement membranes, resulting in increased capillary permeability and inflammatory cell influx [41, 42]. Similar ultrastructural abnormalities have been described in areas of lung from patients with fibrosing alveolitis which are normal to light microscopy [32, 33, 43]. In these studies, patchy swelling and loss of epithelial cells were observed together with equally severe changes of endothelial ultrastructure. The precise nature of these initiating injurious agents has not been defined but, in the context of individuals who are predisposed to developing fibrosing alveolitis, injury results in the activation of host immunological and inflammatory mechanisms, more extensive lung damage ensues and fibrosis results.

Evidence for immune mechanisms

A number of lines of evidence implicate local immunological responses in the pathogenesis of fibrosing alveolitis.

Immunohistochemical studies of open lung biopsy material from patients with fibrosing alveolitis have shown that multiple lymphoid follicles are present within the interstitium [44]. These lymphoid aggregates bear the morphological and immunohistochemical features of secondary follicles with germinal centres. The central core of IgM+, IgD–, BA1–, B cells and occasional CD4+ T cells are found in association with cells expressing the phenotype of dendritic reticulum cells (RF (Royal Free) D3+, RFDR1–, leu-M2–, RFD2–, ACP–, RFD1–) surrounded by a mantle of BA1+ B cells, features which are typical of true germinal centres. Cells within the interstitium of the lung are predominantly macrophages expressing the phenotype of inflammatory cells, but occasional macrophages express the RFD1 surface determinant which is associated with interdigitating cells in normal lymphoid tissue. Most macrophages within the air spaces bear a marker recognized by the monoclonal antibody RFD9 but few macrophages in the interstitium have this phenotype [45]. The significance of this spatial organization is unknown. Lymphocytes in the interstitium are predominantly CD4+ helper/inducer subset cells although variable numbers of CD8+ suppressor cytotoxic cells are also present [46]. The significance of these latter cells in the context of lymphocyte-induced damage is unclear although cytolytic T cells have been demonstrated in lung lavage cell samples from patients with fibrosing alveolitis [47]. Preliminary studies from this organization have shown that a population of T cells within the interstitium of patients with fibrosing alveolitis associated with systemic sclerosis bear the CD45R0 phenotype of committed memory type T cells, and this is consistent with studies which have identified markers of activation on tissue T cells, for example IL-2R [46].

The immunohistochemical data would therefore strongly support the concept that local immune responses occur within the lung in fibrosing alveolitis. The nature of the antigen is unknown. IgG and complement deposition have been observed within alveolar walls and capillaries in some studies but these complexes are not found in most cases, and are rarely identified by ultrastructural studies [48–50]. However, circulating immune complexes and bronchoalveolar lavage immune complexes have been identified by several investigators [50–54]. It is possible that these complexes are formed locally and may be the product of autoimmune mechanisms. A number of features would support this. Autoimmune diseases such as Hashimoto's thyroiditis and pernicious anaemia occur more commonly in patients with fibrosing alveolitis and their relatives [2]. Fibrosing alveolitis is a common feature of 'classic' autoimmune diseases such as systemic sclerosis and rheumatoid arthritis [2, 5]. Approximately one-third of CFA patients have non-organ-specific autoantibodies in their serum (ANA or rheumatoid factor [55-57]); antibodies to DNA topoisomerase II, an enzyme which plays an important role in gene transcription were present in the sera of 37% of patients with CFA in one study [58]. Immunohistochemical studies of open lung biopsies have shown that the epithelial cells within the acini express HLA DR class II major histocompatibility antigen on their surface, a feature seen in other autoimmune disorders such as autoimmune thyroiditis [44, 59].

Studies of bronchoalveolar lavage fluid and peripheral blood support the concept that immunological mechanisms, particularly B cell stimulation, are involved in the pathogenesis of CFA. Concentrations of immunoglobulin, especially IgG, are increased in lung lavage samples [60, 61] and peripheral blood also contains higher levels of one or more classes of immunoglobulin than normal [62]. Further evidence for local immune responses comes from studies of cells obtained by lavage of the lower respiratory tract. Lung lavage cells, evaluated using a reverse haemolytic plaque assay, include immunoglobulin-secreting cells [63] and in some studies these cells have been found actively to synthesize immunoglobulin [64, 65]. Furthermore, lavage cells from patients with CFA spontaneously secrete more B cell growth factor than control lavage cell populations [66]. Taken together, these data provide convincing evidence that B cells are stimulated, locally within the lung, to synthesize and secrete immunoglobulins which may then form immune complexes, resulting in macrophage stimulation and the generation of complement activation products which are chemotactic stimuli for granulocytes. Macrophages obtained by bronchoalveolar lavage bear fewer Fc and C3b receptors than macrophages from normal individuals and contain less lysosomal acid hydrolase than controls [52, 67]. These data are consistent with the known response of macrophages to immune complex stimulation *in vitro* [68, 69].

Cell-mediated immunity may play a role: peripheral blood T cells from patients with CFA (but not normal individuals) release migration inhibition factor in response to stimulation with type I collagen [70]. Soluble markers of T cell activation, IL-2 and soluble CD8 have been identified in serum of patients with CFA [71].

Inflammatory response

Studies of bronchoalveolar lavage and open lung biopsy provide evidence for inflammatory responses being involved in the process of lung damage in CFA. Lung lavage reveals increased numbers of neutrophils and eosinophils [15, 72–74] although relatively few granulocytes are found within lung tissue [75]. These cells can be found in bronchoalveolar lavage fluid at the earliest stages of lung disease identified by high-resolution computed tomography or other non-invasive assessments of lung inflammation such as ^{99m}Tc DTPA clearance from the lung [76]. Each of these investigative techniques has shown that eosinophils and neutrophils are present before extensive lung damage and fibrosis have occurred. In addition to granulocyte traffic, large numbers of cells of the mononuclear phagocyte series are present within both the lung interstitium and the air spaces. All three types of cell have an extensive repertoire of proinflammatory mediators and tissue-damaging potential.

Macrophages

Higher numbers of macrophages are present in bronchoalveolar lavage fluid from patients with fibrosing alveolitis than in controls [3, 61]. The population is heterogeneous, consisting of cells bearing the phenotype of mature alveolar macrophages (RFD7), macrophages bearing markers normally found on interdigitating cells (RFD1), macrophages expressing a molecule identified by RFD9 (also found on the surface of cells within sarcoid granulomas), and macrophages bearing the phenotype of less mature monocyte-like cells (RFD2) [77, 78]. The functional significance of these macrophage subsets is unknown. Other cell-surface receptors which have been less well studied include molecules important in cell–cell interactions (such as ICAM-1) but little is known of these in the context of fibrosing alveolitis.

Functional repertoire of alveolar macrophages

Macrophages have a wide range of functional capacity (Table 11.2). They are present in large numbers on the epithelial surface of the respiratory tract, and play an important first-line role in host defence against inhaled particulate matter, including microbes. Human alveolar macrophages can exhibit anti-tumour activity by direct or antibody-dependent mechanisms [79, 80] and can also present antigen to T cells, albeit less efficiently than other antigen-presenting cells [81–83]. However, it is the capacity of alveolar macrophages to produce a wide variety of mediators which can have important effects on cells within the local milieu, attract inflammatory cells to the sites of inflammation and provide growth signals to cells such as fibroblasts which makes this cell of central importance in the organization of the inflammatory response in fibrosing alveolitis [84]. Of the vast array of molecules that the macrophage is capable of producing, probably the most important to the pathogenesis of CFA are those which are involved in attracting neutrophils and eosinophils to the lung interstitium, modulating endothelial cell function, and providing competence and progression growth factor signals to fibroblasts and other connective tissue matrix cells.

Alveolar macrophages can secrete two distinct factors which are chemoattractant for neutrophils [85, 86]. One, a 400–600 Da factor (which is partially lipid) is produced by normal human alveolar macrophages which have been stimulated by immune complexes or bronchoalveolar lavage-containing immune complexes. The second factor is larger, a 10 kDa protein, and is produced by normal alveolar macrophages stimulated with aggregated IgG or zymosan particles. The exact nature of these factors is not yet clear but evidence is emerging that IL-8 may be one [86, 87]. IL-8 is one of at least ten 8–10 kDa proteins which form the newly defined intercrine supergene family [88]. It is a potent neutrophil chemoattractant and activator (producing degranulation), and can be synthesized by a number of cells including fibroblasts, epithelial cells and macrophages [89–91]. Other potent macrophage cytokines include tumour necrosis factor-α (TNFα), which is synthesized and secreted mainly by macrophages [92] in response to a number of stimuli such as IL-2, interferon-γ and immune complexes [92, 93]. It may have direct effects upon connective tissue matrix cells, neutrophils, lymphocytes and may also act in an autocrine fashion on the macrophage itself [92]. Local release of TNFα may exert

Table 11.2 Macrophage products of relevance to CFA

Factor	*Size* (Da)	*Target**
Neutrophil chemotactic factor 1	500	Neutrophil
Neutrophil chemotactic factor 2	10 000	Neutrophil
IL-8	8–10 000	Neutrophil
GCSF	20 000	Neutrophil
TNFα	17 000	Neutrophil, endothelial cell
IL-1	17 500	T cell, endothelial cell, fibroblast
TGFβ	25 000	Fibroblast
Interferon γ	90–95 000	T cell, macrophage
Fibronectin	440 000	Fibroblast
PDGF	12–36 000	Fibroblast
IGF1	26 000	Fibroblast

*Main target of relevance in CFA

a number of effects on vascular endothelium including cell injury, increasing vascular permeability and modulating cell surface adhesion molecule expression [94, 95]. There is some evidence that macrophages may also secrete interferon-γ, although this is predominantly a lymphocyte-derived cytokine [96]. Finally, alveolar macrophages may synthesize and secrete a number of factors which can influence fibroblast growth and collagen synthesis and secretion. Of these, fibronectin, platelet-derived growth factor (PDGF) and insulin-like growth factor 1 (IGF-1) have been studied extensively, although other factors such as IL-1, IL-6, IL-8 and transforming growth factor β are likely to play important roles.

Evidence for macrophage functional involvement in CFA

Extensive studies of macrophages obtained by lavage from patients with CFA have indicated that the alveolar macrophage has a pivotal influence on disease pathogenesis. CFA macrophages exhibit the morphological features of activation when cultured on glass, spreading avidly [97]. They spontaneously synthesize and secrete a lipid chemotactic factor for neutrophils which has not been characterized but which is possibly LTB4 [98]. Recent studies have also demonstrated that alveolar macrophages contain levels of mRNA for IL-8, a potent neutrophil chemoattractant, higher than those present in normal macrophages [87]. Other macrophage products probably contribute to the attraction of neutrophils and eosinophils to disease sites in CFA. TNFα and IL-1 are produced by alveolar macrophages (AM) from patients with CFA [99-101], and both may exert important effects on the vascular endothelium by increasing the expression of the adhesion molecules ICAM-1, ELAM-1 and VCAM-1 [102–105]. ELAM-1 is now recognized as an adhesion molecule for neutrophils but the corresponding neutrophil ligand is not known; VCAM-1 has been shown to adhere eosinophils [106]. At present there are no immunohistochemical data to confirm the enhanced expression of these adhesion molecules on lung endothelial cells in CFA.

Interferon-γ (ifnγ) has been shown by one group to be produced by alveolar macrophages [96], and work from the same unit has shown that lavage fluid from CFA patients contains more ifnγ than controls [107]. It is a T cell activator which signals IL-2 receptor expression in T cells, stimulates endothelial cells to express ICAM-1 (the specific ligand for the T cell adhesion molecule LFA-1), activates macrophages and is a powerful inducer of class II MHC expression on a number of cells, including antigen-presenting cells, and lung epithelial cells [108].

Best defined of all macrophage functions in CFA is the capacity to provide growth signals for fibroblasts. Alveolar macrophages spontaneously secrete fibronectin [109], PDGF [110] and IGF-1 [111]. These factors provide competence signals (fibronectin and PDGF) to stimulate resting fibroblasts to enter the G1 phase of the growth cycle and progression signals (IGF-1) which stimulate the cell to complete G1 and proceed to cell division.

Alveolar macrophages, by their potential to secrete lysosomal enzymes, proteases and to produce oxygen-derived radicals, may also be involved in tissue damage. Oxygen-derived radicals, including superoxide anion, hydrogen peroxide, hydroxyl radicals and hypohalous acids, are capable of damaging lung epithelial cells [112]. Within the lower respiratory tracts of patients with CFA, macrophages and neutrophils are the cells most likely to generate oxidants [113, 114]: studies of lung lavage cells have demonstrated that oxidants are spontaneously released by these cells and that the neutrophil may be of most importance in this regard. The effect of this spontaneous release of oxidants is magnified by the relative deficiency of glutathione within the lower respiratory tract [115]. Of all known oxidant scavengers, glutathione is present in large amounts in the normal respiratory tract, which implies that this thiol has an important role in protecting epithelial cells from local oxidants [116].

Neutrophils

Neutrophils have the capacity to damage host tissue. They are capable of producing potent oxidant species and can release a wide range of granule-associated proteins, particularly the proteases collagenase and elastase [40]. A number of factors control neutrophil traffic from the blood to sites of disease including neutrophil margination within the pulmonary capillary bed, changes in neutrophil cell membrane characteristics which affect its deformability, adherence to endothelial cells by expressing cell-surface adhesion molecules (particularly the integrin CD18/CD11b and other less-defined mechanisms), and changes in pulmonary haemodynamics [117, 118].

Once the neutrophil has extravasated, it is capable of causing major tissue destruction. Its effects may be mediated by the serine proteases such as neutrophil elastase, which are capable of cleaving a wide range of substrates (including all of the major components of connective tissue matrix), neutrophil collagenase and through the generation of highly reactive oxygen radicals [40, 119, 120]. Neutrophil cell surface triggering with TNFα or interferon-γ increases the production of oxygen free radicals, particularly hydroxyl radicals and hypohalous acids. Hypohalous acids, particularly $HOCl^-$, can have powerful tissue-damaging effects and their synthesis requires the presence of myeloperoxidase (a granule protein found in high concentrations in neutrophils) and halide anions.

Evidence for the role of neutrophils in CFA

Neutrophils are present in increased numbers (up to 15-fold, especially in smokers) in bronchoalveolar lavage fluid from patients with CFA. Although present in lung tissue examined histologically they are relatively sparse by comparison with lavage numbers, which has cast some doubts on their role in disease pathogenesis, but the balance of evidence would support the conclusion that their traffic through the lung into the air spaces is associated with lung injury. Neutrophils are present in individuals at risk of CFA but whose chest radiographs appear normal: it has been shown that patients with rheumatic diseases such as systemic sclerosis and rheumatoid arthritis may have increased numbers of lavage neutrophils [76, 121, 122], suggesting subclinical alveolitis. Neutrophil secretion products are present in lung lavage fluid. Gadek *et al.* found high levels of collagenase and neutral proteinase in epithelial lining fluid [123], and a more recent observation by Hallgren *et al.* of increased myeloperoxidase in the lower respiratory tract would support the concept that neutrophil-mediated damage occurs in CFA [124].

These observations from human studies are supported by animal models of pulmonary fibrosis, in which agents such as bleomycin or asbestos produce epithelial and endothelial cell injury and a neutrophil inflammatory cell response before there is evidence of lung damage and fibrosis [38, 39].

Eosinophils

Eosinophils are found within lung tissue examined after open lung biopsy and in lung lavage sampling of the lower respiratory tract, in which up to 20% of all cells may be eosinophils. In an assessment of the diagnostic significance of a finding of >5% eosinophils in the lower respiratory tract of unselected individuals undergoing bronchoalveolar lavage, 14 of 48 patients (29%) were found to have CFA [125]. Eosinophils contain a number of granule proteins that can damage host tissue, including major basic protein, eosinophil cationic protein and eosinophil peroxidase [126].

Evidence for eosinophil involvement in CFA

There have been few studies of eosinophil function in CFA and the significance of increased eosinophil numbers in CFA is not yet known. However, Davies *et al.* [127] have shown that eosinophils can mediate lung parenchymal cell and tissue matrix injury and Hallgren *et al.* [124] have found increased concentrations of eosinophil cationic protein in the lower respiratory tracts of patients with CFA, which suggests that eosinophil products may contribute to host injury.

Mast cells

Mast cells may be found in lung biopsy material from patients with CFA, particularly in areas where the interstitium contains abundant fibrosis. These appear to be partially degranulated. Consistent with this, levels of histamine in lung lavage fluid from patients with CFA are higher than those in smoking controls [128, 129]. Mast cell degranulation may therefore play a role in amplifying inflammation by releasing vasoactive substances and thus increasing vascular permeability.

The relevance of alveolitis in CFA

There seems no doubt that the cellular components (the alveolitis) of CFA play a major role in directing events leading to tissue damage and fibrosis. All available evidence implicates the lymphocyte, neutrophil, eosinophil and especially the macrophage in the production of lung inflammation, which becomes persistent and results in terminal respiratory failure. An understanding of the cellular mechanisms causing disease is a prerequisite for the development of laboratory investigations which will lead to an understanding of how these mechanisms can be controlled.

Clinical management

Relevance of cell biological studies to clinical management

At present only 20% of patients with fibrosing alveolitis will respond objectively to treatment. One reason for this may be that the disease at presentation has produced sufficient damage and fibrosis to remove the reserve capacity of the lungs. At this stage no treatment regimen will produce any effective benefit: therapeutic strategies should be directed to the inflammatory, 'alveolitic' component of the disease process.

Family studies have shown that alveolitis can occur in the absence of clinical disease and this is confirmed by studies of patients with rheumatic diseases and normal radiographs but who have evidence of alveolitis at the time the chest radiograph is normal. Taken together with the observation that response to treatment is better in those whose disease has features of being early, it is logical to conclude that detection of early lung disease, prediction of those individuals whose disease will progress and the development of more specific disease treatments should be the goal.

One approach would be the identification of a homogeneous population of individuals who are at increased risk from CFA and assessing whether early detection and the prediction of progression are feasible.

A series of studies from the Royal Brompton Hospital has addressed some of these issues. Over 100 patients with systemic sclerosis, a disease characterized by a high prevalence of fibrosing alveolitis, have been evaluated for evidence of lung disease.

Early detection

In an assessment of early detection of disease, patients with normal chest radiographs were found to have evidence of fibrosing alveolitis on high-resolution computed tomography (HRCT), an abnormal bronchoalveolar lavage cell differential count and evidence of increased lung epithelial permeability assessed by ^{99m}Tc DTPA clearance [76]. Taken together with bronchoalveolar lavage studies from elsewhere on patients with rheumatic diseases, there appears to be little doubt that alveolitis can be detected before the patient becomes symptomatic and before the chest radiograph becomes abnormal.

Prediction of disease progression

An association has been found between HLA DR class II haplotype and pulmonary fibrosis in systemic sclerosis [27]. In this study of 42 patients with pulmonary fibrosis, 19 (45%) had the class II MHC haplotype DR3/DRw52a and, strikingly, in only 2 of 33 patients without fibrosing alveolitis was this haplotype present. When the presence of the anti-topoisomerase I antibody Scl-70 was considered, 24 of 42 patients in the fibrosis group had either anti Scl-70 or DR3/DRw 52a. No patient with anti Scl-70 was without pulmonary fibrosis. These observations define an 'at risk' population of patients with systemic sclerosis.

HRCT and ^{99m}Tc DTPA have proved to be reliable tools in the evaluation of disease evolution in systemic sclerosis. The pattern of HRCT abnormality – predominantly reticular, suggestive of predominant fibrosis or a pattern of parenchymal opacification which correlates with more cellularity in the biopsy – can predict the relative degrees of cellularity and fibrosis in open lung biopsy specimens with considerable accuracy for a predominantly fibrotic biopsy, although with less precision in patients whose lung biopsy is found to consist of fibrosis accompanied by less marked cellularity [130–133]. Furthermore, the presence of parenchymal opacification is associated with subsequent disease evolution (progression or improvement) and can indicate a subgroup of patients for whom therapy is indicated [130–133].

When the extent of disease assessed by HRCT is related to lavage cell profiles, a striking observation is made [134]. Lymphocytes are more numerous before any abnormality is seen on imaging (chest radiography or HRCT). As HRCT changes appear high percentages of eosinophils are found and these numbers change little when HRCT changes become more extensive and involve more than 50% of the lungs. By contrast, the highest numbers of neutrophils are found when more than 50% of the lung is involved and fewer neutrophils are present when lung involvement is less than 50% (i.e. higher neutrophil percentages relate to more extensive evidence of lung damage on HRCT). Thus, disease extent correlates with granulocyte traffic into the lungs. It is not clear whether this is the cause of, or a consequence of, tissue damage and fibrosis but the finding of granulocyte secretory products in the lower respiratory tract would suggest that they may be involved in the amplification of disease. If so, further studies need to address the mechanisms which promote granulocyte migration from blood to lung in early disease and a means of blocking the process must be developed.

^{99m}Tc DTPA studies have also provided valuable information relevant to disease pathogenesis and progression: first, in the presence of HRCT evidence of lung fibrosis, an abnormally rapid clearance of DTPA is associated with high percentages of bronchoalveolar lavage eosinophils [135]; secondly, if serial DTPA measurements at approximately 12-month intervals are made, a DTPA trend of an abnormal scan remaining abnormal is associated with progressive deterioration in lung gas transfer (DLCO) [136], but a scan which returns to normal predicts DLCO improvement. Of most importance is the finding that no patient whose DTPA trend remained normal suffered subsequent gas transfer loss.

These studies have identified patients at risk of developing fibrosis, those with early fibrosing alveolitis and those whose disease is more likely to progress. Further studies of these patients, the progressors and the non-progressors, should aid our understanding of the cellular biological and molecular biological mechanisms which are responsible for more progressive disease.

Treatment of CFA

Standard treatment for fibrosing alveolitis generally consists of corticosteroids or corticosteroids and immunosuppression with cyclophosphamide or azathioprine. Corticosteroids exert their anti-inflammatory effects through a number of mechanisms which can suppress activation of macrophages, lymphocytes and neutrophils in addition to influencing neutrophil and mononuclear cell migration to disease sites. This wide range of anti-inflammatory activity is, however, matched by the equally extensive range of side-effects which are experienced by some patients taking corticosteroids. In patients with CFA who are treated with corticosteroids and respond, this response is matched by a fall in neutrophil percentages in bronchoalveolar lavage [137]. This is not a non-specific effect of corticosteroid therapy *per se* because patients whose disease remains stable or deteriorates show no similar fall in neutrophil percentages.

Combination therapy of low-dose corticosteroids with cyclophosphamide or azathioprine may also be effective in CFA. Immunosuppression modulates lymphocyte function, mononuclear phagocyte function and also bone marrow cell production. The most significant side-effects are those related to opportunistic infection which can be life-threatening. A response to cyclophosphamide therapy is associated with an improvement in lung lavage granulocyte numbers [137, 138].

New treatments for CFA

Studies of the cellular and molecular mechanisms which produce inflammation in fibrosing alveolitis have identified areas which might be explored fruitfully in the development of new treatments for fibrosing alveolitis. The best general approach to new therapies would be the identification of events at the initiation of the disease process. Knowledge of the triggering mechanisms is so limited that at present prevention of exposure to likely agents is an unfruitful avenue. However, it is likely that local immune processes are involved at the inductive phase. Antigen is recognized by CD4+ T cells only when presented as a complex with class II MHC molecules. In the context of class II HLA DR MHC restriction in a homogeneous population of patients with systemic sclerosis [27], it seems possible that there may exist a bias in the local T cell antigen receptor repertoire which identifies the antigen class/II MHC complex as the first step in mounting an immune response to the presented antigen. If so, early disease could be modulated using immunotherapeutic approaches, for example by depleting the family of T cells bearing the relevant T-cell antigen receptor variable region or inducing tolerance using tolerogens such as superantigen. This approach would be productive only if patients were treated at the earliest phase of disease; this would be ethical only if a significantly 'at risk' population were identifiable.

The observation that bronchoalveolar lavage granulocyte numbers relate to disease extent assessed by HRCT and the presence of granulocyte products in epithelial lining fluid support the concept that granulocytes are involved in tissue damage, and implies that treatment which limits the migration of granulocytes to disease sites or prevents the release of toxic granulocyte products such as oxidants might provide innovative approaches to management. Mechanisms of granulocyte adhesion and passage through endothelial barriers into the lung interstitium and airways including macrophage-derived chemotactic factors and vascular endothelial molecule expression are the subjects of active research in our unit. Pharmaceutical agents which block adhesion molecule function are currently being developed.

Glutathione levels in the lower respiratory tracts of patients with CFA are reduced and inflammatory cells in the lungs of patients with CFA produce more oxidants than in normal lungs. Based on this knowledge, a recent clinical trial using inhaled glutathione to augment the epithelial lining fluid defence mechanisms in patients with CFA has shown that glutathione levels can be significantly elevated through this route. Targeting lower respiratory disease via inhaled therapy, using smaller dosages than would be needed for systemic treatment, is a highly attractive approach, particularly when the disease process is in an early, relatively asymptomatic phase, when side-effects of therapy are less acceptable. Other methods of local administration of therapy to limit tissue damage will undoubtedly evolve once the underlying mechanisms are defined more precisely.

Finally, methods which limit fibroblast proliferation and connective tissue matrix deposition may hold promise. There are no formal trials of D-penicillamine (which blocks collagen cross-linking) or colchicine (which prevents alveolar macrophage fibroblast growth factor release) but anecdotal reports have indicated that they are occasionally successful in limiting disease [139, 140]. Interferon α (a powerful immunomodulatory agent) is capable of blocking collagen transcription: preliminary studies of skin thickness in systemic sclerosis are encouraging and pilot studies of lung fibrosis are now being undertaken. Inhibitors of prolyl hydroxylase (which catalyses the hydroxylation of proline to hydroxyproline, an essential step in collagen synthesis) are being developed but are not yet available for human studies.

Only through an increased detailed knowledge of the cellular and molecular mechanisms of disease pathogenesis in CFA will novel treatments be developed. Studies are urgently needed for patients whose median survival from diagnosis is less than 5 years.

References

1. Scadding JG. Fibrosing alveolitis. *BMJ* 1964; **2:** 686.
2. Turner-Warwick M. *Immunology of the Lung*. London: Edward Arnold, 1978; 165.
3. Crystal RG, Bitterman PB, Rennard ST, Hance AJ, Keogh BA. Interstitial lung diseases of unknown cause: disorders characterized by chronic inflammation of the lower respiratory tract. *N Engl J Med* 1984; **310:** 154–165, 235–244.
4. Davison AG, Haslam PL, Corrin B *et al*. Interstitial lung disease and asthma in hard-metal workers: bronchoalveolar lavage, ultrastructural, and analytical findings and results of bronchial provocation tests. *Thorax* 1983; **38:** 119–128.
5. Alton E, Turner-Warwick M. Lung involvement in scleroderma. In: Jayson MIV, Black CM, eds. *Systemic Sclerosis: Scleroderma*. London: John Wiley & Sons Ltd, 1988; 181.
6. Gibson GJ. Adverse pulmonary effects of drugs and radiation. In: Brewis RAL, Gibson GJ, Geddes DM, eds. *Respiratory Medicine*. London: Baillière Tindall, 1990; 1149.
7. Pepys J. Hypersensitivity disease of the lungs due to fungi and other organic dusts. *Monogr Allergy* 1969; **4:** 1–145.

8. Reynolds HY. Hypersensitivity pneumonitis: Correlation of cellular and immunologic changes with clinical phases of disease. *Lung* 1988; **166:** 189–208.
9. du Bois RM. Cryptogenic fibrosing alveolitis. In: Brewis RAL, Gibson GJ, Geddes DM, eds. *Respiratory Medicine*. London: Baillière Tindall, 1990; 1088.
10. Johnston I, Britton J, Kinnear W, Logan R. Rising mortality from cryptogenic fibrosing alveolitis. *BMJ* 1990; **301:** 1017–1020.
11. Turner-Warwick M, Burrows B, Johnson A. Cryptogenic fibrosing alveolitis: response to corticosteroid treatment and its effect on survival. *Thorax* 1980; **35:** 593–599.
12. Johnson MA, Kwan S, Snell NJC, Nunn AJ, Darbyshire JH, Turner-Warwick M. Randomised controlled trial comparing prednisolone alone with cyclophosphamide and low dose prednisolone in combination in cryptogenic fibrosing alveolitis. *Thorax* 1989; **44:** 280–288.
13. Turner-Warwick M, Burrows B, Johnson A. Cryptogenic fibrosing alveolitis: clinical features and their influence on survival. *Thorax* 1980; **35:** 171–180.
14. Carrington CB, Gaensler EA, Coutu RE, Fitzgerald MX, Gupta RG. Natural history and treated course of usual and desquamative interstitial pneumonia. *N Engl J Med* 1978; **298:** 801–809.
15. Haslam PL, Turton CWG, Lukoszek A *et al*. Bronchoalveolar lavage fluid cell counts in cryptogenic fibrosing alveolitis and their relation to therapy. *Thorax* 1980; **35:** 328–339.
16. Watters LC, King TE, Schwartz MI, Waldron JA, Stanford RE, Cherniak RM. A clinical, radiographic, and physiologic scoring system for the longitudinal assessment of patients with idiopathic pulmonary fibrosis. *Am Rev Respir Dis* 1986; **133:** 97–103.
17. Vergnon JM, De The G, Weynants P, Vincent M, Mornex JF, Brune J. Fibrosing alveolitis and Epstein–Barr virus: an association? *Lancet* 1984; **ii:** 768–771.
18. Kuwano K, Hayashi S, Mackenzie A, Hogg JC. Detection of adenovirus DNA in paraffin-embedded lung tissues from patients with bronchiolitis obliterans and organising pneumonia (BOOP) using *in situ* hybridization. *Am Rev Respir Dis* 1990; **141:** A319.
19. Scott J, Johnston I, Britton J. What causes cryptogenic fibrosing alveolitis? A case-control study of environmental exposure to dust. *BMJ* 1990; **301:** 1015–1017.
20. Bitterman PB, Rennard SI, Keogh BA, Wewers MD, Adelberg S, Crystal RG. Familial idiopathic pulmonary fibrosis. Evidence of lung inflammation in unaffected family members. *N Engl J Med* 1986; **314:** 1343–1347.
21. Hoste P, Williams J, Devriendt J, Lamont H, Van der Straeten M. Familial diffuse interstitial pulmonary fibrosis associated with oculocutaneous albinism. Report of two cases with a family study. *Scand J Respir Dis* 1979; **60:** 128–134.
22. Turton CWG, Morris LM, Lawler SD, Turner-Warwick M. HLA in cryptogenic fibrosing alveolitis. *Lancet* 1978; **i:** 507-508.
23. Libby DM, Gibofsky A, Fotino M, Waters J, Smith JP. Immunogenetic and clinical findings in IPF: association with the B-cell alloantigen HLA-DR2. *Am Rev Respir Dis* 1983; **127:** 618–622.
24. Fulmer JD, Sposovska MS, Von Gal ER, Mittal KK. Distribution of HLA antigens in idiopathic pulmonary fibrosis. *Am Rev Respir Dis* 1978; **118:** 141-147.
25. Musk AW, Zilko PJ, Manners P, Kay PH, Kamboh MI. Genetic studies in familial fibrosing alveolitis: Possible linkage with immunoglobulin allotypes (Gm). *Chest* 1986; **89:** 206–210.
26. Welsh KI. HLA associations in fibrotic disease. In: *CIBA Foundation Symposium 114. Fibrosis*. London: Pitman, 1985; 164.
27. Briggs DC, Vaughan RW, Welsh KI, Myers A, du Bois RM, Black CM. Immunogenetic prediction of pulmonary fibrosis in systemic sclerosis. *Lancet* 1991; **338:** 661–662.
28. Scadding JG, Hinson KFW. Diffuse fibrosing alveolitis (diffuse interstitial fibrosis of the lungs). *Thorax* 1967; **22:** 291–304.
29. Heard BE. Pathology of interstitial lung diseases, with particular reference to terminology, classification and trephine lung biopsy. **Chest** 1976; **69** (Suppl.): 252–253.
30. Liebow AA, Definition and classification of interstitial pneumonias in human pathology. In: Basset F, Georges R, eds: *Progress in Respiration Research*. New York: Karger, 1975; 1-33.
31. Crystal RG, Fulmer JD, Roberts WC, Moss ML, Line BR, Reynolds HY. Idiopathic pulmonary fibrosis: clinical, histologic, radiographic, physiologic, scintigraphic, cytologic and biochemical aspects. *Ann Intern Med* 1976; **85:** 769–788.
32. Corrin B, Dewar A, Rodriguez-Roisin R, Turner-Warwick M. Fine structural changes in cryptogenic fibrosing alveolitis and asbestosis. *J Pathol* 1985; **147:** 107–119.
33. Harrison NK, Myers AR, Soosay G *et al*. Structural features of interstitial lung disease in systemic sclerosis. *Am Rev Respir Dis* 1991; **144:** 706–713.
34. Vrako R. Signficance of basal lamina for regeneration of injured lung. *Virchows Arch Pathol (Pathol Anat)* 1972; **355:** 264–274.
35. Low RB. Bronchoalveolar lavage lipids in idiopathic pulmonary fibrosis. *Chest* 1989; **95:** 3–5.

36. Hughes DA, Haslam PL. Changes in phosphatidylglycerol in bronchoalveolar lavage fluids from patients with cryptogenic fibrosing alveolitis. *Chest* 1989; **95:** 82–89.
37. Robinson PC, Watters LC, King TE, Mason RJ. Idiopathic pulmonary fibrosis. Abnormalities in bronchoalveolar lavage fluid phospholipids. *Am Rev Respir Dis* 1988; **137:** 585–591.
38. McCullough B, Collins JF. Bleomycin-induced diffuse interstitial pulmonary fibrosis in baboons. *J Clin Invest* 1978; **61:** 79–88.
39. Snider GL, Hayes JA, Korthy AL. Chronic interstitial pulmonary fibrosis produced in hamsters by endotracheal bleomycin: pathology and stereology. *Am Rev Respir Dis* 1978; **177:** 1009–1108.
40. Weiss SJ. Tissue destruction by neutrophils. *N Engl J Med* 1989; **320:** 365–376.
41. Rinaldo JE, Rogers RM. Adult respiratory distress syndrome. *N Engl J Med* 1986; **315:** 578–579.
42. Brigham KL, Meyrick B. Endotoxin and lung injury. *Am Rev Respir Dis* 1986; **133:** 913–927.
43. Kawanami O, Ferrans VJ, Crystal RG. Structure of alveolar epithelial cells in patients with fibrotic lung disorders. *Lab Invest* 1982; **46:** 39–53.
44. Campbell DA, Poulter LW, Janossy G, du Bois RM. Immunohistological analysis of lung tissue from patients with cryptogenic fibrosing alveolitis suggesting local expression of immune hypersensitivity. *Thorax* 1985; **40:** 405–411.
45. Noble B, du Bois RM, Poulter LW. The distribution of phenotypically distinct macrophage subsets in the lungs of patients with cryptogenic fibrosing alveolitis. *Clin Exp Immunol* 1989; **76:** 41–46.
46. Haslam PL. Evaluation of alveolitis by studies of lung biopsies. *Lung* 1990; **168** (Suppl): 984–992.
47. Karpel JP, Norin AJ. Association of activated cytolytic lung lymphocytes with response to prednisolone therapy in patients with idiopathic pulmonary fibrosis. *Chest* 1989; **96:** 794–798.
48. Turner-Warwick M, Haslam P, Weeks J. Antibodies in some fibrosing lung diseases. II. Immunofluorescent studies. *Clin Allergy* 1971; **1:** 209–219.
49. Nagaya H, Elmore M, Ford CD. Idiopathic interstitial pulmonary fibrosis. An immune complex disease? *Am Rev Respir Dis* 1973; **107:** 826–830.
50. Dreisin RB, Schwarz MI, Theofilopoulos AN, Stanford RE. Circulating immune complexes in the idiopathic interstitial pneumonias. *N Engl J Med* 1978; **298:** 353–357.
51. Haslam PL, Thompson B, Mohammed I *et al*. Circulating immune complexes in patients with cryptogenic fibrosing alveolitis. *Clin Exp Immunol* 1979; **37:** 381–390.
52. Hunninghake GW, Gadek JE, Lawley TJ, Crystal RG. Mechanisms of neutrophil accumulation in the lungs of patients with idiopathic pulmonary fibrosis. *J Clin Invest* 1981; **68:** 259–269.
53. Dall'Aglio PP, Pesci A, Bertorelli G, Brianti E, Scarpa S. Study of immune complexes in bronchoalveolar lavage fluids. *Respiration* 1988; **54** (Suppl. 1): 36–41.
54. Gosset P, Perez T, Lassalle P *et al*. Increased TNF-α secretion by alveolar macrophages from patients with rheumatoid arthritis. *Am Rev Respir Dis* 1991; **143:** 593–597.
55. Turner-Warwick M, Doniach D. Autoantibody studies in interstitial pulmonary fibrosis. *BMJ* 1965; **1:** 886–891.
56. Turner-Warwick M, Haslam P. Antibodies in some chronic fibrosing lung diseases. I. Non organ specific antibodies. *Clin Allergy* 1971; **1:** 83–95.
57. Haslam P, Turner-Warwick M, Lukoszek A. Antinuclear antibody and lymphocyte responses to nuclear antigens in patients with lung disease. *Clin Exp Immunol* 1975; **20:** 379–395.
58. Meliconi R, Bestagno M, Sturani C *et al*. Autoantibodies to DNA topoisomerase II in cryptogenic fibrosing alveolitis and connective tissue disease. *Clin Exp Immunol* 1989; **76:** 184–189.
59. Londei M, Lamb JR, Bottazzo GF, Feldmann M. Epithelial cells expressing aberrant MHC class II determinants can present antigen to cloned human T-cells. *Nature* 1984; **312:** 639–641.
60. Reynolds HY, Fulmer JD, Kazmierowski JA, Roberts WC, Frank MM, Crystal RG. Analysis of bronchoalveolar lavage fluid from patients with idiopathic pulmonary fibrosis and chronic hypersensitivity pneumonitis. *J Clin Invest* 1977; **59:** 165–175.
61. Weinberger SE, Kelman JA, Elson NA *et al*. Bronchoalveolar lavage in interstitial lung disease. *Ann Intern Med* 1978; **89:** 459–466.
62. Hobbs JR, Turner-Warwick M. Assay of circulating immunoglobulins in patients with fibrosing alveolitis. *Clin Exp Immunol* 1967; **2:** 645–652.
63. Hance AJ, Saltini C, Crystal RG. Does *de novo* immunoglobulin synthesis occur on the epithelial surface of the human lower respiratory tract? *Am Rev Respir Dis* 1988; **137:** 17–24.
64. Lawrence EC, Martin RR, Blaese RM *et al*. Bronchoalveolar IgG secreting cells in interstitial lung diseases. *N Engl J Med* 1980; **302:** 1186–1188.
65. Hunninghake GW, Crystal RG. Mechanisms of hypergammaglobulinemia in pulmonary sarcoidosis: site of increased antibody production and role of T-lymphocytes. *J Clin Invest* 1981; **67:** 86-92.
66. Emura M, Nagai S, Takeuchi M, Kitaichi M, Izumi T. *In vitro* production of B-cell growth factor and B-cell differentiation factor by peripheral blood mononuclear cells and bronchoalveolar lavage T lymphocytes from patients with idiopathic pulmonary fibrosis. *Clin Exp Immunol* 1990; **82:** 133–139.

67. du Bois RM, Townsend PJ, Cole PJ. Alveolar macrophage lysosomal enzyme and C3b receptors in cryptogenic fibrosing alveolitis. *Clin Exp Immunol* 1980; **40:** 60–65.
68. Borok Z, Trapnell BC, Crystal RG. Neutrophils and the pathogenesis of idiopathic pulmonary fibrosis. In: Baggiolini M, Pozzi E, Semenzato G, eds. *Pathophysiology of Pulmonary Cells: Neutrophils and Lymphocytes*. Milan: Masson Italia, 1990; 111.
69. Cardella CJ, Davies P, Allison AC. Immune complexes induce selective release of lysosomal hydrolases from macrophages. *Nature* 1974; **247:** 46–48.
70. Kravis TC, Ahmed A, Brown TE, Fulmer JD, Crystal RG. Pathogenic mechanisms in pulmonary fibrosis: collagen-induced migration inhibition factor production and cytotoxicity mediated by lymphocytes. *J Clin Invest* 1976; **58:** 1223–32.
71. Meliconi R, Lalli E. Borzi RM *et al.* Idiopathic pulmonary fibrosis: can cell mediated immunity markers predict clinical outcome? Thorax *1990;* **45:** 536–540.
72. Watters LC, Schwarz MI, Cherniack RM *et al.* Idiopathic pulmonary fibrosis. Pretreatment bronchoalveolar lavage cellular constituents and their relationships with lung histopathology and clinical response to therapy. *Am Rev Respir Dis* 1987: **135:** 696–704
73. Allen JN, Davis BW, Pacht ER. Diagnostic significance of increased bronchoalveolar lavage fluid eosinophils. *Am Rev Respir Dis* 1990; **142:** 642–647.
74. Bronchoalveolar lavage constituents in healthy individuals, idiopathic pulmonary fibrosis and selected comparison groups. The BAL cooperative group steering committee. *Am Rev Respir Dis* 1990; **141** (Suppl. 5): 5188–5192.
75. Haslam P, Turton CWG, Heard B *et al.* Bronchoalveolar lavage in pulmonary fibrosis: comparison of cells obtained with lung biopsy and clinical features. *Thorax* 1980; **35:** 9–18.
76. Harrison NK, Glanville AR, Strickland B *et al.* Pulmonary involvement in systemic sclerosis: the detection of early changes by thin section CT scan, bronchoalveolar lavage and ^{99m}Tc DTPA clearance. *Respir Med* 1989; **83:** 403–414.
77. Campbell DA, Poulter LW, du Bois RM. Phenotypic analysis of alveolar macrophages in normal subjects and in patients with interstitial lung disease. *Thorax* 1986; **41:** 429–434.
78. Campbell DA, Poulter LW, du Bois RM. Immunocompetent cells in bronchoalveolar lavage reflect the cell populations in transbronchial biopsies in pulmonary sarcoidosis. *Am Rev Respir Dis* 1985; **132:** 1300–1306.
79. Johnson WJ, Somers SD, Adams DO. Activation of macrophages for tumour cytotoxicity. *Contemp Top Immunobiol* 1983; **14:** 127–146.
80. Nathan C, Cohn Z. Role of oxygen-dependent mechanisms in antibody-induced lysis of tumour cells by activated macrophages. *J Exp Med* 1980; **152:** 198–208.
81. Unanue ER. Antigen-presenting function of the macrophage. *Ann Rev Immunol* 1984; **2:** 395–428.
82. Lem VM, Lipscomb MF, Weissler JC *et al.* Bronchoalveolar lavage cells from sarcoid patients demonstrate enhanced antigen presentation. *J Immunol* 1985; **135:** 1766–1771.
83. Venet A, Hance AJ, Saltini C, Robinson WS, Crystal RG. Enhanced alveolar macrophage-mediated antigen-induced T lymphocyte proliferation in sarcoidosis. *J Clin Invest* 1985; **75:** 293–301.
84. Kelley J. Cytokines of the lung. *Am Rev Respir Dis* 1990; **141:** 765–788.
85. Merrill WW, Naegel GP, Matthay RA, Reynolds HY. Alveolar macrophage derived chemotactic factor. Kinetics of *in vitro* production and partial characterization. *J Clin Invest* 1980; **65:** 268–276.
86. Hunninghake GW, Gadek JE, Fates HM, Crystal RG. Human alveolar macrophage-derived chemotactic factor for neutrophils. *J Clin Invest* 1980; **66:** 473–483.
87. Carre PC, Mortenson RL, King TE, Noble PW, Sable CL, Riches DWH. Overexpression of the interleukin 8 gene by alveolar macrophages from patients with idiopathic pulmonary fibrosis. *Am Rev Respir Dis* 1991; **143:** A396.
88. Oppenheim JJ, Zachariae COC, Mukaida N, Matsushima K. Properties of the novel proinflammatory supergene 'intercrine' cytokine family. *Ann Rev Immunol* 1991; **9:** 617–648.
89. Yoshimura TK, Matsushima K, Oppenheim JJ, Leonard EJ. Neutrophil chemotactic factor produced by lipopolysaccharide (LPS)-stimulated human blood mononuclear leukocytes: Partial characterization and separation from interleukin 1 (IL-1). *J Immunol* 1987; **139:** 788–793.
90. Schroeder J-M, Sticherling M, Henicke HH, Preissner WC, Christophers E. IL 1α or tumour necrosis factor α stimulate release of three NAP-1/IL-8-related neutrophil chemotactic proteins in human dermal fibroblasts. *J Immunol* 1990; **144:** 2223–2232.
91. Nakamura H, Yoshimura K, Jaffy HA, Crystal RG. Transcriptional regulation of interleukin-8 gene expression by tumour necrosis factor alpha in bronchial epithelial cells. *Am Rev Respir Dis* 1991; **143:** A201.
92. Schollmeier K. Immunologic and pathophysiologic role of tumour necrosis factor. *Am J Respir Cell Mol Biol* 1990; **3:** 11–12.
93. Strieter RM, Remick DG, Lynch JP, Spengler RN, Kunkel SL. Interleukin-2-induced tumour necrosis

factor-alpha (TNF-α) gene expression in human alveolar macrophages and blood monocytes. *Am Rev Respir Dis* 1989; **139:** 335–342.
94. Gamble JR, Harlan JM, Klebanoff SJ, Vadas MA. Stimulation of the adherance of neutrophils to umbilical vein endothelium by human recombinant tumour necrosis factor. *Proc Natl Acad Sci USA* 1985; **82:** 8667–8671.
95. Montefort S, Holgate ST. Adhesion molecules and their role in inflammation. *Respir Med* 1991; **85:** 91–99.
96. Robinson BWS, McLemore TL, Crystal RG. Gamma interferon is spontaneously released by alveolar macrophages and lung T lymphocytes in patients with pulmonary sarcoidosis. *J Clin Invest* 1985; **75:** 1488–1495.
97. du Bois RM, Townsend PJ, Haslam PL, Turner-Warwick M. Bronchoalveolar macrophages in sarcoidosis and cryptogenic fibrosing alveolitis. *Clin Allergy* 1981; **11:** 409–419.
98. Martin TR, Raugi G, Merritt TL, Henderson WR Jr. Relative contribution of leukotriene B_4 to the neutrophil chemotactic activity produced by the resident human alveolar macrophage. *J Clin Invest* 1987; **80:** 1114–1124.
99. Galve-de Rochemonteix B, Nicod LP, Junod AF, Dayer J-M. Characterization of a specific 20- to 25-kD interleukin-1 inhibitor from cultured human lung macrophages. *Am J Respir Cell Mol Biol* 1990; **3:** 355–361.
100. Nagai S, Aung H, Takeuchi M, Kusume K, Izumi T. IL-1 and IL-1 inhibitory activity in the culture supernatants of alveolar macrophages from patients with interstitial lung diseases. *Chest* 1991; **99:** 674–680.
101. Gosset P, Perez T, Lassalle P *et al.* Increased TNFα secretion by alveolar macrophages from patients with rheumatoid arthritis. *Am Rev Respir Dis* 1991; **143:** 593–597.
102. Bierer BE, Burakoff SJ. T-cell adhesion molecules. *FASEB J* 1988; **2:** 2584–2590.
103. Stoolman LM. Adhesion molecules controlling lymphocyte migration. *Cell* 1989; **56:** 907–910.
104. Berman JS, Beer DJ, Theodore AC, Kornfeld H, Bernardo J, Center DM. Lymphocyte recruitment to the lung. *Am Rev Respir Dis* 1990; **142:** 238–257.
105. Ruosiahti E. Integrins. *J Clin Invest* 1991; **87:** 1–5.
106. Walsh GM, Mermod JJ, Hartnell A, Kay AB, Wardlaw AJ. Human eosinophil but not neutrophil adherence to IL-1 stimulated HUVEC is α4B1 (VLA-4) dependent. *J Immunol* 1991; **146:** 3419–3423.
107. Robinson BW, Rose AH. Pulmonary gamma interferon production in patients with fibrosing alveolitis. *Thorax* 1990; **45:** 105–108.
108. Saltini C, Richeldi L, Holroyd KJ, du Bois RM, Crystal RG. Lymphocytes. In: Crystal RG, West JB, eds. *The Lung: Scientific Foundations.* New York: Raven Press, 1991; 459.
109. Yamauchi K, Martinet Y, Crystal RG. Modulation of fibronectin gene expression in human mononuclear phagocytes. *J Clin Invest* 1987; **80:** 1720–1727.
110. Martinet Y, Rom WM, Grotendorst GR, Martin GR, Crystal RG. Exaggerated spontaneous release of platelet-derived growth factor by alveolar macrophages from patients with idiopathic pulmonary fibrosis. *N Engl J Med* 1987; **317:** 202–209.
111. Rom WN, Basset P, Fells GA, Nukiwa T, Trapnell BC, Crystal RG. Alveolar macrophages release an insulin-like growth factor 1-type molecule. *J Clin Invest* 1988; **82:** 1685–1693.
112. Cross CE, Halliwell B, Borish ET *et al.* Oxygen radicals and human disease. *Ann Intern Med* 1987; **107:** 526–545.
113. Cantin AM, North SL, Fells GA, Hubbard RC, Crystal RG. Oxidant-mediated epithelial cell injury in idiopathic pulmonary fibrosis. *J Clin Invest* 1987; **79:** 1665–1673.
114. Strausz J, Mueller-Quernheim J, Steppling H, Ferlinz R. Oxygen radical production by alveolar inflammatory cells in idiopathic pulmonary fibrosis. *Am Rev Respir Dis* 1990; **141:** 124–128.
115. Cantin AM, Hubbard RC, Crystal RG. Glutathione deficiency in the epithelial lining fluid of the lower respiratory tract in idiopathic pulmonary fibrosis. *Am Rev Respir Dis* 1989; **139:** 370–372.
116. Borok Z, Buhl R, Grimes GJ *et al.* Effect of glutathione aerosol on oxidant-antioxidant imbalance in idiopathic pulmonary fibrosis. *Lancet* 1991; **338:** 215–216.
117. MacNee W, Selby C. Neutrophil kinetics in the lungs. *Clin Sci* 1990; **79:** 97–107.
118. Hogg JC. Neutrophil kinetics and lung injury. *Physiol Rev* 1987; **67:** 1249–1295.
119. Bieth JG. Elastases: catalytic and biological properties. In: Mecham R ed. *Regulation of Matrix Accumulation.* San Diego: Academic Press, 1986; 217–320.
120. Ward PA. Overview of the processes of cellular injury in interstitial lung disease. *Chest* 1991; **100:** 230–232.
121. Rossi GA, Bitterman PB, Rennard SI, Crystal RG. Evidence for chronic inflammation as a component of the interstitial lung disease associated with progressive systemic sclerosis. *Am Rev Respir Dis* 1985; **131:** 612–617.
122. Garcia JGN, Parhami N, Garcia PL. Keogh BA. Bronchoalveolar lavage fluid evaluation in rheumatoid arthritis. *Am Rev Respir Dis* 1986; **133:** 450–454.

123. Gadek JE, Kelman JA, Fells G *et al*. Collagenase in the lower respiratory tract of patients with idiopathic pulmonary fibrosis. *N Engl J Med* 1979; **301:** 737–742.
124. Hallgren R, Bjermer L, Lundgren R, Venge P. The eosinophil component of the alveolitis in idiopathic pulmonary fibrosis. Signs of eosinophil activation in the lung are related to impaired lung function. *Am Rev Respir Dis* 1989; **139:** 373–377.
125. Allan JN, Davies WB, Pacht ER. Diagnostic significance of increased bronchoalveolar lavage fluid eosinophils. *Am Rev Respir Dis* 1991; **42:** 642–647.
126. Hoidal JR. The eosinophil and acute lung injury. *Am Rev Respir Dis* 1990; **142:** 1245–1246.
127. Davies WB, Fells GA, Sun XH, Gadek JE, Venet A, Crystal RG. Eosinophil mediated injury to parenchymal cells and interstitial matrix. A possible role for eosinophils in chronic inflammatory disorders of the lower respiratory tract. *J Clin Invest* 1984; **74:** 269–278.
128. Haslam PL, Cromwell O, Dewar A, Turner-Warwick M. Evidence of increased histamine levels in lung lavage fluids from patients with cryptogenic fibrosing alveolitis. *Clin Exp Immunol* 1981; **44:** 587–593.
129. Kawanami O, Ferrans VJ, Fulmer JD, Crystal RG. Ultrastructure of pulmonary mast cells in patients with fibrotic lung disorders. *Lab Invest* 1979; **40:** 717–734.
130. Muller NL, Millar RR, Webb WR, Evans KG, Ostrow DN. Fibrosing alveolitis: CT – pathologic correlation. *Radiology* 1986; **160:** 585–588.
131. Muller NL, Staples CA, Millar RR, Vedal S, Thurlbeck WM, Ostrow DN. Disease activity in idiopathic pulmonary fibrosis: CT and pathologic correlation. *Radiology* 1987; **165:** 731–734.
132. Wells AU, Hansell DM, Corrin B *et al.* High resolution computed tomography as a predictor of lung histology in systemic sclerosis. *Thorax* 1992; **47:** 508–512.
133. Hansell DM, Kerr IH. The role of high resolution computed tomography in the diagnosis of interstitial lung disease. *Thorax* 1991; **46:** 77–84.
134. Wells AU, Hansell DM, Haslam PL, Cullinan P, Black CN, du Bois RM. Bronchoalveolar lavage cell profiles and high resolution computed tomography in systemic sclerosis; a correlation. *Eur Respir J* 1991; **4:** 254S.
135. Wells AU, Lawrence R, Black CM, du Bois RM. Inhaled ^{99m}Tc DTPA clearance as a marker of pulmonary disease activity in progressive systemic sclerosis (PSS). *Thorax* 1991; **46:** 302.
136. Wells AU, Lawrence R, Black CM, Harrison NK, du Bois RM. Enhanced ^{99m}Tc DTPA clearance is a predictor of declining gas transfer in systemic sclerosis. *Am Rev Respir Dis* 1991; **143:** A52.
137. Turner-Warwick M, Haslam P. The value of serial bronchoalveolar lavages in assessing the clinical progress of patients with cryptogenic fibrosing alveolitis. *Am Rev Respir Dis* 1987; **135:** 26–34.
138. O'Donnell K, Keogh B, Cantin A, Crystal RG. Pharmacologic suppression of the neutrophil component of the alveolitis in idiopathic pulmonary fibrosis. *Am Rev Respir Dis* 1987; **136:** 288–292.
139. Goodman M, Turner-Warwick M. Pilot study of penicillamine therapy in corticosteroid failure patients with widespread pulmonary fibrosis. *Chest* 1978; **74:** 338.
140. Rennard SI, Bitterman PB, Ozaki T, Rom WN, Crystal RG. Colchicine suppresses the release of fibroblast growth factors from alveolar macrophages *in vitro*: the basis of a possible therapeutic approach to the fibrotic disorders. *Am Rev Respir Dis* 1988; **137:** 181–185.

12
Home ventilation

A.K. Simonds

Introduction

The delivery of high technology care in the home is now a realistic proposition in a wide variety of conditions. Technical advances and growing indications for home-care, together with the pressures of cost containment and consumer choice are likely to ensure that the field will expand rapidly. Home ventilation is one of the longest established domiciliary-based services, having evolved over 30 years ago to cater for poliomyelitis patients with respiratory insufficiency. This considerable experience means that the provision of domiciliary ventilation can act as a useful model for the delivery of other forms of complex home care.

Current research on home ventilation centres on four main areas:

1. The development of new, more versatile ventilatory methods.
2. Establishing guidelines for patient selection.
3. Assessing outcome by evaluating the effects on physiological indices, quality of life and mortality.
4. Analysis of the cost-effectiveness of home care.

In this chapter, particular consideration will be given to innovations in non-invasive ventilation, potential new indications for treatment and recent research on underlying mechanisms of action. Clinical and economic outcome will be surveyed, and as funding remains a crucial issue, the scheme for the provision and finance of domiciliary ventilation in the UK will be compared to programmes elsewhere in Europe and the USA.

Ventilatory techniques (Figure 12.1)

Almost all positive pressure and negative pressure ventilatory techniques used in hospital can be applied in the home, but simplicity and portability are an advantage. Non-invasive techniques are preferable for patients with minimal bronchial secretions and intact bulbar reflexes, but for individuals who require ventilatory support for more than 16 h a day, intermittent positive-pressure ventilation (IPPV) via tracheostomy is

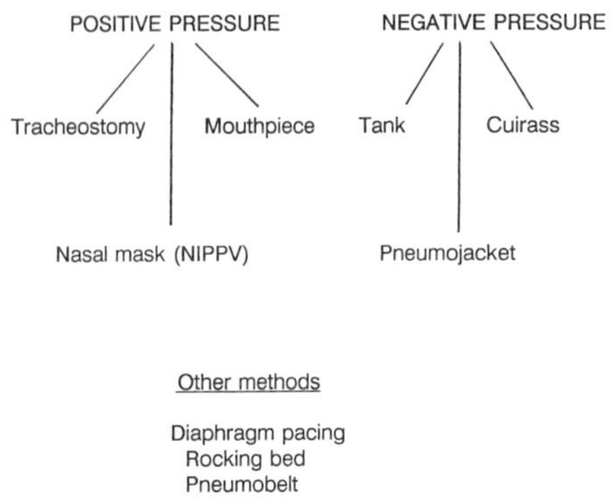

Figure 12.1 Ventilatory techniques

usually required. Following the introduction of nasal intermittent positive-pressure ventilation (NIPPV), there has been a marked shift in preference from external negative pressure to nasal positive-pressure systems over the past 5 years.

Negative-pressure apparatus

The prototype negative-pressure device is the tank ventilator or iron lung. Domiciliary iron lungs are still in use in the UK [1], predominantly for individuals with post-poliomyelitis respiratory muscle weakness. More portable negative-pressure systems such as the cuirass or jacket ventilator were the subject of renewed attention in the 1980s, with detailed exploration of their role in respiratory failure due to chest wall disorders and chronic obstructive pulmonary disease (COPD). The cuirass and jacket ventilators apply negative pressure over a smaller surface area of chest wall than the tank ventilator and so tend to generate a lower tidal volume. Mechanical efficiency can be further compromised by desynchronization between the fixed rate negative-pressure pump and the patient's spontaneous breathing, and by upper airway obstruction during sleep [2] (see below). Most patients receiving domiciliary negative-pressure treatment have neuromuscular disorders or restrictive chest wall defects. For the latter group, negative-pressure devices need to be constructed individually, so it is inevitable that use of these methods will remain limited to the small number of centres which can offer this expertise.

The rocking bed uses gravity-assisted movement of the abdominal contents to enhance diaphragmatic excursion. This can be helpful in patients with diaphragm weakness, but the augmentation of tidal volume may be small, and patient mobility is severely limited. Alexander *et al.* [3] note that motion sickness is not a problem as the bed rotates through a single plane.

Positive-pressure techniques

Positive pressure can be delivered through a tracheostomy, nasal mask, full face mask, or mouth piece. Intermittent positive-pressure ventilation via tracheostomy has never been widely employed in the UK except in cases of bulbar insufficiency and/or extreme ventilator dependence (e.g. high spinal cord injury), but until recently in

France tracheostomy-IPPV was the ventilatory method of choice in patients with respiratory insufficiency secondary to COPD.

The introduction of nasal intermittent positive ventilation has been a major influence on the development and availability of home ventilation. The technique has evolved from continuous positive airway pressure (CPAP) therapy and utilizes the same nasal masks. This has led to some confusion between the techniques, despite the fact that the physiological principles of CPAP and NIPPV are different. During nasal CPAP the patient breathes at a self-determined rate and depth with airway pressure maintained above atmospheric level e.g. 5–15 cmH_2O. In contrast, during NIPPV the patient's minute volume is augmented by preset pressure or volume-cycled equipment. Pressure support is a newer form of ventilatory assistance which can be delivered by nasal mask. Here each spontaneous breath is assisted by a constant positive pressure applied for the duration of inspiration. Respiratory rate is determined by the patient, and cycling to expiration occurs once inspiratory flow rate falls below a fixed percentage of peak flow rate. Positive pressure can be applied during expiration at a lower level than inspiratory positive pressure (bilevel positive pressure or BiPAP).

Some authorities recommend customized nasal masks, but many patients can be adequately served by commercially produced standard-size silicone nasal masks. These masks are usually well tolerated, the main drawbacks being nasal bridge ulceration and mouth leaks. A newer alternative is the Adam circuit nasal pillows (Puritan-Bennett) which consist of silicone plugs which sit in the nares. Although originally designed for CPAP use, recent work has shown that NIPPV can be satisfactorily delivered using this system [4].

The administration of assisted ventilation via mouthseal is not common in the UK and elsewhere in Europe, but Alba's group in New York have had considerable success in treating individuals with post-poliomyelitis respiratory insufficiency with this method [5]. Disadvantages include dental injury, leaks from around the mouthseal and nose, and disconnection of the patient from the delivery system during sleep.

A final method that utilizes positive pressure is the pneumobelt. This comprises an expandable bladder sealed within an abdominal corset which can be inflated to a pressure of 50 cmH_2O. The resulting abdominal displacement causes active expiration and facilitates passive inspiration. The device allows mobility and can be used to provide daytime ventilatory assistance in wheelchair-bound individuals.

Diaphragm pacing

The main indications for electrophrenic pacing are quadriplegia with a spinal cord lesion rostral to C3, and central alveolar hypoventilation [6]. In both conditions normal functioning of the phrenic nerve and diaphragm is an absolute prerequisite, and the technique is unlikely to be successful in the presence of additional pulmonary or chest wall pathology.

Despite the technical advances and an improved understanding of diaphragmatic response to stimulation, electrophrenic pacing may produce inadequate ventilation so that patients require a back up ventilatory system. In addition, upper airway obstruction may be precipitated by the dissociation of diaphragm and upper airway muscle activation requiring treatment with tracheostomy [7]. The cost outstrips that of a non-invasive ventilator by at least a factor of five.

The choice of ventilatory technique and appropriate matching of equipment performance to the patient's ventilatory needs are considered in detail below.

Patient selection

Long-term assisted ventilation is indicated in patients with chronic hypercapnic respiratory failure who are unresponsive to optimal conventional measures, and in whom reasonable benefit can be expected from the intervention. Suitability for home ventilation will depend on the wishes of the patient and his or her family, psychological and social factors plus the overall level of disability of the individual.

Spencer has classified respiratory disability into four categories:

Grade 1. Mechanical ventilation required only after illness or operation.
Grade 2. Mechanical ventilation required regularly during sleep.
Grade 3. Mechanical ventilation required during sleep and for some parts of the day.
Grade 4. Mechanical ventilation required continuously.

Grade 4 patients are relatively few in number and include those with high spinal cord injury and profound respiratory muscle weakness. Severe motor disability, and impaired glottic function are common in this group. The care of these patients in the home is complex and clearly requires a more comprehensive range of facilities and services than is necessary for the other levels of disability.

The vast majority of patients for whom home ventilation is appropriate fall into Grades 2 and 3. Here the most frequent underlying conditions are chest wall disorders and non-progressive neuromuscular disease, but potential indications for non-invasive ventilation have grown to include patients with parenchymal lung disease (Table 12.1). In all these conditions a precarious balance between ventilatory demand and capacity is disrupted by sleep, resulting in nocturnal hypoventilation. A combination of reduction in central drive [8], impaired ability to compensate for respiratory muscle load [9], and decrease in intercostal and accessory muscle activity predisposes to arterial desaturation and CO_2 retention, particularly during rapid eye movement (REM) sleep [10]. The resulting rise in CSF bicarbonate and fragmented sleep pattern depress chemosensitivity and arousal reflexes further [11]. If unchecked, these nocturnal derangements in blood gas tensions can progress to diurnal respiratory failure, pulmonary hypertension, and ultimately cor pulmonale.

Symptoms of nocturnal hypoventilation often evolve insidiously and include morning headaches, disturbed sleep pattern, diurnal somnolence and general lassitude. These symptoms should be sought specifically in high-risk patients, e.g. in patients with vital capacity less than 30% of predicted, and those with respiratory muscle weakness and/or central drive disorders. If they are present, measurement of arterial blood gas tensions and nocturnal monitoring of arterial oxygen saturation and, preferably, transcutaneous P_{CO_2} is essential. A trace with features characteristic of nocturnal hypoventilation and the response to NIPPV is shown in Figure 12.2.

Table 12.1 Indications for home ventilation

Treatment of hypercapnic respiratory failure due to

- Chest wall disease
  - — Scoliosis
  - — Thoracoplasty
  - — Fibrothorax
- Respiratory muscle disorders
  - — Old poliomyelitis
  - — Myopathies
  - — Muscular dystrophies
- Neurological disorders
  - — Primary alveolar hyperventilation
  - — Central sleep apnoea
  - — Brainstem lesions
  - — Cervical spinal cord injury
  - — Phrenic nerve lesions, polyneuropathy

Possible indications (see text):

- COPD
- Bronchiectasis
- Rapidly progressive neuromuscular disorders

Physiological effects of home ventilation

Recent work has been helpful in clarifying the mechanisms of action of nocturnal assisted ventilation. Effects on arterial blood gas tensions, ventilatory drive, respiratory muscle function and lung/chest wall mechanics are important, but information on the relative contribution of each of these effects and differences in efficiency between negative- and positive-pressure techniques in various conditions is emerging.

Negative pressure

Restrictive chest wall/neuromuscular disease

Numerous studies have confirmed that negative-pressure ventilation can correct arterial blood gas tensions in patients with scoliosis [12], thoracoplasty [13] and non-progressive neuromuscular disorders [14], and these improvements can be maintained in the long term. For individuals with nocturnal hypoventilation, assisted ventilation at night can control arterial blood gas tensions adequately by day [12, 15, 16]. This sustained effect is partly attributable to the resetting of arterial $P\text{CO}_2$ and bicarbonate levels resulting in enhanced hypercapnic ventilatory response. Patients often comment on improved sleep quality once nocturnal hypoventilation has been corrected, in spite of encumbrance with apparatus at night. This subjective impression has been confirmed by studies of sleep architecture and number of arousals before and after the introduction of nocturnal negative-pressure treatment [16].

As indicated above, upper airways obstruction may reduce the efficiency of negative-pressure ventilation. This tendency is produced by the absence of concurrent activation of upper airway abductor muscles and diaphragm [16, 17]. Upper airway

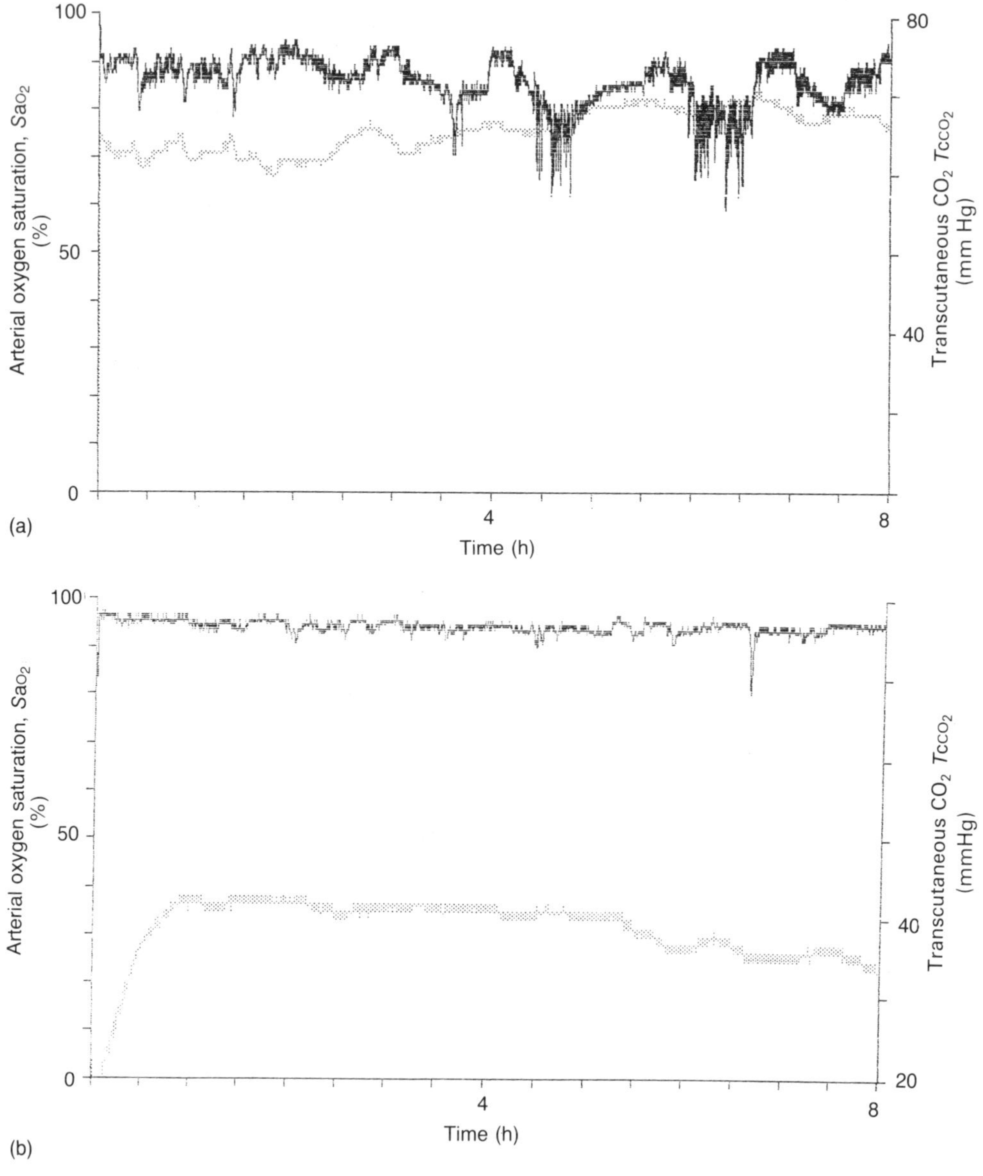

Figure 12.2 Trace showing arterial oxygen saturation (Sa_{O_2}) and transcutaneous CO_2 (Tc_{CO_2}) during sleep in a patient with Marfan's syndrome and scoliosis. (a) While breathing spontaneously, demonstrating nocturnal hypoventilation; (b) receiving nasal intermittent positive-pressure ventilation

obstruction may be diminished by the tricyclic agent protriptyline which reduces REM sleep-related episodes [18] and increases upper airway muscle tone [19]. As with diaphragm pacing, desynchronization of the patient's spontaneous respiratory effort with the fixed-rate applied cycle of the negative-pressure pump can be a problem, especially during REM sleep when respiratory rate is more erratic [1].

If these difficulties limit the effectiveness of treatment, triggering of the negative-pressure pump using a sensor placed in the airway is possible. In practice, however, a switch to a more mechanically effective system such as NIPPV is usually required.

In 20 consecutive patients with chest wall disorders or stable neuromuscular disease treated with negative pressure in a tank ventilator for 2 weeks in this unit, mean vital capacity increased from 750 ml (range 200–1150) to 960 ml (range 350–1700) while ambulant diurnal arterial oxygen tension rose from a mean of 5.8 (range 3.0–8.5) kPa to 7.4 (range 5.5–10.1) kPa. Mean arterial $P\text{CO}_2$ fell from 7.4 (range 5.9–8.6) kPa to 6.1 (range 5.2–7.2) kPa and maximum inspiratory mouth pressure (PI_{max}) doubled, with a rise in maximum expiratory mouth pressure (PE_{max}) by around 40%. Others [13, 14] have shown improvements in arterial blood gas tensions of similar magnitude, with little difference in results between patients with idiopathic scoliosis, paralytic disorders or thoracoplasty.

Early improvements in respiratory muscle strength which precede significant changes in arterial blood gas tensions have been documented [20]. This evidence suggests that in the patient group with restrictive disorders, assisted ventilation acts to off-load ventilatory muscles which may be functioning close to fatigue level. Rochester and coworkers [21] have demonstrated a fall in diaphragm surface electromyogram (EMG) activity to 9% of the level during spontaneous breathing in patients treated with a tank ventilator. Improvements in global respiratory muscle strength unrelated to changes in arterial $P\text{CO}_2$ were seen, accompanied by a reduction in dyspnoea. A comparable reduction in dyspnoea was produced in normal subjects who were treated in the tank ventilator while their respiratory muscles were loaded by added airway resistance.

In patients commencing negative-pressure ventilation an early diuresis is commonly observed in the absence of any alteration in diuretic therapy. This is likely to reflect increased renal blood flow and oxygenation [22], and improved cardiac function. Garay and colleagues [12] have shown a significant decrease in pulmonary artery pressure in a small series of patients with idiopathic scoliosis and/or respiratory muscle weakness. However, large-scale trials examining the action of negative-pressure ventilation on pulmonary hypertension and cardiac performance have not been undertaken.

Chronic obstructive pulmonary disease

Studies of domiciliary negative-pressure ventilation in patients with hypercapnic respiratory failure due to COPD have produced mixed results, despite early encouraging reports of successful use in hospital [23, 24]. More recently, short-term treatment with a pneumojacket 4 h/day for 2 weeks in inpatients with hypercapnic COPD has been shown to produce a significant reduction in diaphragm EMG activity during treatment, and improvements in vital capacity, PI_{max} and 12-min walking distance compared with a control group who received conventional therapy [25]. Gutierrez and colleagues [26] treated a similar group of COPD patients with a weekly 8-h session of negative-pressure ventilation over 4 months and report objective improvements in arterial blood gas tensions, PI_{max}, exercise tolerance and quality of life. These workers suggest that only COPD patients with severe inspiratory muscle weakness (PI_{max} < 50 cmH_2O) are likely to benefit from weekly negative-pressure ventilation. Other research groups have been unable to replicate these beneficial effects in patients with severe airflow obstruction treated with a weekly regime of 8 h nasal positive-pressure ventilation [27].

Delivery of negative-pressure ventilation in the home in COPD patients has proved more problematical. For practical reasons most studies have employed the pneumojacket or pneumowrap. Two controlled trials [28, 29] have failed to demonstrate improvement although there is some evidence that, despite lack of benefit in the group as a whole, patients with severe hypercapnia may have been helped. Macklem and coworkers (as described by Martin [30]) have carried out a double-blind randomized study, using sham negative-pressure ventilation in the control group. Again, no significant objective improvement was seen in the treatment group, although it is not clear how effectively the respiratory muscles were rested. This seems to be a crucial issue, as Rodenstein *et al.* [31] have shown that reduction in diaphragm EMG during negative-pressure ventilation is variable, and is produced most effectively in patients who are acclimatized to the technique.

Finally, negative-pressure ventilation was developed primarily as a pump substitute for patients with ventilatory failure, but with normal lungs. Not unexpectedly, therefore, although it is able to redress the effects of diurnal and nocturnal hypoventilation, it lacks the flexibility and efficiency to remedy concurrent ventilation/perfusion mismatch and diffusion defects in subjects with parenchymal lung disease.

Positive-pressure techniques

Restrictive chest wall/neuromuscular disorders

Home ventilation with tracheostomy-IPPV is used rarely in the UK for patients with restrictive or obstructive disorders. In a large French series Bertrand and Milane [32] have shown that the best results with this technique are obtained in patients with RCWD and that outcome in COPD patients was little improved over conventional regimes. Early mortality is high and usually related to the tracheostomy [33]. Tracheostomy-related morbidity was also a major limiting factor in Hoeppner's study of nocturnal IPPV in scoliosis [15].

The use of non-invasive positive-pressure systems circumvents some of these airway-related problems. Control of nocturnal hypoventilation using nasal IPPV was originally described in patients with chest wall or neuromuscular diseases [34–36]. Significant improvements in nocturnal and diurnal arterial blood gas tensions have been demonstrated accompanied by reduction in inspiratory muscle workload [37]. Long-term effects of NIPPV on respiratory muscle function, lung/chest wall mechanics, ventilatory drive, pulmonary artery pressure, and right heart function have not been determined, although studies are in progress. Early data suggest that significant improvements in respiratory muscle strength and an increase in chest wall compliance may occur. The latter is consistent with a study of intermittent positive-pressure hyperinflation delivered via mouthpiece in patients with RCWD [38]: here hyperinflation of the chest with a delivered volume of roughly double the spontaneous tidal volume resulted in a significant increase in vital capacity, and respiratory muscle endurance, but no change in accessible alveolar volume – suggesting a volume history-determined effect on alveolar surface tension forces and long-term effect on the elastic properties of the chest wall.

COPD

Elliott and coworkers [39] have carried out a pilot study of domiciliary NIPPV in 12 patients with chronic stable hypercapnic respiratory failure secondary to severe COPD. Their approach has differed from other studies in that NIPPV was used specifically to treat nocturnal hypoventilation, although effects on respiratory muscle indices were also monitored. Patients were taught to use the equipment during an acclimatization period in hospital. Eight patients completed 6 months of treatment with nocturnal NIPPV, and full polysomnography showed improved nocturnal arterial oxygen saturation and transcutaneous $P\text{CO}_2$. Total sleep time and sleep efficiency increased overall, dispelling the notion that sleep quality is inevitably disrupted by ventilatory equipment. NIPPV was associated with improved diurnal arterial blood gas tensions, decreased gas trapping and a trend to improved quality of life. An analysis of the mechanisms responsible for these changes has been performed [40]. Following 6 months' NIPPV, an increase in FEV_1 and reduction in gas trapping was accompanied by a fall in arterial $P\text{CO}_2$ and increase in dynamic compliance. This evidence of improvement in small airway function may be a consequence of reduction in pulmonary venous engorgement and indicates a reduction in load on the ventilatory pump. In addition, improvement in central drive occurred, as demonstrated by an increase in minute volume in response to hypercapnia. Interestingly, no consistent improvement in any indices of diaphragm or global respiratory muscle strength was seen, suggesting that control of nocturnal hypoventilation and reduction in load on the respiratory system are more important than respiratory muscle 'rest' in patients with end-stage COPD.

Three of the 12 patients discontinued treatment because they were unable to sleep with the apparatus and one subject with very severe airflow obstruction died after only a short period of NIPPV. In contrast, Strumpf *et al.* [41] found no significant alterations in diurnal arterial blood gas tensions, pulmonary function, mouth pressures or sleep efficiency in a cross-over study of 3 months' NIPPV in patients with severe COPD, although neuropsychiatric functioning improved. Seven patients withdrew due to poor tolerance of apparatus, but six patients completed the study. It is notable that this study and the previous trial [39] differ in several important respects. Patients recruited by Strumpf *et al.* were less hypercapnic than those in Elliot's study (mean diurnal $P\text{CO}_2$ 6.5 kPa compared with 7.7 kPa) and were not, in general, admitted to hospital for familiarization with the equipment. From these studies, COPD patients with moderate to severe hypercapnia and significant sleep disturbance associated with nocturnal derangement of blood gas tensions seem most likely to benefit from NIPPV. An adequate period teaching the patient and family how to use the ventilator and initial familiarization in hospital will probably improve compliance rates. Further work is required to compare NIPPV with the gold-standard treatment of long-term oxygen therapy in COPD.

Progressive neuromuscular disease

The implementation of assisted ventilation in patients with progressive disease poses difficult ethical problems: quality of life, symptom relief, patient choice and the retention of autonomy are the central issues. A number of workers have examined whether the advantages of assisted ventilation in terms of symptom relief outweigh the obvious disadvantages of increased dependency and prolongation of an inevitable decline in function.

Many of the studies describing the use of home ventilation in progressive neuromuscular disorders include patients treated with negative and positive pressure methods. Mohr and colleagues [42] followed a series of patients with Duchenne muscular dystrophy for an average of 39 months. Arterial $P\text{CO}_2$ remained stable, but vital capacity fell by 33%. Mean requirement for ventilatory support increased from 8 to 18 h a day, although symptom control remained good. Comparable findings emerged from a study by Curran *et al.* [43], with overall length of survival increasing from 19 years 9 months to 25 years 9 months. Heckmatt and coworkers [44] have used domiciliary nocturnal non-invasive ventilation in patients aged 2–28 years with neuromuscular disease and symptomatic nocturnal hypoventilation. For some patients NIPPV was more effective than negative-pressure ventilation, although four of the five youngest patients were unable to cope with the nasal mask. Successful use of NIPPV has been reported in a 6-year-old child with central hypoventilation [34], but it seems that children under this age are best managed by alternative methods. A trial comparing negative-pressure ventilation, tracheostomy-IPPV and NIPPV in Duchenne muscular dystrophy is in progress.

Few patients with motor neurone disease are appropriate candidates for home ventilation, but for selected individuals who present with early respiratory muscle involvement and preserved bulbar function ventilatory failure can be reversed and distressing respiratory symptoms relieved by non-invasive ventilatory support [45]. Transient improvement in pulmonary function was seen in a French series of such patients treated with nasal-buccal or tracheostomy IPPV and all patients were discharged home [46]. There is limited physiological information on patients with progressive neuromuscular conditions.

Bronchiectasis

The extensive French multicentre series of patients receiving home ventilation [47] includes a small subgroup with respiratory failure due to bronchiectasis of varying aetiology. Of all forms of chronic obstructive lung disease, treatment of diffuse bronchiectasis with tracheostomy-IPPV appears to produce the worst results. Benhamou *et al.* [48] report modest improvements in arterial blood gas tensions in patients with diffuse bronchiectasis receiving NIPPV and supplemental oxygen therapy. In the UK there is growing experience of the use of NIPPV as a bridge to heart–lung transplantation in patients with cystic fibrosis and intractable ventilatory failure. Stabilization of arterial blood gas status can be achieved with no apparent deleterious effects on sputum clearance and improved early results following transplantation [49].

Matching ventilatory technique to the patient

In some clinical situations, e.g. Grade 4 patients with bulbar weakness there is little option but to use tracheostomy-IPPV. However, in Grade 2 and 3 patients a number of issues need to be considered when deciding which ventilatory system to employ.

Negative- versus positive-pressure methods

Several studies have compared the mechanical efficiency of negative- and positive-pressure ventilatory apparatus. In a cross-over trial [50] 15 chest wall disease patients maintained on negative-pressure ventilation (ten cuirass, three pneumojacket, two portable tank ventilator) for an average of 38 months were transferred to NIPPV. Patients used volume-cycled ventilators (eight Lifecare PLV 100, four BromptonPac, three Monnal D) with standard silicone nasal masks and were followed for an average of 32.7 months. Arterial blood gas tensions improved significantly on NIPPV (Figure 12.3) and hospital admission rates were reduced following the transfer. The majority of patients felt less breathless on NIPPV and 10 of the 15 were less fatigued. No patient requested a return to negative-pressure ventilation and the more compact positive-pressure apparatus facilitated a greater degree of patient mobility.

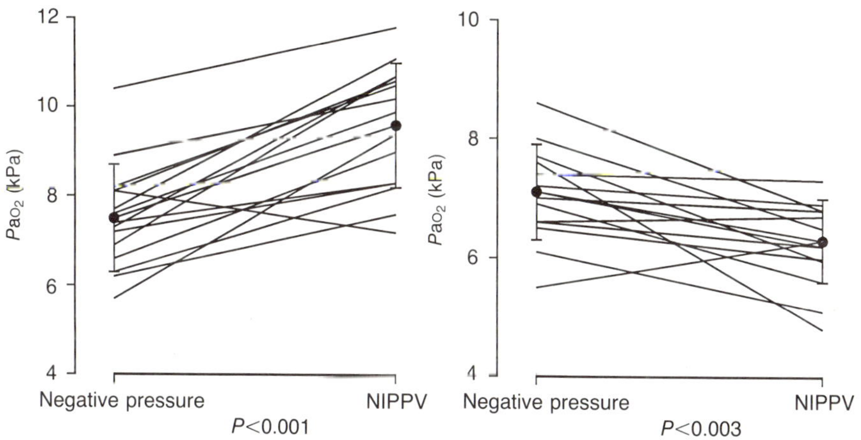

Figure 12.3 Arterial blood gas tensions in patients with restrictive chest wall disease on negative-pressure ventilation and after transfer to nasal intermittent positive-pressure ventilation (NIPPV)

Heckmatt and colleagues [44] have also demonstrated that NIPPV is preferable to other ventilatory methods in some patients with neuromuscular disease and preserved bulbar function. In four patients converted from negative-pressure ventilation to NIPPV, nocturnal and diurnal arterial blood gas tensions improved and lifestyle was enhanced in that foreign travel became feasible. Similarly, Ellis *et al.* [34] have shown that while negative-pressure ventilation enhanced oxygenation in non-REM sleep, it did not prevent REM sleep-related desaturation in a group with neuromuscular disease – largely due to the induction of upper airway obstruction. By contrast, NIPPV produced adequate arterial blood gas tensions in all stages of sleep.

Jackson *et al.* [50] have reported comparable clinical outcomes in two groups of patients matched for age, sex and primary diagnosis treated with either negative-pressure ventilation or NIPPV. Patients were not randomized to each form of treatment, however, and baseline arterial oxygen level appeared lower in the NIPPV group.

Overall, the use of negative-pressure ventilation is likely to remain limited, although it has a place in the management of patients with neuromuscular and chest wall disease, young children, and individuals who cannot tolerate nasal or face masks.

Volume-cycled versus pressure-preset positive-pressure systems

Most of the positive-pressure systems originally developed for NIPPV are volume-cycled flow generators. As discussed above, pressure-preset or pressure-limited systems are now available. Theoretically, volume-cycled ventilators offer more stable alveolar ventilation in the face of changing pulmonary characteristics, but compensate for leaks poorly. Pressure-preset equipment compensates for leaks, but will deliver a reduced minute volume in the presence of increased airways resistance or decreased lung compliance [52].

To examine the advantages and limitations of volume-cycled and pressure-preset ventilation the BiPAP pressure support system (Respironics Inc.) has been compared to a volume-cycled flow generator system in a cross-over study [53] of nine subjects receiving NIPPV for hypercapnic respiratory failure due to a range of pulmonary pathologies (three COPD, three early-onset idiopathic scoliosis, two paralytic scoliosis, one kyphosis). All subjects were experienced NIPPV users, stable on a volume-cycled flow generator ventilator (VCF). Polysomnography was carried out on the VCF and repeated on the BiPAP system after 7–14 nights' acclimatization. In subjects requiring an inflation pressure of more than 25 cmH_2O indices of nocturnal arterial oxygen saturation and Pco_2 were lower using the BiPAP machine, whereas in subjects with an inflation pressure below 25 cmH_2O nocturnal oxygenation was similar or improved on BiPAP compared with VCF (Figure 12.4). This suggests that the BiPAP machine is best suited to individuals with relatively low thoracic impedance (less than 25 cmH_2O). Patients with high thoracic impedance who require inflation pressures of greater than 25 cmH_2O are probably served better by a VCF or pressure-preset system with an inspiratory airway pressure provision higher than the present BiPAP maximum of 20 cmH_2O.

Assist/control pattern of ventilation

In conscious subjects, spontaneous breathing is most comfortably augmented by use of the 'assist' mode of positive-pressure ventilation, in which each breath is triggered by the subject. However, in clinical situations where the patient is incapable of respiratory effort, automatic cycling or 'control' mode is necessary to secure adequate gas exchange. Most patients who require nocturnal ventilation benefit from the combined advantages of the 'assist/control' mode which promotes patient synchrony with the ventilator during wakefulness, but will provide back-up cycling during sleep when apnoeic or profound hypopnoeic episodes may supervene (Figure 12.5).

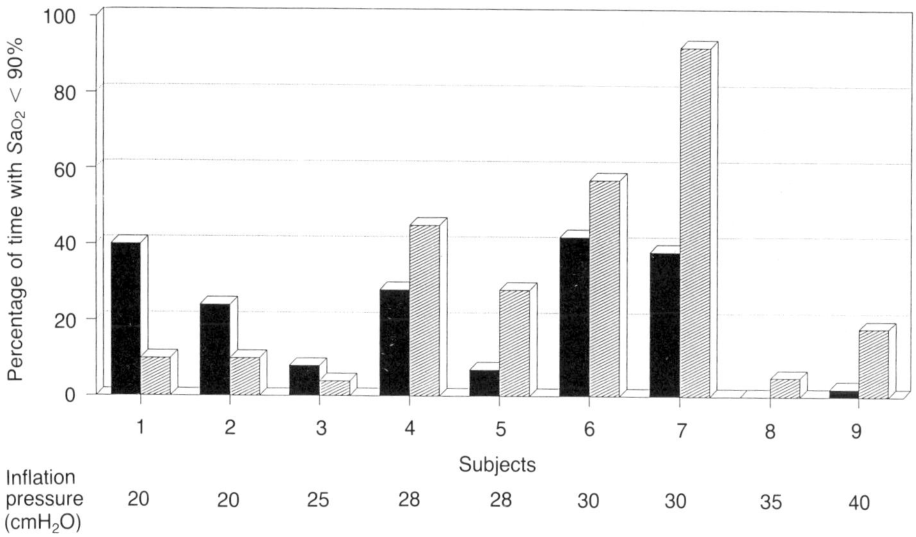

Figure 12.4 Nocturnal arterial oxygen saturation (percentage of time saturation < 90%) on volume-cycled flow generator and BiPAP ventilator

The characteristics of the trigger are important. In order to reduce inspiratory muscle work the trigger threshold should be low, with a short response time. A period in the respiratory cycle during which the trigger is refractory is also required so that successive respiratory efforts do not produce breath 'stacking' and consequent hyperinflation [54]. In some individuals with COPD, severe airflow obstruction produces continued positive pressure in the airway at end-expiration, so-called auto-PEEP. This increases the work required to trigger the next breath and may be eased by matching the ventilator expiratory positive airway pressure (EPAP) setting to the level of auto-PEEP [55].

Some authorities prefer to use the control mode in all patients in an effort maximally to rest the respiratory muscles. A disadvantage of this, apart from desynchronization with the patient's respiratory efforts, is that controlled cycling in patients with low minute volume requirements can produce marked hyperventilation. Delguste *et al.* [56] have recently reported upper airway obstruction occurring in a female with myopathy receiving controlled-mode NIPPV. Active glottic closure during sleep appears to be a mechanism provoked by hypocapnia, which limits further hyperventilation.

Long-term outcome of home ventilation

It is important that the results of home ventilation are judged on quality of life as well as on morbidity and mortality rates, but, unfortunately this information is lacking in many trials. Overall the British, American and French programmes now encompass 20–30 years of experience with home ventilation.

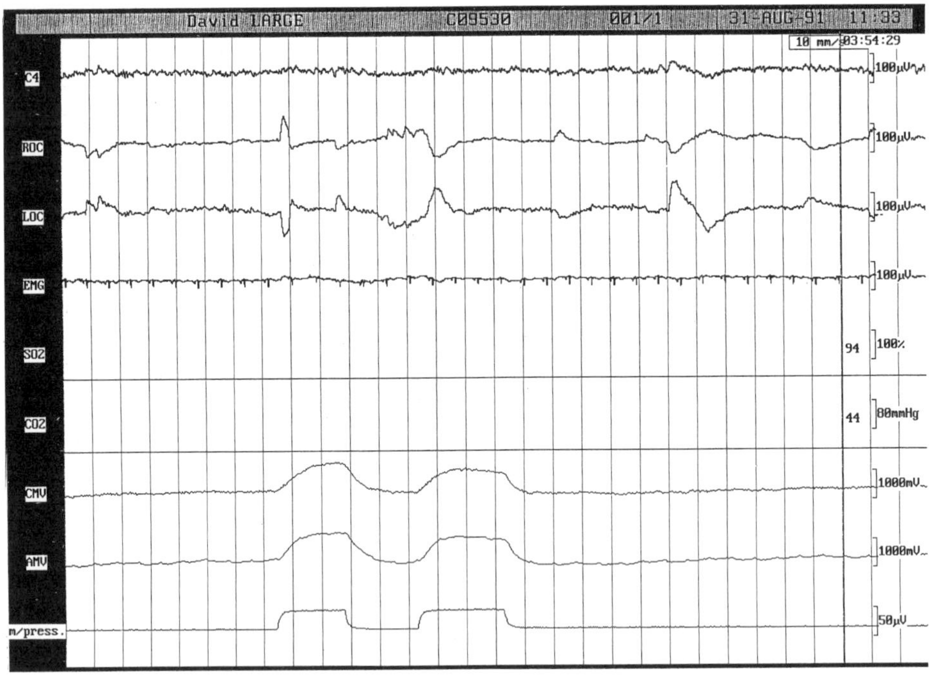

Figure 12.5 30-Second epoch of polysomnography trace, showing inadequate ventilatory rate during triggered pressure support ventilation. CMV, ribcage movement; AMV, abdominal movement; m/press, mask pressure

A number of large studies have been published detailing survival in these patients. The most extensive longitudinal data concerns the use of tracheostomy-IPPV and negative-pressure ventilation, as NIPPV was not introduced until 1986. Splaingard and coworkers [14, 57] have demonstrated survival rates of 80% and 67%, at 5 and 10 years respectively, in patients with stable neuromuscular disease treated with negative-pressure ventilation. It proved possible to care for 93% of these individuals entirely at home.

In France about 4500 people receive home ventilation, with 50% using tracheostomy-IPPV and 50% NIPPV. The proportion receiving NIPPV has grown rapidly over the last 5 years and very few French patients are now treated with negative-pressure ventilation. Follow-up data from the Lyon/Paris/Dijon/Nancy Co-operative study [47] show 1-year survival rates of 91% for patients with scoliosis (n=112), 86% for patients with sequelae of pulmonary tuberculosis (n=88), 76% for patients with stable neuromuscular disorders (n=55) and 74% in patients with COPD (n=118): 3-year survival rates are 80%, 75%, 62% and 61%, respectively.

In a study in the UK Sawicka *et al.* [58] examined the clinical outcome in patients receiving predominantly negative-pressure ventilation for respiratory failure secondary to skeletal or neuromuscular diseases. Improvements in exercise tolerance and breathlessness were reported in all patients. Of the patients with skeletal deformities 71% were able to return to work, and 46% of those with stable or slowly progressive neuromuscular disorders returned to full-time employment. Details on hospital admission rates were not available on all patients, but the average admission rate fell to 0.44/year. Outcome was independent of the degree or chronicity of cardio-respiratory failure, and was largely determined by the rate of progression of the underlying pathology. All patients with progressive neuromuscular disease continued to deteriorate and died a median of 13 months after initiation of treatment. It is notable that in this study the efficiency of negative-pressure ventilation was limited by upper airway obstruction in 11 patients requiring treatment with protriptyline or by tracheostomy – with resultant deleterious effects on their quality of life.

Clinical outcome, quality of life and economic activity have been monitored in 74 patients at the Royal Brompton National Heart and Lung Hospital receiving domiciliary NIPPV [59]. Of these, 67 had respiratory failure secondary to neuromusculoskeletal disorders and seven had COPD. Mean age for the group was 50.2 (range 19–74) years, with an average follow-up period on NIPPV of 24.9 (range 1–48) months. In response to a self-administered quality of life questionnaire 73% of subjects felt less fatigued on NIPPV, 44% experienced less breathlessness and 91% felt more in control of their health after starting NIPPV. Symptomatic improvement was most marked in those with early-onset idiopathic scoliosis, and least well demonstrated in patients with intrapulmonary disease or progressive pathology. Eleven individuals had retired and six had taken early retirement; 63% of the remaining subjects are in full or part-time employment, 26% receive long-term sickness benefit and 11% classify themselves as housewives (Figure 12.6).

A substantial proportion of patients on home ventilation remain economically active; this is particularly true of those with restrictive chest wall and stable neuromuscular disease. This level of functioning is achieved despite additional handicaps such as limb weakness and wheelchair dependence due to old poliomyelitis.

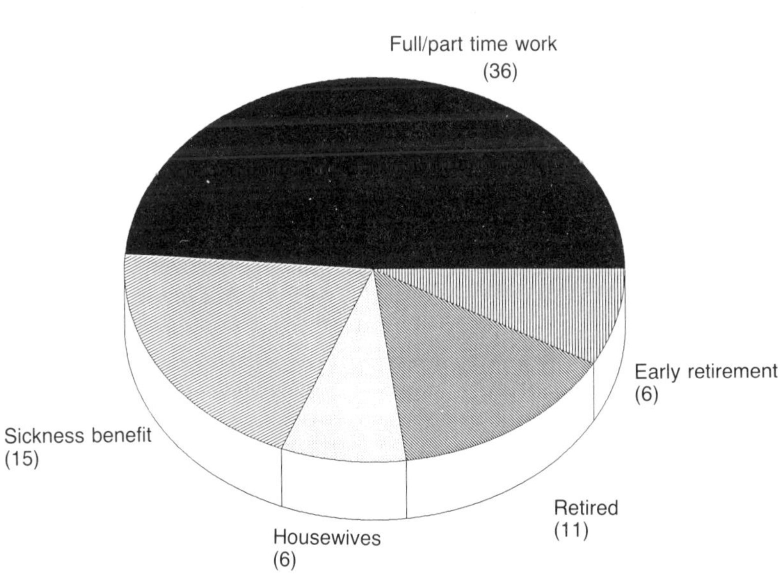

Figure 12.6 Economic activity in 74 NIPPV users (67 with restrictive chest wall disease, 7 with COPD)

Homecare ventilatory support organization

The pivotal importance of providing coordinated medical and technical back-up for domiciliary ventilator-dependent individuals has long been recognized [60]. This includes easy access to medical advice, an emergency breakdown service, routine maintenance of ventilatory equipment, and provision of consumables (masks, suction catheters, oxygen etc.). The level of home support required will vary considerably, with highly ventilator-dependent patients needing care 24 h/day. In contrast, the vast majority of individuals requiring nocturnal ventilation are able to care for themselves. Good communication between the hospital, general practitioner and community services is vital.

Home ventilatory care in the UK is provided at present by three large centres with 100–200 patients each, and 15–20 units caring for smaller numbers of patients. The pioneer programme for highly ventilator-dependent patients is the Responaut scheme based at St Thomas' Hospital, London [61], although other centres can now offer this level of care.

Approximately 600 patients in the UK are treated with home ventilation. Of these, 50–100 are Grade 4 ventilator-dependent, 100 use negative-pressure systems and fewer than ten have phrenic nerve pacemakers (J. Shneerson, 1992, personal communication).

World perspective

It has been estimated that around 8000 persons worldwide receive long-term domiciliary ventilation for several hours each day [62]. Data are difficult to obtain and this figure is almost certainly an underestimate. The major reported activity is in France, USA and the UK, with marked variations in the pattern and organization of care between countries.

France

The French programme offers a highly organized, model approach to home respiratory care [63, 64]. It has grown from a series of regional centres, which were originally set up in the 1960s to cater for the local needs of post-polio ventilator-dependent patients. Activities subsequently increased to include the provision of long-term oxygen therapy. In 1981 a French National Home Care Association for Chronic Respiratory Insufficiency (ANTADIR) was created. This body has unified the activities of the regional associations with the aim of coordinating a national network, facilitating centralized purchase of equipment and reimbursement, providing social assistance and organizing data collection and research. The usual practice is for a French physician to issue a prescription for home ventilatory apparatus. This is installed by the local regional association which is also responsible for technical back-up. ANTADIR figures show that, by 1990, 1800 patients were receiving non-invasive ventilation and 2200 tracheostomy-IPPV. A far higher proportion of patients receiving home ventilation in France have end-stage COPD than in the UK treatment population. Average daily cost per patient for respiratory homecare is reported to be £4–5, which represents a total expenditure of £1630 per patient per year [64]. In addition to this centrally sponsored scheme, a private system has emerged over the last few years, but at present this is mainly responsible for delivery of long-term oxygen therapy.

USA

Despite a long tradition of home ventilation, and the production of guidelines [65] and a consensus report [66] on the management of ventilator-dependent individuals, there is no national policy, administrative structure or system for funding long-term ventilation in the USA [62]. It is estimated that 4000 patients are receiving home ventilation, many as a result of failure to wean from conventional IPPV following an acute episode of decompensation. This means that the patient population differs from that in France and the UK, with more American patients being Grade 4 ventilator-dependent. Pierson [62] lists the most common indications for long-term ventilatory assistance as high cervical cord lesions due to road traffic accidents, gunshot wounds, or sports injuries; primary neurological or neuromuscular disorders; and COPD or other chronic lung disease. Some rehabilitation centres thrive [67] and there is special expertise in using negative-pressure ventilation and electrophrenic pacing. However, lack of any established funding system and administrative difficulties means that many ventilator-dependent individuals who could be cared for at home remain in hospital [68].

Other countries

Growing domiciliary ventilation programmes exist in Australia, Sweden and Germany among other countries, but are difficult to quantify. There is a major need for comprehensive data collection in this area.

Economic impact of homecare

Hospital-oriented delivery of health care has long been the norm in the National Health Service. Interest in home-based treatment has arisen in an attempt to reduce the social and psychological disadvantages of institutional care, and to cut costs. Some economic analyses cover the whole gamut of homecare, including early discharge schemes, terminal care and physical therapy at home. This is misleading, as the savings which accrue from domiciliary high-technology care are likely to be considerably greater than those from rehabilitative schemes [69, 70].

The efficacy and efficiency of home ventilation, particularly in chest wall disease and stable neuromuscular conditions, have been demonstrated. Marks [71] suggests that an ideal cost-effectiveness study comparing home and hospital long-term ventilation should include measurements of mortality, morbidity, disability, discontent and discomfort, as well as analysing economic and psychosocial effects, and non-monetary costs to the carers and community. Not surprisingly, no such study has been undertaken, and some of the work that exists suffers from selection bias, unobjective reporting and incomplete cost analysis [72].

Creese and Fielden [73] have carried out a valuable analysis of the cost of home and hospital care for Responaut patients from St Thomas' Hospital, London. Taking into account recurrent and capital costs for these highly dependent individuals, 1 year of ventilatory care in the home cost two-thirds the total for an equivalent period of hospital care. Others have cited savings of 50–90% for patients receiving home ventilation [71], and Goldberg *et al.* [68] describe an initial cost reduction of 70% in a paediatric ventilatory homecare programme. These examples relate to relatively ventilator-dependent groups. Savings may be greater still in Grade 2 and 3 patients as a proportion of these return to work.

Summary

The clinical and physiological benefits of home ventilation have been established in chest wall and neuromuscular disease, and information on cost-effectiveness is emerging. The newer technique of NIPPV will allow greater dissemination of the treatment and the advantages and limitations of this intervention now should be determined in patients with respiratory failure due to parenchymal lung disease and progressive neuromuscular disorders.

Thoracic physicians need to incorporate domiciliary ventilation into a unified programme of home respiratory care. Nationwide coordination of the provision of home ventilation in the UK with centralized purchase of equipment should increase cost effectiveness and facilitate data collection and the organization of multicentre trials, which are needed to clarify the indications for home therapy [74].

References

1. Schneerson JM. Non-invasive and domiciliary ventilation: negative pressure techniques. *Thorax* 1991; **46:** 131–135.
2. Simonds AK, Branthwaite MA. Efficiency of negative pressure ventilatory equipment. *Thorax* 1985; **40:** 213.
3. Alexander MA, Johnson EW, Petty J, Staunch D. Mechanical ventilation of patients with late stage Duchenne muscular dystrophy. *Arch Phys Med Rehabil* 1979; **60:** 289–292.
4. Simonds AK, Cramer D, Wedzicha J. Nasal plugs (Adam circuit) for the delivery of CPAP and nasal intermittent positive pressure ventilation. *Thorax* 1991; **46:** 291P.
5. Bach JR, Alba A, Bohatiuk G, Saporito L, Lee M. Mouth intermittent positive pressure ventilation in the management of postpolio respiratory insufficiency. *Chest* 1987; **91:** 859–864.
6. Glenn WWL, Holcomb WG, Shaw RK, Hogan JF, Holschuh KR. Long-term ventilatory support by diaphragm pacing in quadriplegia. *Ann Surg* 1976; **183:** 566–577.
7. Hyland RH, Hutcheon MA, Peri A *et al.* Upper airway occlusion induced by diaphragm pacing for primary alveolar hypoventilation: implications for the pathogenesis of obstructive sleep apnoea. *Am Rev Respir Dis* 1981; **124:** 180–185.
8. Phillipson EA. Control of breathing during sleep. *Am Rev Respir Dis* 1978; **118:** 909–939.
9. Badr MS, Skatrud JB, Dempsey JA, Begle RL. Effect of mechanical loading on expiratory and inspiratory muscle activity during NREM sleep. *J Appl Physiol* 1990; **68:** 1195–1202.
10. Sawicka EH, Branthwaite MA. Respiration during sleep in kyphoscoliosis. *Thorax* 1987; **42:** 801–808.
11. Bowes G, Woolf GM, Sullivan CE, Phillipson EA. Effect of sleep fragmentation on ventilatory and arousal responses of sleeping dogs to respiratory stimuli. *Am Rev Respir Dis* 1980; **122:** 899–908.
12. Garay SM, Turing GM, Goldring RM. Sustained reversal of chronic hypercapnia in patients with

alveolar hypoventilation syndrome. *Am J Med* 1981; **70:** 269–274.
13. Sawicka EH, Branthwaite MA, Spencer GT. Respiratory failure after thoracoplasty: treatment by intermittent negative pressure ventilation. *Thorax* 1983; **38:** 433–435.
14. Splaingard ML, Frates RC, Jefferson LS, Rosen CL, Harrison GM. Home negative pressure ventilation: report of 20 years of experience in patients with neuromuscular disease. *Arch Phys Med Rehabil* 1985; **66:** 239–242.
15. Hoeppner VH, Cockroft DW, Dosman JA, Cotton DJ. Nighttime ventilation improves respiratory failure in secondary kyphoscoliosis. *Am Rev Respir Dis* 1984; **129:** 240–243.
16. Goldstein RS, Molotiu N, Skrastins SL *et al.*Reversal of sleep-induced hypoventilation and chronic respiratory failure by nocturnal negative pressure ventilation in patients with restrictive ventilatory impairment. *Am Rev Respir Dis* 1987; **135:** 1049–1055.
17. Levy RD, Bradley D, Newman SL, Macklem PT, Martin JG. Negative pressure ventilation: effects on ventilation during sleep in normal subjects. *Chest* 1989; **95:** 95–99.
18. Brownell LG, West P, Acres JC, Kryger MH. Protriptyline in obstructive sleep apnea – a double blind trial. *N Engl J Med* 1982; **307:** 1037–1042.
19. Bonora M, St John WM, Bledsoe TA. Differential elevation by protriptyline and depression by diazepam of upper airway respiratory motor activity. *Am Rev Respir Dis* 1985; **131:** 41–45.
20. Braun NMT, Marino WD. Effect of daily intermittent rest of respiratory muscles in patients with severe chronic airflow limitation. *Chest* 1984; **85:** 59S.
21. Rochester DF, Braun NMT, Laine S. Diaphragmatic energy expenditure in chronic respiratory failure. The effect of assisted ventilation with body respirators. *Am J Med* 1977; **63:** 223–232.
22. Baudouin SV, Bott J, Deane C, Ward A. Is oxygen a renal vasodilator? *Thorax* 1990; **45:** 787.
23. Bourteline-Young HJ, Whittenberger JL. The use of artificial respiration in pulmonary emphysema accompanied by high carbon dioxide levels. *J Clin Invest* 1951; **30:** 838–844.
24. Marks A, Bodes J, Morganti L. A new ventilatory assistor for patients with respiratory acidosis. *N Engl J Med* 1963; **268:** 61–68.
25. Ambrosino N, Montagna T, Nava S *et al.* Short term effect of intermittent negative pressure ventilation in COPD patients with respiratory failure. *Eur Respir J* 1990; **3:** 502–508.
26. Gutierrez M, Berioza T, Contreras G *et al.* Weekly cuirass ventilation improves blood gases and inspiratory muscle strength in patients with chronic airflow limitation and hypercarbia. *Am Rev Respir Dis* 1988; **138:** 617–623.
27. Bott J, Keilty SEJ, Jenkins SC *et al.* Weekly nasal positive pressure ventilation does not improve arterial blood gas tensions, exercise tolerance, pulmonary function and sensation of breathlessness in patients with stable severe chronic obstructive pulmonary disease (COPD). *Am Rev Respir Dis* 1991; **143:** A74.
28. Zibrak JD, Hill NS, Federman S *et al.* Evaluation of intermittent long-term negative pressure ventilation in patients with severe chronic obstructive pulmonary disease. *Am Rev Respir Dis* 1988; **138:** 1515–1518.
29. Celli B, Lee H, Criner G *et al.* Controlled trial of external negative pressure ventilation in severe chronic airflow obstruction. *Am Rev Respir Dis* 1989; **140:** 1251–1256.
30. Martin JG, Levy RD. Respiratory muscle rest. *Probl Respir Care* 1990; **3:** 534–541.
31. Rodenstein DO, Stanescu DC, Cutita G *et al.* Ventilatory and diaphragmatic EMG responses to negative pressure ventilation in airflow obstruction. *J Appl Physiol* 1988; **65:** 1621–1626.
32. Bertrand A, Milane J. La ventilation assiste à domicile des insuffisants respiratoires chroniques dans le région Languedoc-Roussillon. *Rev Franc Mal Respir* 1979; **7:** 341–352.
33. Parent B, Paramelle B, Demetriou R *et al.* Tracheotomie pour ventilation assistée au long cours. A propos de 22 observations d'insuffisance respiratoire chronic et grave. *Rev Franc Mal Respir* 1979; **7:** 356–358.
34. Ellis ER, Bye PTB, Bruderer JW. Treatment of respiratory failure during sleep in patients with neuromuscular disease. *Am Rev Respir Dis* 1987; **135:** 148–152.
35. Kerby GR, Mayer LS, Pingleton SK. Nocturnal positive pressure ventilation via nasal mask. *Am Rev Respir Dis* 1987; **135:** 738–740.
36. Carroll N, Branthwaite MA. Control of nocturnal hypoventilation by nasal intermittent positive pressure ventilation. *Thorax* 1988; **43:** 349–353.
37. Carrey Z, Gottfried SB, Levy RD. Ventilatory muscle support in respiratory failure with nasal positive pressure ventilation. *Chest* 1990; **97:** 150–158.
38. Simonds AK, Parker RA, Branthwaite MA. The effect of intermittent positive pressure hyperinflation in restrictive chest wall disease. *Respiration* 1989; **55:** 136–143.
39. Elliott MW, Simonds AK, Carroll MP *et al.* Domiciliary nocturnal nasal intermittent positive pressure ventilation in hypercapnic respiratory failure due to COPD. *Thorax* 1992; **47:** 342–348.

40. Elliott MW, Mulvey D, Moxham J *et al*. Domiciliary nocturnal nasal intermittent positive pressure ventilation in COPD: mechanisms underlying changes in arterial blood gas tensions. *Eur Respir J* 1991; **4:** 1044–1052.
41. Strumpf DA, Carlisle CC, Millman RP *et al*. Therapy of severe COPD with nocturnal nasal positive pressure ventilation. *Am Rev Respir J* 1990; **141:** A322.
42. Mohr CH, Hill NS. Long-term follow-up of nocturnal ventilatory assistance in patients with respiratory failure due to Duchenne-type muscular dystrophy. *Chest* 1990; **97:** 91–96.
43. Curran FJ, Colbert AP. Ventilator management in Duchenne muscular dystrophy and postpoliomyelitis syndrome; twelve years experience. *Arch Phys Med Rehabil* 1989; **70:** 180–185.
44. Heckmatt JZ, Loh L, Dubowitz V. Night time nasal ventilation in neuromuscular disease. *Lancet* 1990; **335:** 579–582.
45. Howard RS, Wiles CM, Loh L. Respiratory complications and their management in motor neurone disease. *Brain* 1989; **112:** 1155–1170.
46. Goulon M, Goulon-Goeau C. Sclerose lateral amyotrophique et assistance respiratoire. *Rev Neurol (Paris)* 1989; **145:** 293–298.
47. Leger P, Bedicam JM, Cornette A. Long term follow up of severe chronic respiratory insufficiency patients (*n*=373) treated by home nocturnal non-invasive nasal IPPV (cooperative study Lyon/Paris/Nancy/Dijon). *Am Rev Respir Dis* 1991; **143:** A73.
48. Benhamou D, Faure C, Heliot P *et al*. Nasal intermittent positive pressure ventilation (NIPPV) in patients with severe diffuse bronchiectasis (DB) and chronic respiratory failure (CRF). 1991 Abstract; International Conference on Pulmonary Rehabilitation and Home Ventilation: 103.
49. Hodson ME, Madden BP, Steven MH *et al*. Non-invasive nasal ventilation in cystic fibrosis patients – a potential bridge to transplantation. *Eur Respir J* 1991; **4:** 524–527.
50. Simonds AK, Elliott MW, Carroll N *et al*. Improved control of hypercapnic respiratory failure in patients transferred from negative pressure ventilation to nasal intermittent positive pressure ventilation. *Am Rev Respir Dis* 1991; **143:** A586.
51. Jackson M, Hockley S, King MA, Shneerson JM. A comparison of results of treatment with NIPPV or cuirass ventilation. *Am Rev Respir Dis* 1991; **143:** A585.
52. Sassoon CSH. Positive pressure ventilation. Alternate modes. *Chest* 1991; **100:** 421–429.
53. Simonds AK, Elliott MW. Use of the BiPAP ventilator for non-invasive ventilation: advantages and limitations. *Am Rev Respir Dis* 1991; **143:** A585.
54. Branthwaite MA. Non-invasive and domiciliary ventilation: positive pressure techniques. *Thorax* 1991; **46:** 208–212.
55. Elliott MW, Aquilina R, Steven MH, Simonds AK. Effects of expiratory positive airway pressure in patients with chronic airflow limitation and neuromusculo-skeletal disorders receiving nasal intermittent positive pressure ventilation. *Am Rev Respir Dis* 1992; **145:** A527.
56. Delguste P, Aubert-Tulkens G, Rodenstein DO. Upper airway obstruction during nasal intermittent positive pressure hyperventilation in sleep. *Lancet* 1991; **338:** 1295–1297.
57. Splaingard ML, Jefferson LS, Harrison GM. Survival of patients with neuromuscular disease treated at home with negative pressure ventilation (NPV). *Am Rev Respir Dis* 1982; **125:** 139.
58. Sawicka EH, Loh L, Branthwaite MA. Domiciliary ventilatory support: an analysis of outcome. *Thorax* 1988; **43:** 31–35.
59. Simonds AK, Elliott MW, Carroll N, Branthwaite MA. Long term intermittent positive pressure ventilation: clinical, physiological and economic outcome. *Am Rev Respir Dis* 1991; **143:** A586.
60. Dunkin LJ. Home ventilatory assistance. *Anaesthesia* 1983; **38:** 644–649.
61. Goldberg AI, Faure EAM. Home care for life-supported persons in England: the Responaut programme. *Chest* 1984; **86:** 910–914.
62. Pierson DJ. Home respiratory care in different countries. *Eur Respir J* 1989; **2:** 630S–636S.
63. Goldberg AI. Home care for life-supported persons. Is a national approach the answer? *Chest* 1986; 90: 744–748.
64. Muir J-F. Home mechanical ventilation (HMV) organisation and costs (France). In: Marini JJ, Roussos C eds. *Ventilatory Failure. Update in Intensive Care and Emergency Medicine 15*. Heidelberg: Springer-Verlag, 1991.
65. Long term mechanical ventilation. Guidelines for management in the home and at alternate community sites. Report of the *ad hoc* committee, Respiratory care section, American College of Chest Physicians. *Chest* 1986; **90:** 1S–37S.
66. Plummer AL, Donohue WJ, Petty TL. Consensus report: Conference on problems in home mechanical ventilation. *Am Rev Respir Dis* 1989; **140:** 555–560.
67. Make B, Gilmartin M, Brody JS, Snider GL. Rehabilitation of ventilator-dependent subjects with lung diseases. The concept and initial experience. *Chest* 1984; **86:** 358–365.

68. Goldberg AI, Faure EAM, Vaughn CJ *et al*. Home care for life-supported persons: an approach to programme development. *J Pediatr* 1984; **104:** 785–795.
69. Hammond J. Home health care cost effectiveness: an overview of the literature. *Public Health Rep* 1979; **94:** 305–311.
70. Fox DM, Anderson KS, Benjamin AE, Dunatov LJ. Intensive home health care in the United States. Financing as technology. *Int J Technol Assess Health Care* 1987; **3:** 561–573.
71. Marks L. *Home and Hospital Care: Redrawing the Boundaries*. London: Kings Fund Institute, 1991; 31–37.
72. Hedrick SC, Inui TS. The effectiveness and cost of home care: an information synthesis. *Health Serv Res* **1986;** 20: 851–880.
73. Creese AL, Fielden R. Hospital or home care for the severely disabled: a cost comparison. *Br J Prev Soc Med* 1977; **31:** 116–121.
74. Branthwaite MA. Mechanical ventilation at home. *BMJ* 1989; **298:** 1409.

13

Respiratory muscles in health and disease

M. Green and J. Moxham

Weakness

Muscle weakness is common and when present will usually involve the respiratory muscles (Table 13.1). Severe respiratory muscle weakness may, of itself, cause ventilatory failure (e.g. myasthenia gravis) but most commonly weakness is one of several factors contributing to ventilatory failure (e.g. patients in an intensive care unit with weaning difficulties). Respiratory muscle weakness is often overlooked. For a particular patient, respiratory symptoms and signs, ranging from breathlessness on exertion to severe ventilatory failure, reflect the balance between the load imposed on the respiratory muscles by the disease process, and the capacity of the respiratory muscle pump. (Figure 13.1). When the imposed load is high small degrees of impairment of capacity may have important clinical consequences.

The load: capacity relationship is frequently more complex than that expressed by the balance between lung disease and respiratory muscle strength. The capacity of the respiratory muscle pump to lower intrathoracic pressure can be reduced by factors other than muscle weakness; for example, in patients with airways obstruction, hyperinflation leads to shortening of the inspiratory muscles and a reduction in pressure-generating capacity. Similarly, the load on the respiratory muscle pump (limiting its capacity to effect volume change) may be increased by factors other than intrinsic lung disease (e.g. kyphoscoliosis, in which the chest wall is rigid).

In some patients a number of factors may simultaneously act to increase the load on the respiratory muscle pump and at the same time cause respiratory muscle weakness or impair the translation of inspiratory pressure to volume change, for example patients with severe chronic airways obstruction precipitated into ventilatory failure by respiratory infection after abdominal surgery (Table 13.2).

Diagnosis and assessment of respiratory muscle weakness

Symptoms and signs

Severe respiratory muscle weakness causes breathlessness but moderate impairment may cause few problems, particularly in patients with neuromuscular disease who have

Table 13.1 Causes of respiratory muscle weakness

Neurological	
	Polyneuropathy
	Motor neurone disease
	Charcot–Marie–Tooth
	Phrenic nerve trauma/palsy
	Neuralgic amyotrophy
	Poliomyelitis
	Multiple sclerosis
	Traumatic tetraplegia
	Acute porphyria
Neuromuscular transmission	
	Myasthenia gravis
	Eaton–Lambert myasthenic syndrome
Muscle	
	Muscle wasting
	Muscular dystrophy
	Inflammatory myopathies
	Biochemical abnormalities (e.g. acidosis, hypokalaemia, hypophosphataemia)
	Myotonia
	Systemic lupus erythematosus
	Thyroid myopathy
	Acid maltase deficiency

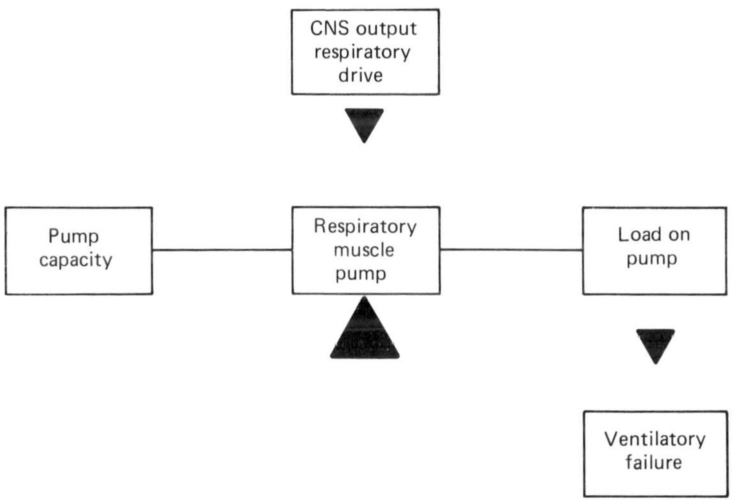

Figure 13.1 Scheme to illustrate the central importance of the respiratory muscle pump and the crucial balance between load and capacity. When the ratio of load to capacity is high, respiratory symptoms, and eventually ventilatory failure, occur

limited exercise capacity. In such patients overt problems may develop only when the load on the respiratory muscle pump is increased (e.g. by respiratory inflection). The onset of ventilatory failure as a consequence of respiratory muscle weakness is frequently gradual and hypoventilation first develops during sleep. Such patients present with

Table 13.2 Factors reducing respiratory muscle force and generation

Muscle shortening (length–tension relationship)
Diaphragm flattening (law of Laplace)
Increased inspiratory flow rate (force–velocity relationship)
Weakness (including neuromuscular block)
Metabolic abnormalities
Hypophosphataemia
Hypomagnesaemia
Hypokalaemia
Hyper- and hypothyroidism
Steroid therapy
Other drugs (e.g. myasthenic syndromes)
Hypoxia
Hypercapnia
Fatigue

characteristic problems of disordered sleep: daytime tiredness, impaired concentration, and eventually cor pulmonale. Some patients with neuromuscular diseases have bulbar dysfunction which predisposes to aspiration. Abdominal muscles are also frequently weak and this impairs cough. The combination of bulbar problems and impaired cough predisposes to repeated and increasingly severe respiratory infections.

The most important ventilatory muscle is the diaphragm. If respiratory muscle weakness spares the diaphragm, ventilatory failure is unlikely. Alternatively, respiratory muscle weakness that includes the diaphragm is likely to be symptomatic. Severe weakness of the diaphragm causes orthopnoea; when the patient is supine the weakened diaphragm is unable to prevent the abdominal contents being sucked up into the thorax during inspiration. Patients with bilateral paralysis of the diaphragm are unable to lie flat. When upright, inspiration is assisted by gravity acting upon the abdominal contents, thereby facilitating diaphragm descent. At rest, patients with isolated diaphragm paralysis are not breathless when standing although they are dyspnoeic on exertion. In normal subjects lying supine, the descent of the diaphragm during inspiration displaces the abdominal contents and moves the anterior abdominal wall outwards. In patients with severe diaphragm weakness the sucking upwards of the diaphragm and abdominal contents into the thorax results in the anterior abdominal wall moving inwards. This paradoxical inward motion of the abdominal wall is an important physical sign of diaphragm paralysis or severe weakness. Severe orthopnoea and obvious abdominal paradox occur only when the strength of the diaphragm is reduced to approximately 25% of normal. Thus, even patients with considerable weakness will not have this symptom or sign [1].

Paralysis of one hemidiaphragm may cause breathlessness, which is usually transient unless there is pre-existing respiratory disease. Not uncommonly, hemidiaphragmatic paralysis is asymptomatic [2].

Radiology

In patients who have near-normal pulmonary compliance, weakness of the respiratory muscles must be severe to reduce lung volume on chest radiograph. The diaphragm is elevated in cases of paralysis or severe weakness and there may be paradoxical movement during inspiration. When screening the diaphragm patients are best kept supine (or as near supine as possible) and should be asked to make a short, sharp, sniff.

Lung function tests

Weakness of both inspiratory and expiratory muscles reduces vital capacity. The measurement of vital capacity is therefore an excellent, simple, test for detecting respiratory muscle weakness. However, because relatively small pressures are required to inflate the normal lung, substantial falls in vital capacity occur only when respiratory muscle weakness is moderately severe. For a given degree of respiratory muscle weakness the reduction in vital capacity will also be determined by the compliance of the lung and chest wall. Furthermore, vital capacity will be reduced by many other co-existent respiratory disorders (e.g. COPD). Thus, vital capacity can be a rather insensitive, inaccurate and non-specific measurement of respiratory muscle weakness. However, in routine clinical practice it is still a useful observation and one that should be undertaken in all patients in whom respiratory muscle weakness is a possible diagnosis (Figure 13.2). In patients with substantial diaphragm weakness, vital capacity falls in the supine posture. The measurement of the change in vital capacity is therefore of considerable clinical value (Figure 13.3). A marked reduction in supine vital capacity occurs in those patients who also have orthopnoea and abdominal paradox [1]. In patients with bilateral diaphragm paralysis, the fall in vital capacity is approximately 50% [4].

Although the measurement of vital capacity has limitations in the assessment of

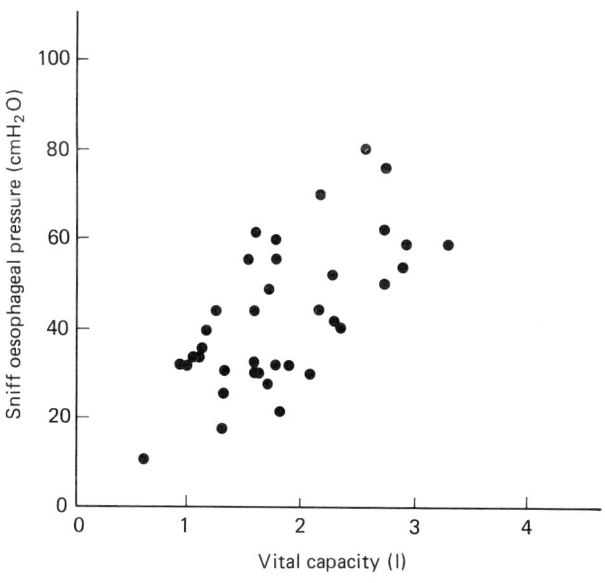

Figure 13.2 Relationship between vital capacity and global inspiratory muscle strength as judged by sniff oesophageal pressure in patients with isolated neuromuscular disease. (From [3], with permission)

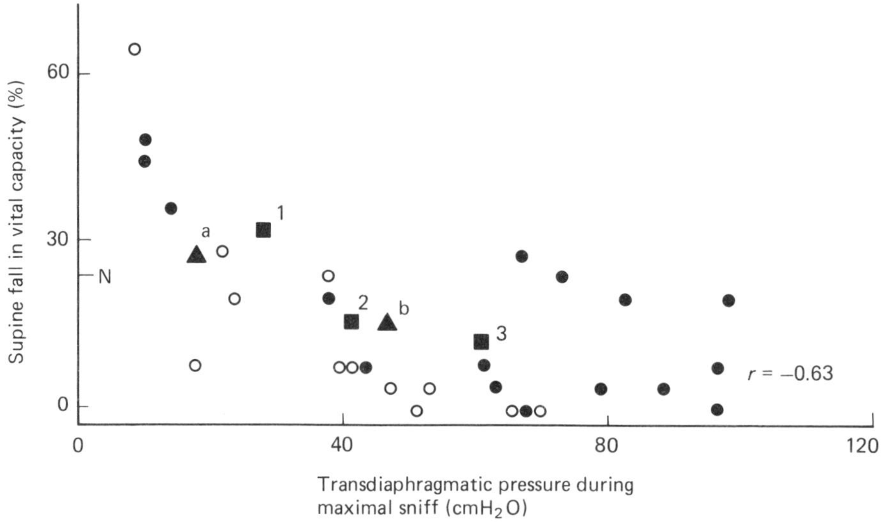

Figure 13.3 Relationship between percentage fall in vital capacity on adopting the supine posture and transdiaphragmatic pressure during maximal sniffs. The two sequences (■ 1–3 and ▲ a and b) represent two male patients studied as their clinical condition improved. (After [1], with permission)

respiratory muscle weakness, the demonstration of a normal supine vital capacity indicates that a patient does not have substantial respiratory muscle weakness and, in the absence of excessive respiratory loading, any undetected weakness is unlikely to be clinically significant.

The restrictive ventilatory defect caused by respiratory muscle weakness reduces overall gas transfer (DLCO), but increases the transfer coefficient (KCO). An elevated KCO in a patient with a restrictive ventilatory defect is a useful pointer to the possibility of respiratory muscle weakness (Table 13.3).

Arterial blood gases

Ventilatory failure occurs only when respiratory muscle weakness is severe and generalized. Isolated bilateral diaphragm paralysis rarely causes ventilatory failure [4]. In the absence of excessive loading, hypercapnia will not normally develop until respiratory muscle strength is reduced to less than 30% of normal [5]. Initially hypercapnia occurs only during sleep and sleep studies are therefore an important part of assessment. From a clinical standpoint it is important to note that the presence of hypercapnia implies severe weakness – and substantial weakness is still possible despite normal levels of blood gases.

Respiratory pressures

The strength and weakness of the respiratory muscles is conventionally measured by documenting their capacity to generate pressure.

Table 13.3 Lung function in six patients with severe isolated diaphragm weakness

Patient no.	*Vital capacity (litres, % predicted)*	*Supine vital capacity (% fall)*	*FEV_1 (litres, % predicted)*	*Total lung capacity (% predicted)*	*Residual value (% predicted)*	*Diffusing capacity (% predicted) DLCO*	*Krogh constant (% predicted) KCO*
1	2.2, 45	36	1.7, 47	64	85	78	142
2	2.5, 56	35	1.9, 54	63	139	65	122
3	2.2, 45	55	1.7, 50	79	101	59	101
4	3.2, 69	37	2.5, 74	83	124	75	101
5	1.7, 40	30	1.3, 38	59	90	44	137
6	1.5, 36	30	1.5, 45	54	83	71	167
Mean	2.1, 48	37	1.8, 51	67	104	65	128
s.d.	0.7, 12	9	0.4, 12	11	23	12	26

From [4], with permission

Mouth pressures

The strength of the expiratory muscles (PE_{max}) can be measured by recording the pressure at the mouth when the patient makes a maximum expiratory effort, against a closed airway from total lung capacity. The strength of the inspiratory muscles (PI_{max}) can be assessed by recording the mouth pressure during a maximum effort from residual volume or functional residual capacity. The measurement of maximum static mouth pressures has the great advantage of being more specific for respiratory muscle strength than the measurement of vital capacity. When mouth pressure measurements are performed well (by both the patient and the operator) the information is very useful for assessing respiratory muscle weakness. Maximum effort by the patient is crucial and many points of detail require attention. The results also depend upon the type of mouthpiece used, and this is an important point when comparing the result for a particular patient with published normal values [6] (Table 13.4). Hitherto, measurements of mouth pressure have usually been undertaken in specialist laboratories but meters for measuring mouth pressures are now portable and suitable for use in respiratory clinics or at the bedside (Figure 13.4).

Table 13.4 Reference normal ranges for PE_{max} and PI_{max}*

No.	PE_{max}	PI_{max}	*Reference no.*	*Mouthpiece design*
Male				
106	23.4(4.5)	12.7(3.1)	7	Tube
60	22.8(4.1)	12.1(2.1)	8	Tube
80	21.2(4.4)	12.4(2.7)	9	Tube
325	15.1(8.0)	11.1(3.5)	10	Flanged
80	14.5(3.3)	10.4(3.0)	11	Flanged
46	13.7(3.7)	10.3(2.5)	12	Flanged
Female				
94	16.1(2.9)	9.6(2.4)	7	Tube
60	14.9(2.6)	8.5(1.5)	8	Tube
121	13.5(6.7)	8.9(2.4)	9	Tube
480	9.2(3.2)	7.0(2.6)	10	Flanged
87	9.1(1.6)	7.2(2.1)	11	Flanged
60	8.7(2.3)	6.9(2.3)	12	Flanged

*kPa = 10.19 cmH_2O. PE_{max}, maximum static expiratory pressure; PI_{max}, maximum static inspiratory pressure.
Values in parentheses are s.d. From [6] with permission

A PI_{max} more negative than 80 cmH_2O excludes clinically significant inspiratory muscle weakness. Unless respiratory load is excessive it is unusual for patients to develop ventilatory failure unless maximum respiratory pressures are reduced to less than 30% of normal [5] (Figure 13.5).

Oesophageal pressures

When vital capacity (sitting and supine) is near normal and maximum mouth pressures are high, respiratory muscle weakness can be excluded. However, vital capacity is frequently reduced because of co-existing lung disease and low mouth pressures can often be due to poor patient effort or difficulty with the technique. In these circumstances identification and quantitation of respiratory muscle weakness are frequently

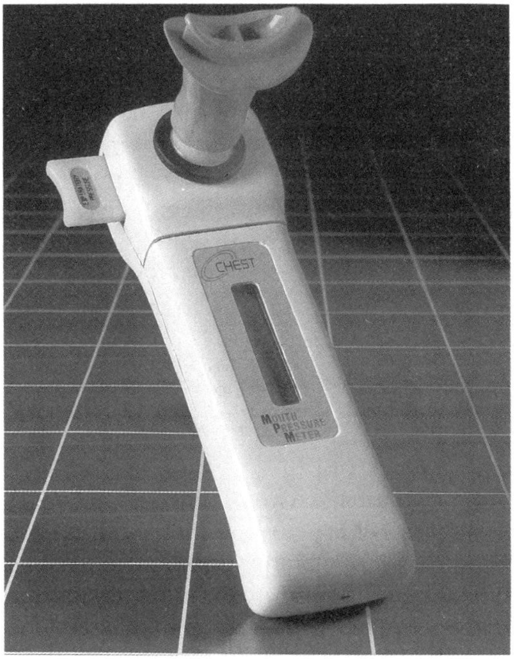

Figure 13.4 Meter for measurement of mouth pressures. (Precision Medical Ltd, Pickering, Yorkshire,UK)

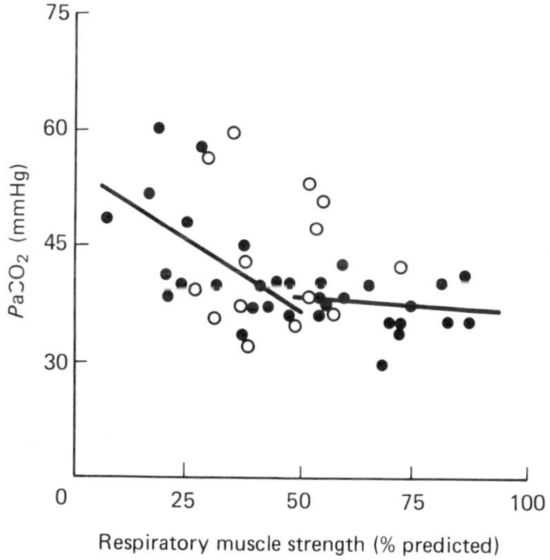

Figure 13.5 Relationship between arterial carbon dioxide tension ($Paco_2$) and respiratory muscle strength in 33 patients with uncomplicated myopathy (●, regression line) and 14 patients with myopathy plus chronic lung disease (○). Respiratory muscle strength is the sum of inspiratory and expiratory maximum static mouth pressure, expressed as a percentage of normal and divided by two. (Reproduced from [5], with permission)

impossible using these tests and the measurement of oesophageal pressure then becomes a useful tool. Oesophageal pressure during a static maximum inspiratory effort is very similar to pressure generated at the mouth, and in patients who have difficulty in making this static manoeuvre it is equally misleading. However when patients perform a maximum sniff they commonly generate larger oesophageal pressures [13] (Figure 13.6). Oesophageal sniff pressure has a narrower normal range than static measurements and is more reproducible. The superiority of the sniff manoeuvre is most likely a reflection of it being a natural inspiratory effort – the mouth and lips are closed but the nose is not clipped. The clinical use of oesophageal sniff pressure has demonstrated that many patients that would be judged to be weak by static measurements have normal respiratory muscle strength (Figure 13.6).

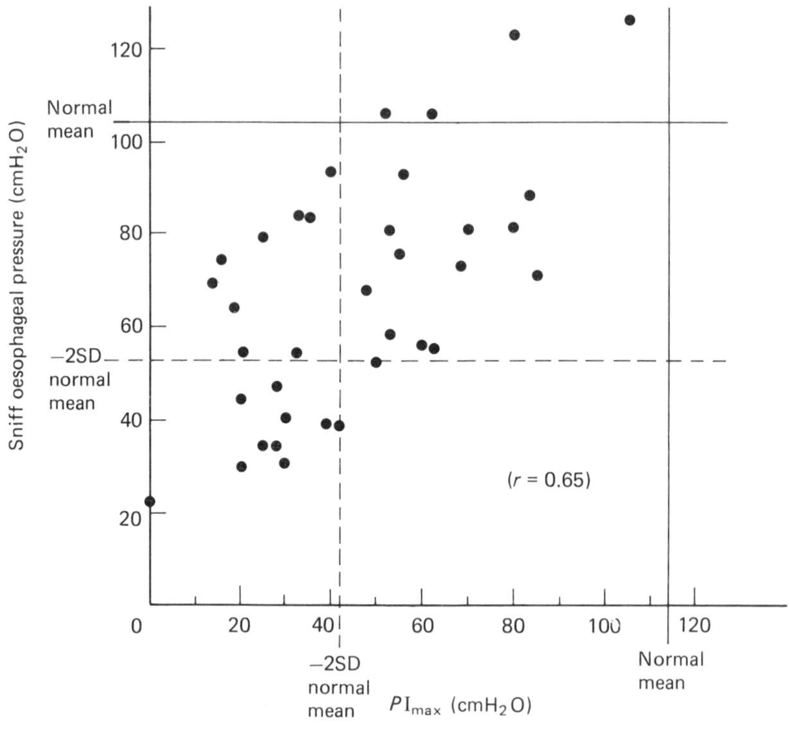

Figure 13.6 Maximum static inspiratory mouth pressure versus maximum sniff oesophageal pressure in 36 male patients investigated for respiratory muscle weakness. (Reproduced from [13], with permission)

Nasopharyngeal pressure

During a maximum sniff manoeuvre the nose narrows and nasal flow is greatly limited [14], thereby facilitating the generation of high oesophageal pressures. Pressures are high at all points beyond the flow-limiting segment of the nose, and pressures are therefore high in the nasopharynx. To measure nasopharyngeal pressure (*P*np) a conventional balloon catheter is advanced 10 cm from the anterior nares after applying local anaesthesia to the nose. The 10 cm oesophageal balloon has its proximal 5 cm taped leaving a distal 5 cm balloon into which 0.7 ml of air is introduced. Nasopharyngeal balloons are well tolerated by patients and during a sniff manoeuvre the pressure recorded in the nasopharynx is close to the intrathoracic pressure and therefore gives a good index of inspiratory muscle strength [15]. In some patients a balloon catheter placed in the mouth (with the lips closed) records a sniff pressure (*P*mo)similar to that in the nasopharynx and oesophagus [15] (Figure 13.7). Occasionally, patients find it less easy to sniff with a mouth balloon than with one in the nasopharynx. Sniff oesophageal, nasopharyngeal or mouth pressure can provide a very accurate measurement of inspiratory muscle strength, and in practice a pressure more negative than 60 cmH_2O excludes substantial weakness; a pressure less negative than this indicates that respiratory muscle weakness is likely and further investigations are required.

Transdiaphragmatic pressure

The diaphragm is the major muscle of inspiration and it is often helpful specifically to measure its strength. Furthermore, in patients with weakness (as determined by low inspiratory mouth, nasopharyngeal or oesophageal pressures) it is helpful to partition that weakness between the diaphragm and other inspiratory muscles. Diaphragm strength can be specifically assessed by measuring transdiaphragmatic pressure (*P*di) with balloon catheters positioned in the oesophagus and in the stomach. When the diaphragm contracts oesophageal pressure (*P*oes) becomes negative and gastric pressure becomes positive; the transdiaphragmatic pressure is the difference between the two. The best manoeuvre for assessing transdiaphragmatic pressure is a maximum, 'natural' sniff [16] (Figure 13.8). Historically, *P*di has been measured for a maximum static inspiratory effort but the sniff manoeuvre is easier for patients to perform, generates more reproducible results, and the normal range is narrower. Sniff *P*di is therefore a better measurement when diaphragm weakness is

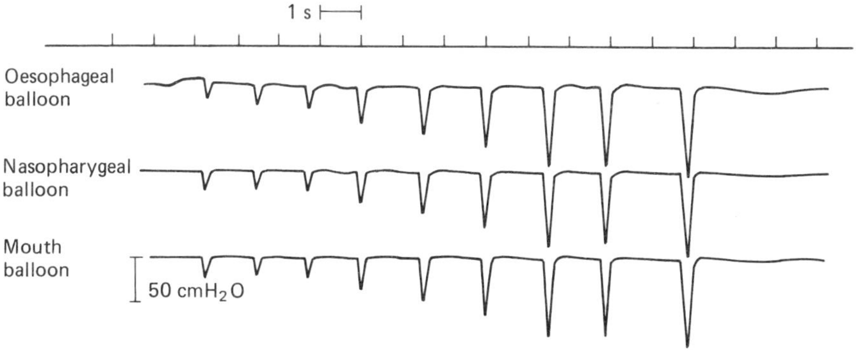

Figure 13.7 Simultaneous pressure waveforms from oesophageal, nasopharyngeal and mouth balloons in a single normal subject performing sniffs of increasing effort. Paper speed was 10 mm/s. (Reproduced from [15], with permission)

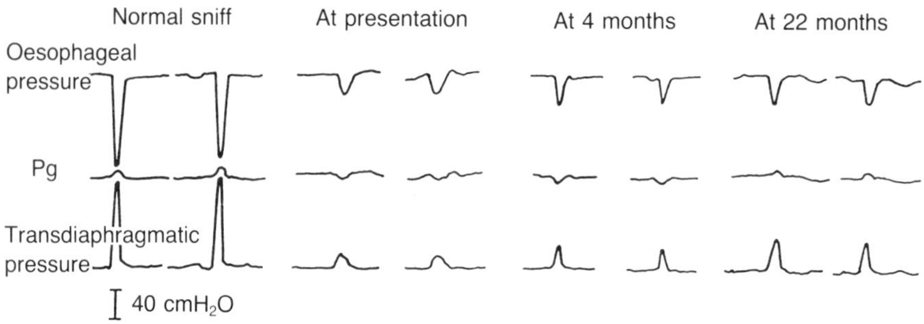

Figure 13.8 Sniff transdiaphragmatic pressure in a normal subject (top left) and a patient with weakness due to phrenic nerve trauma. The diaphragm weakness gradually improved over a 22-month period

being investigated. A sniff *P*di greater than 100 cmH_2O in males and 70 cmH_2O in females excludes important diaphragm weakness; values much below these strongly support the diagnosis. The measurement of sniff *P*di has been useful in identifying diaphragm weakness in a wide range of patients, including those with thyroid disease [17], myasthenia gravis [18], Addison's disease [19], Charcot–Marie–Tooth disease [20], Eaton–Lambert myasthenic syndrome [21] and neuralgic amyotrophy [22]. The precise quantification of diaphragm weakness has also enhanced our understanding of the symptoms and signs of diaphragm weakness: orthopnoea and abdominal paradox [1] (Figure 13.9).

Volitional versus non-volitional tests of strength

A major disadvantage of maximum mouth, nasopharyngeal, oesophageal and transdiaphragmatic pressures for the assessment of respiratory muscle strength is that the manoeuvres are volitional. Many patients find it difficult to make truly maximum efforts and it is not always possible for the operator to be sure that maximum efforts have been made. If the pressures generated are high it is likely that effort has been maximal (or nearly so), and respiratory muscle weakness is excluded. However, if pressures are low, doubt often remains as to whether the respiratory muscles are weak. Although repeated measurements and close observation of the pressure traces can reduce uncertainty, doubt frequently remains. In these cases a non-volitional test of respiratory muscle strength would be of great value. The strength of limb muscles can be investigated by electrical stimulation techniques and, although similar techniques cannot be applied to all of the muscles of respiration, the diaphragm can be stimulated via its phrenic nerve supply.

Phrenic nerve stimulation

The phrenic nerves can be electrically stimulated using surface or needle electrodes [23]. The results achieved by the two techniques are similar but surface electrodes are more acceptable. Phrenic nerve function can be assessed by measuring the conduction time from the stimulus artefact to the diaphragm evoked action potential record-

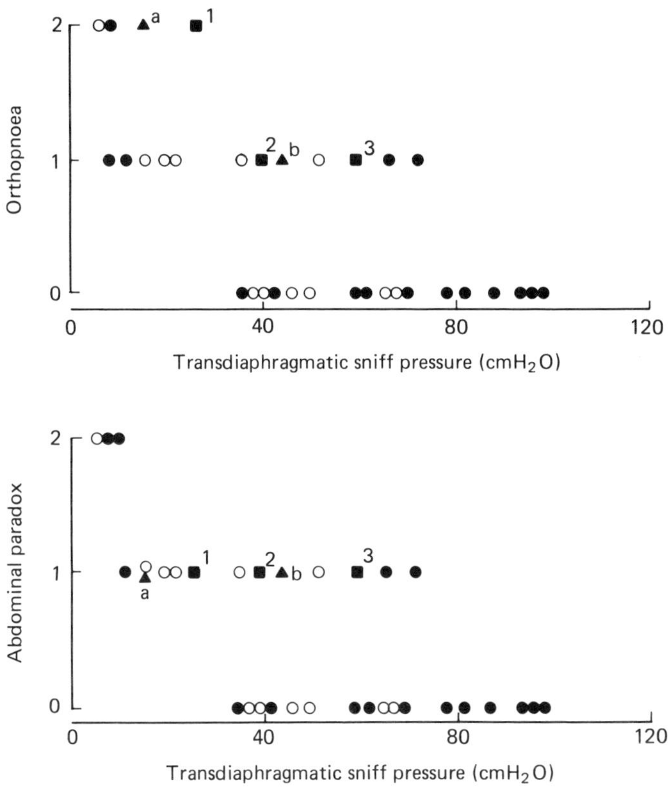

Figure 13.9 Association between grade of orthopnoea (upper panel) and degree of abdominal paradox (lower panel), and transdiaphragmatic pressure during maximal sniffs. The two sequences (■ 1–3 and ▲ a and b) represent two male patients studied as their clinical condition improved. (Reproduced from [1], with permission)

ed by surface electrodes. Phrenic nerve conduction time is less than 9.5 ms in normal subjects. The transdiaphragmatic pressure twitch response (twitch *P*di) following phrenic nerve stimulation gives a useful objective measurement of diaphragm contractility. Phrenic nerves can be stimulated unilaterally and bilaterally and normal values have been reported. Supramaximal bilateral phrenic nerve stimulation generates a twitch *P*di of approximately 25–30 cmH_2O. The electrical stimulation technique usually works well for normal subjects being studied in the laboratory but it is less satisfactory when applied to patients, many of whom find the electrical technique uncomfortable, particularly when attempts are made to achieve bilateral supramaximal stimulation. Furthermore, in many clinical situations (for example in the intensive care unit) practical problems are considerable. For these reasons the electrical stimulation technique has been of limited clinical value.

The technique of magnetic stimulation [24] of the phrenic nerve roots has considerable advantages compared with electrical phrenic nerve stimulation. The method is less uncomfortable and it is frequently easier to activate the diaphragm. The magnetic coil is placed over the cervical spine at the level of C6–C7 with the neck flexed.

The twitch *P*di elicited is highly reproducible and similar to that produced by supramaximal bilateral electrical stimulation [25] (Figure 13.10). This technique represents an important advance in the diagnosis and accurate measurement of diaphragm weakness. It is likely that diaphragm function will now be studied in a variety of clinical circumstances in which measurements were not hitherto possible.

Scheme for patient assessment

Patients are usually referred for assessment with two questions in mind: is there weakness of the respiratory muscles? If such weakness is present, how severe is it? An appropriate history and examination followed by the application of the tests of respiratory muscle strength outlined above will usually answer these questions [26] (Table 13.5).

The balance of respiratory muscle capacity and load

The clinical importance of respiratory muscle weakness depends not only on the severity of that weakness but also on the respiratory load imposed on the muscle pump. Thus, the balance between load and capacity is more important than either of these two factors in isolation (Figure 13.1). It is now possible to assess respiratory muscle strength and weakness with considerable precision and therefore provide accurate data on respiratory muscle pump capacity. However, the load on the muscle pump is less easily measured. This load is reflected in the pressure that the inspiratory muscles generate during ventilation. Laboratory-based experimental work has demonstrated that when the mean inspiratory pressure (*P*m) becomes a high fraction of maximum pressure (i.e. Pm/PI_{max} = 0.15–0.2) the load cannot be sustained and ventilation fails [27]. Similarly, studies on patients in the intensive care unit have demonstrated that during failure to wean from mechanical ventilation this load: capacity ratio is greater than 0.15 whereas for patients weaning successfully the ratio is below this value [28]. It should be stressed that some patients with greatly reduced capacity due to respiratory muscle weakness have a low load: capacity ratio because the load is also low and these patients wean successfully. In contrast, some patients with less weak respiratory muscles nevertheless fail to wean because the load is excessively high.

Respiratory muscle fatigue

Conceptually it appears entirely reasonable that when the load imposed on the respiratory muscle pump is excessive compared to its capacity, the respiratory muscles could develop fatigue and precipitate ventilatory failure. The notion of respiratory muscle fatigue has attracted great scientific interest over the last decade, and much effort has been expended in an attempt to detect fatigue in the clinical context [29]. One problem has been to define exactly what is meant by 'fatigue'. Recently a NHLBI Workshop defined fatigue as the loss of capacity to develop force and/or velocity, in response to a load, that is reversible by rest [30]. A further complexity is

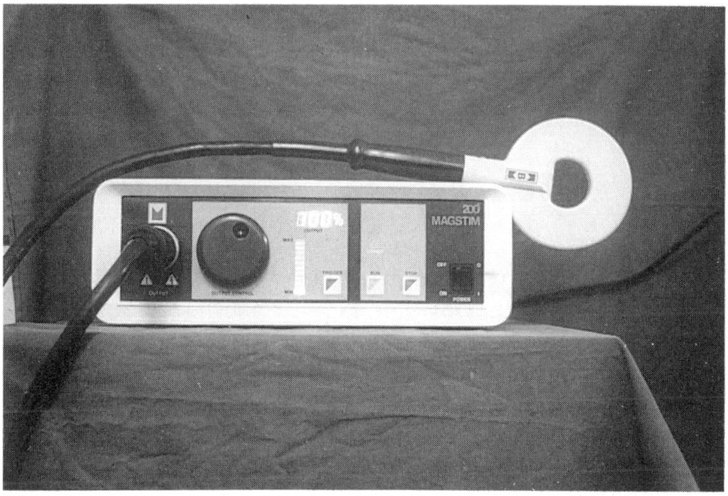

Figure 13.10 Magnetic stimulator (Magstim Co. Ltd., Whitland,Dyfedd, UK). When applied to the flexed neck at the level of C6–C7 the coil activates the phrenic nerve roots

Table 13.5 Sequential assessment of patients with possible respiratory muscle weakness

History and examination	Respiratory muscle involvement is likely in any patient with a neurological or muscle disorder
Sitting and supine vital capacity	Normal supine vital capacity excludes important respiratory muscle weakness
Lung function, including KCO	The combination of reduced TLC and normal or raised KCO in a patient with reduced lung volumes suggests respiratory muscle weakness
Arterial (or arterialized ear lobe) blood gas analysis	Hypoxaemia due to weakness implies moderately severe disease: hypercapnia indicates severe weakness
PI and PE_{max}	PI_{max} more negative than 60–80 cmH_2O excludes important inspiratory muscle weakness
If PI_{max} low, measure sniff, mouth or nasopharyngeal pressures	Sniff *Pmo* or *Pnp* more negative than 60 cmH_2O excludes important inspiratory muscle weakness
If sniff *Pmo* or *Pnp* low (or if significant co-existing lung disease) measure sniff oesophageal pressure	Sniff *Poes* nore negative than 60 cmH_2O excludes important inspiratory muscle weakness
If sniff *Poes* low and/or specific assessment is required of diaphragm weakness, measure transdiaphragmatic pressure	Sniff *Pdi* of 70–100 cmH_2O excludes important diaphragm weakness
If sniff *Pdi* low (or in patients unable to perform voluntary maoneuvres) stimulate phrenic nerves electrically or magnetically and measure *Pdi* and nerve conduction time	Conduction time is normally 9.5 ms. Twitch *Pdi* of 10.5 (right), 8.8 (left) and 20.7 cmH_2O(bilateral) exclude important diaphragm weakness

From [26], with permission

that any loss of tension generation in muscle could be due to failure of any of the links in the chain of physiological events involved in tension generation, from the central nervous system to the peripheral contractile machinery [31]. By convention, failure within the central nervous system is termed 'central fatigue' and failure beyond the central nervous system is termed 'peripheral fatigue'.

Central fatigue

When normal subjects undertake maximum voluntary contractions all motor units can be fully activated and under these circumstances a superimposed electrical stimulus produces no augmentation of force. However, if individuals are sub-maximally activating peripheral muscle despite their best efforts, the interpolation of an electrical stimulus produces an increase in force. Electrical stimulation can therefore provide a test of whether central activation is maximal or whether there is an element of central fatigue. Studies of limb and respiratory muscles have clearly demonstrated that when normal subjects are set endurance tasks it is possible to demonstrate substantial central fatigue in some individuals [32, 33]. However, it is also clear that central fatigue is dependent on the task involved and is more likely to occur in prolonged low-intensity exercise protocols. Such studies are tedious for the subjects and it is not certain that the central fatigue that can be detected in the laboratory necessarily implies that central fatigue occurs in patients during ventilatory failure.

Peripheral fatigue

Fatigue due to failure of peripheral neuromuscular processes is conventionally divided into *high-frequency fatigue*, which is due to failure of excitation at the neuromuscular junction or the muscle cell membrane, and *low-frequency fatigue*, in which excitation processes are not impaired and force failure is due to impaired performance of the intramuscular contractile machinery.

High-frequency fatigue can be produced in the laboratory easily by electrically stimulating muscle via its nerve supply at high frequencies [34]. When this is done there is rapid force loss and an associated decline in the electromyogram. The force loss is a consequence of failure of excitation. This type of fatigue can also be demonstrated following high-intensity ischaemic voluntary contractions. Although it is possible to demonstrate high-frequency fatigue during these physiological studies on normal subjects in the laboratory, it is, again, not clear whether such fatigue occurs in clinical ventilatory failure. Most investigators regard high-frequency fatigue as an unlikely explanation of task failure except in laboratory studies [35]. One study in the literature has demonstrated excitation failure in the respiratory muscles of rabbits subjected to exhaustive inspiratory loading [36], but as yet it has not been possible to detect this type of fatigue in patients. High-frequency fatigue produces rapid force loss and if this type of fatigue were to develop in the respiratory muscles, there would be 'catastrophic' force loss and dramatic failure of the respiratory muscle pump [37].

Given that the task facing the individual is to optimize force generation (and minimize fatigue) it could be argued that central excitation must be sufficient to minimize submaximal activation (central fatigue) but not be so high as to precipitate excitation failure (high-frequency fatigue). Experimental work on limb muscle contractions in normal subjects strongly supports the hypothesis that the central nervous system is capable of modulating central output to optimize force generation. During a prolonged fatiguing maximum voluntary effort, for example, there is a progressive and gradual reduction in central firing frequency which serves to optimize force generation and minimize fatigue [34]. If at any point central nervous system output were to rise the result would be the precipitation of high-frequency fatigue. If central nervous system output were to fall inappropriately there would be central fatigue and further force loss (Figure 13.11). The central nervous system appears to exert a 'central wisdom' which avoids both central fatigue and high-frequency fatigue. Although, as yet, there is no information from patients to substantiate the concept of central wisdom, respiratory drive is high in patients in respiratory failure [38] and it therefore appears

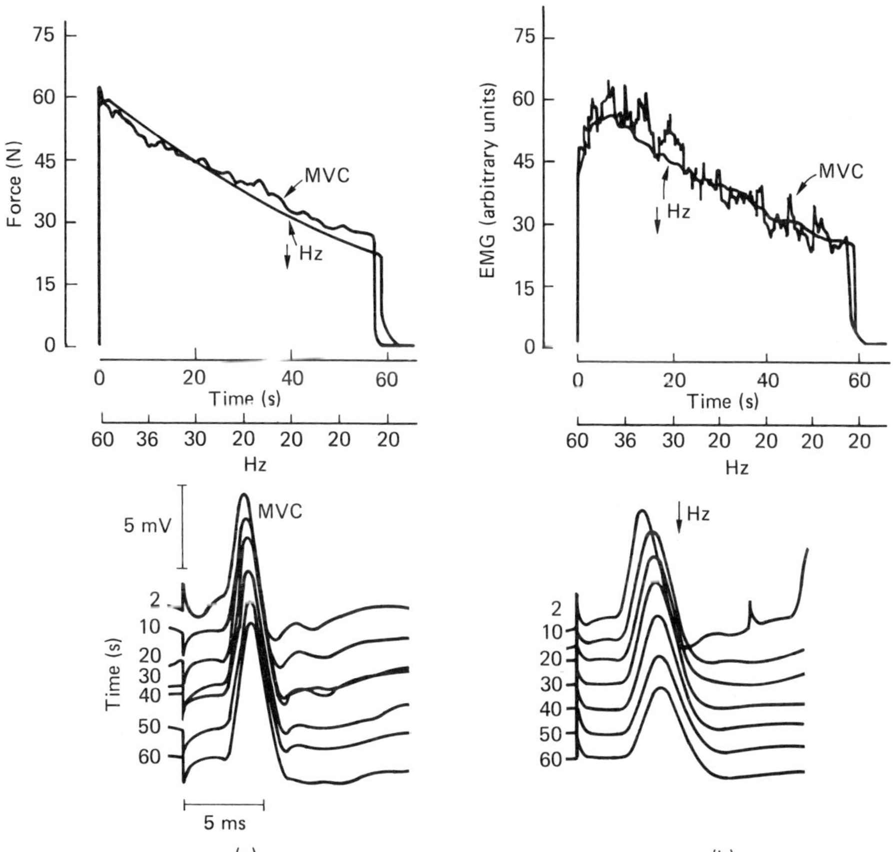

Figure 13.11 Top: Maximum voluntary contractions (MVC) of the adductor pollicis muscle, sustained for 60 s. (a) During an electrically stimulated contraction, the force of the MVC is matched by initial stimulation at 60 Hz, followed by progressive reduction of the stimulation frequency to 20 Hz; (b) the surface EMGs for voluntary and stimulated contractions are closely matched. Bottom: The EMG M-waves during MVC and stimulated contractions are well maintained. (Reproduced from [34], with permission)

unlikely that the respiratory muscles are sub-optimally driven. Indeed, evidence from studies of patients undergoing weaning from mechanical ventilation strongly suggests that central fatigue does not occur [39] (see below). Because the onset of high-frequency fatigue leads to catastrophic and rapid force loss, it would appear to be a highly inappropriate strategy for patients in ventilatory failure to drive peripheral respiratory muscle into such a fatigue state.

When muscle develops low-frequency fatigue the force response is markedly reduced when the muscle is electrically stimulated at low frequencies whereas the force response is relatively well maintained with stimulation at higher frequencies. The frequency force curve for the muscle is thus shifted to the right (Figure 13.12). This type of contractile failure has been extensively studied in respiratory and limb muscles [41, 42]. Laboratory-based studies have consistently documented that low-frequency fatigue develops only when muscle is subjected to very severe and prolonged loading. These studies have also demonstrated that low-frequency fatigue can persist for many hours and is associated with substantial muscle damage [43]. Because low-frequency fatigue is detected by electrical stimulation techniques it has been difficult to study this type of fatigue in patients with ventilatory failure. Although a few studies have detected such fatigue in patients it remains uncertain as to how important low-frequency fatigue is in the clinical situation [42, 44]. The development of low-frequency fatigue implies that to sustain a given ventilatory load there must be an increase in motor neurone firing frequency which would then almost certainly lead to greater fatigue, necessitating a further increase in firing frequency and a progressively fatiguing situation. Furthermore, because progressive increases in motor neurone firing frequency will precipitate high-

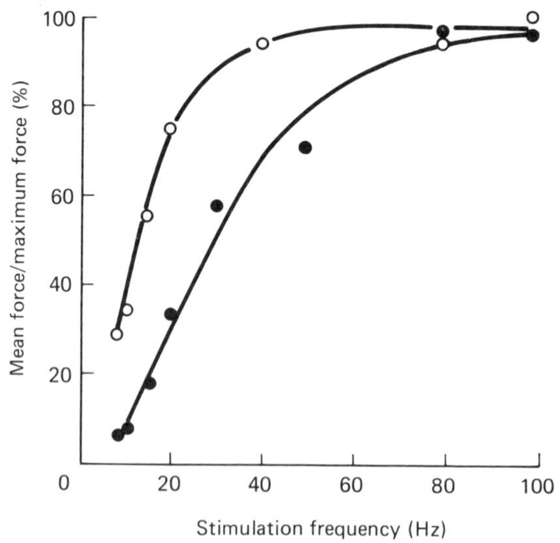

Figure 13.12 Control frequency/force curve of the sternomastoid of a normal subject (○). The subject then breathed through an inspiratory resistance generating 70% of his maximum inspiratory mouth pressure for 200 breaths. The resulting frequency/force curve (●) shows a marked shift to the right with low-frequency fatigue. (Reproduced from [40], with permission)

frequency fatigue (but failure to increase frequency will result in task failure), low-frequency fatigue is likely to be inherently unstable and inconsistent with a steady state (e.g. stable chronic ventilatory failure).

Is fatigue important in chronic ventilatory failure?

In recent years some investigators have suggested that in patients with chronic ventilatory failure the respiratory muscles could be chronically fatigued [45]. This suggestion appears intuitively unlikely given the dynamic nature of fatigue. From what we know about central fatigue, peripheral high- and low-frequency fatigue, they are unlikely to be persistent and stable. In some studies of patients with chronic ventilatory failure maximum respiratory pressures have increased following prolonged periods of respiratory muscle 'rest' by assisted ventilation [46]. These improvements in respiratory muscle strength have been attributed to the reversal of chronic fatigue by rest. However, there have been no adequately controlled studies and improved performance following assisted ventilation could equally well represent either improved effort on behalf of patients, or a learning effect improving their ability to perform strength tests. Furthermore, some studies have failed to demonstrate improvements in respiratory muscle strength [47] (Figure 13.13).

Although there is little evidence to support the notion of chronic central or high-frequency fatigue, the possibility of chronic low-frequency fatigue has not, as yet,

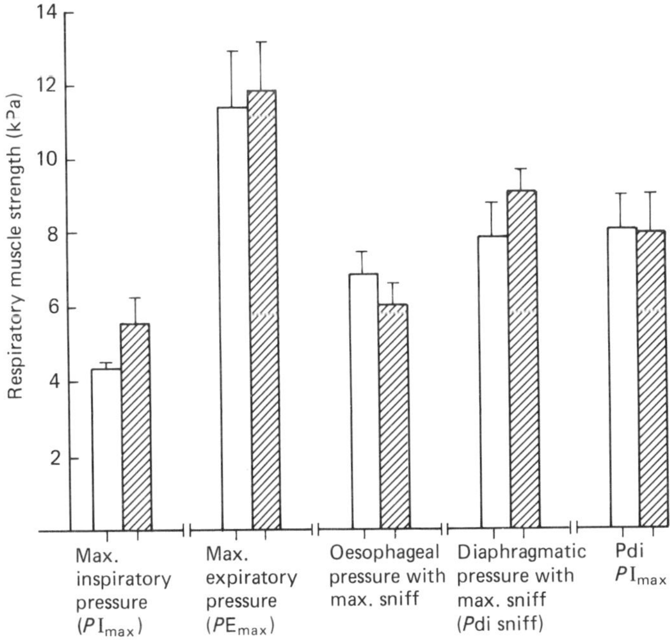

Figure 13.13 Indices of respiratory muscle strength before (■) and after (▨) 6 months' nasal intermittent positive-pressure ventilation. Results are expressed in kPa as mean ± s.e. (Reproduced from [47], with permission)

been excluded. This issue could be addressed by studying respiratory muscle contractility (diaphragm strength in terms of transdiaphragmatic pressure) using phrenic nerve stimulation techniques. Such studies could be possible in patients with chronic ventilatory failure using the new technique of magnetic stimulation.

Overall, there is little information to support the concept of chronic respiratory muscle fatigue, and unless further data become available to support this hypothesis the possibility of such fatigue should not influence clinical management. On the data currently available it seems more likely that hypercapnia develops as a result of relative hypoventilation of the respiratory system in response to the respiratory load being excessive in relation to capacity – the central nervous system adjusting respiratory centre output to avoid overt fatigue; that is, the central nervous system exerts central wisdom.

Does fatigue occur in acute ventilatory failure?

A useful clinical model of acute ventilatory failure is provided by patients who are undergoing weaning trials on the intensive care unit and who subsequently develop ventilatory failure, hypercapnia, and weaning failure. It is possible in these patients to measure the load imposed on the respiratory muscle pump (in terms of intrathoracic pressures and tidal volumes) and also the capacity of the respiratory muscles (in terms of maximum pressure-generating capacity). In this way the ratio of load to capacity can be documented. Studies of patients weaning from ventilation show that when the load is high in relation to capacity weaning will fail and when the ratio is more favourable, weaning will succeed [28]. However, weaning failure does not necessarily imply respiratory muscle fatigue. It is equally plausible that the respiratory system is responding to excessive loading by reducing ventilation through the mechanism of reducing central respiratory drive. The question arises as to whether there is any good evidence that the respiratory muscles develop fatigue during weaning failure? Many of the techniques necessary to study central and peripheral fatigue are exceptionally difficult to apply to patients undergoing weaning trials. However, there are aspects of the fatiguing 'process' that are amenable to study.

The 'process' of fatigue

Muscle fatigue, in the sense of failure to achieve tension, can be understood as the end result of a continuous 'process' that is initiated whenever a muscle is subjected to a sufficiently large load. Fatigue is thus a normal and predictable physiological response to excessive load and is associated with many complex alterations of physiological function affecting all aspects of the events involved in a voluntary contraction. Although tension generation decreases during fatigue, energy depletion sufficient to produce rigor and irreversible muscle damage, and excitation failure (which would precipitate catastrophic force loss) do not normally occur because of adaptive reduction of central drive. Hypercapnic ventilatory failure can be viewed as the response of the respiratory system to excessive loading whereby respiratory drive is reduced to avoid fatigue. Alternatively, hypercapnia can be viewed as the response of the respiratory system to the onset of the fatigue process prior to the development of overt and damaging fatigue events. The difference between these two views is subtle but important [48], not least because it may be possible to detect the onset of the fatigue process.

Can the fatigue process be detected early?

The rate at which tension declines following active muscle contraction can be measured as the maximum relaxation rate (MRR). The relaxation of muscle is an active energy-consuming process and MRR is affected by temperature, thyroid status, the inherent speed of muscle (i.e. muscle fibre types) and fatigue. When skeletal muscle is subjected to an excessive load there is an early slowing of MRR and this physiological change can be viewed as an early signal of the fatiguing process. The MRR of the respiratory muscles is similar to that of other skeletal muscles and it has been demonstrated that MRR slows following exhaustive inspiratory loading in normal subjects [49] (Figure 13.14). Although MRR can be measured for voluntary and electrically stimulated contractions, in practice the easiest way to measure MRR is to record oesophageal or transdiaphragmatic pressures during sharp submaximal sniff manoeuvres. When respiratory muscle MRR is slowed by exhaustive inspiratory loading the time course of recovery during rest is rapid, exponential, and closely similar to the recovery rate of MRR in fatigued limb muscle. The observations that the MRR of respiratory muscles is numerically similar to limb muscle, slows with exhaustive inspiratory loading, and recovers with the expected time course all strongly suggest that respiratory muscle MRR measured from respiratory pressures is indeed reflecting the relaxation rate of the respiratory muscles. Furthermore, the observation that MRR measured from twitch *P*di behaves similarly to that recorded from voluntary diaphragm contractions supports the hypothesis that changes in MRR reflect an alteration in peripheral diaphragm function.

In studies on intubated patients on the intensive care unit MRR has been measured from sniff-like inspiratory manoeuvres before and during weaning [39]. Using balloon catheters MRR was measured for both oesophageal and transdiaphragmatic

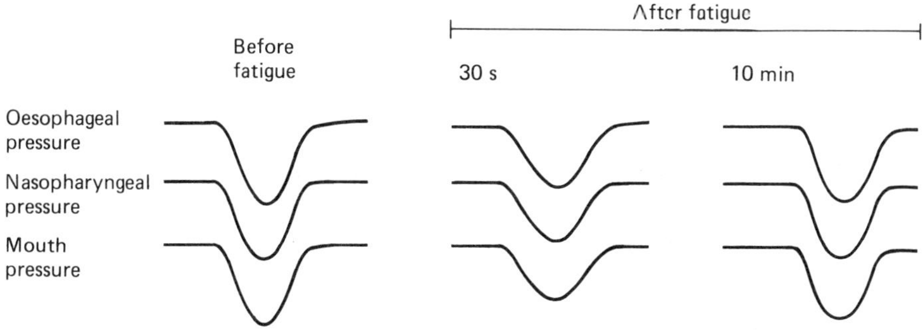

Figure 13.14 Pressure measured in the oesophagus, nasopharynx and mouth during a sniff manoeuvre in a normal subject before, 30 s and 10 min after inspiratory resistive loading to exhaustion. Note the reduced slope of the pressure wave with fatigue (reflecting the slowing of muscle contraction and relaxation) and the subsequent recovery. (Reproduced from [49], with permission)

pressures. Sequential measurements of MRR demonstrated that in patients who weaned successfully MRR remained unchanged whereas in patients failing to wean MRR slowed. Subsequently, when patients who had failed to wean were reventilated MRR returned rapidly to normal. These studies also demonstrated that, in patients who failed to wean and in whom MRR slowed, the load on the respiratory system was excessively high in relation to respiratory muscle capacity [28]: in patients who weaned successfully this ratio was more favourable. These data strongly suggest that in this model of acute ventilatory failure a fatigue process is initiated peripherally in the respiratory muscles.

When normal subjects undertake sustained maximum voluntary ventilation for 2 minutes there is a progress reduction in the ventilation and also a progressive slowing of MRR, measured from submaximal sniff oesophageal or transdiaphragmatic pressure [50]. Thus, in these studies, undertaken in trained respiratory physiologists, the data suggest that sustained maximum voluntary ventilation leads to the onset of a peripheral fatigue process in the respiratory muscles. It is of interest that when subjects undertaking sustained maximum voluntary ventilation slightly reduced their ventilation MRR returned towards normal. This observation suggests that when highly motivated subjects perform maximally MRR slows but when they perform slightly submaximally MRR returns towards normal. It is therefore likely that when slowing of MRR was observed in the patients who were weaning from mechanical ventilation central respiratory drive was maximal and failure of weaning was not due to central fatigue.

The integrated fatigue process

Fatigue is best considered as an integrated response of muscle to excessive loading. It is unlikely that fatigue is due to a failure of one link in the complex chain of events of a voluntary contraction. A plausible hypothesis is that when the respiratory muscles are excessively loaded in relation to their capacity the fatigue process is initiated (as indicated by the slowing of relaxation rate). With the onset of the peripheral fatigue process there is a modification of central drive which reduces ventilation and serves to avoid overt peripheral fatigue and excessive force loss; in this way ventilation is best maintained (Figure 13.15). The integrated system maximizes ventilatory performance whilst minimizing overt fatigue. However if loading is sufficient the optimizing of ventilation will nevertheless be insufficient to avoid hypercapnia, acidosis and even death. It is an interesting observation, consistent with the above hypothesis, that many patients on the intensive care unit who fail to wean from mechanical ventilation adopt a rapid and shallow pattern of ventilation which reduces ventilatory work, although at the expense of hypercapnia and eventual weaning failure [51].

Some respiratory investigators have advocated the use of assisted ventilation to 'rest' the respiratory muscles that they presume to be fatigued. The hypothesis (as discussed above) that ventilatory failure is an integrated response of the respiratory system to excessive loading casts doubt on the value of respiratory muscle rest therapy. When the load on the respiratory muscles is excessive, muscle rest by assisted ventilation will avoid ventilatory failure but will not importantly improve muscle contractility (because the integrated system will not push peripheral muscle into a state of overt fatigue). Thus when rest is withdrawn (assisted ventilation is stopped) the respiratory

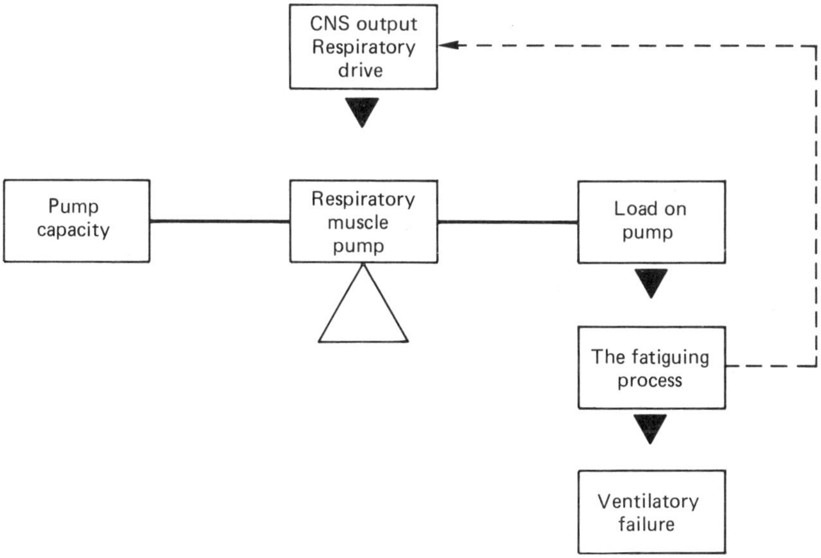

Figure 13.15 In acute ventilatory failure the ratio of load to capacity is high. Fatigue could develop but overt high-frequency or low-frequency fatigue may be averted by adaptation of central drive. (Modified from [29], with permission)

system is subjected to the same excessive load and undergoes the same adaptive response. The correct therapeutic approach to ventilatory failure is therefore not to direct treatment at presumed respiratory muscle fatigue but to alter the balance of load and capacity towards a ratio that is sustainable. Meanwhile, of course, assisted ventilation may be necessary in some patients to control progressive hypercapnia.

Summary

The respiratory muscles constitute a crucial pump. We are now much better at assessing the strength of this pump as a pressure generator. The adequacy of the respiratory muscle pump in producing appropriate ventilation is determined not only by its capacity, but also by the load imposed upon it. The measurement of load is possible but complex. Respiratory muscle fatigue may be relevant to acute ventilatory failure but 'fatigue' is an integrated process, initiated when load is excessive relative to capacity. In the management of acute ventilatory failure therapeutic strategies should be directed not at fatigue itself but at the excessive load or impaired capacity that has precipitated the fatiguing process and the consequent central nervous system adaptive response.

References

1. Mier A, Brophy C, Moxham J, Green M. Assessment of diaphragm weakness. *Am Rev Respir Dis* 1988; **137:** 877–833.
2. Laroche C, Mier AK, Moxham J, Green M. Diaphragm strength in patients with recent hemidiaphragm paralysis. *Thorax* 1988; **43:** 170–174.
3. Laroche CM, Moxham J, Green M. Respiratory muscle weakness and fatigue. *Q J Med* 1989; **71:** 373–397.

4. Laroche C, Carroll N, Moxham J, Green M. Clinical significance of severe isolated diaphragm weakness. *Am Rev Respir Dis* 1988; **138:** 862–866.
5. Braun NMT, Arora NS, Rochester DF. Respiratory muscle and pulmonary function in polymyositis and other proximal myopathies. *Thorax* 1983; **38:** 616–623.
6. Koulouris N, Mulvey D, Laroche CM, Green M, Moxham J. Comparison of two different mouthpieces for the measurement of PI_{max} and PE_{max}in normal and weak subjects. *Eur Respir J* 1988; **1:** 863–866.
7. Ringqvist T. The ventilatory capacity in healthy subjects. An analysis of causal factors with special reference to the respiratory forces. *Scand J Clin Lab Invest* 1966; **88:** 1–23.
8. Black LF, Hyatt RE. Maximal respiratory pressures: Normal values and relationships to age and sex. *Am Rev Respir Dis* 1969; **99:** 698–702.
9. Rochester DF, Arora NS. Respiratory muscle failure. *Med Clin North Am* 1983; **67:** 573–598.
10. Leech JA, Ghezzo H, Stevens D, Becklake MR. Respiratory pressures and function in young adults. *Am Rev Respir Dis* 1983; **128:** 17–23.
11. Wilson SH, Cooke NT, Edwards RHT, Spiro SG. Predicted normal values for maximal respiratory pressures in Caucasian adults and children. *Thorax* 1984: **39:** 535–538.
12. Vincken W, Ghezzo H, Cosio MG. Maximal static respiratory pressures in adults: Normal values and their relationship to determinants of respiratory function. *Bull Eur Physiopathol Respir* 1987; **23:** 435–439.
13. Laroche CM, Mier AK, Moxham J, Green M. Measurement of sniff oesophageal pressures to assess global inspiratory muscle strength. *Am Rev Respir Dis* 1988; **138:** 598–603.
14. Bridger GP, Proctor DF. Maximum nasal inspiratory flow and nasal resistance. *Am Otol Rhinol Laryngol* 1970; **79:** 481–488.
15. Koulouris N, Mulvey D, Laroche CM, Sawicka E, Green M, Moxham J. The measurement of inspiratory muscle strength by sniff oesophageal, nasopharyngeal, and mouth pressures. *Am Rev Respir Dis* 1989; **139:** 641–646.
16. Miller JM, Moxham J, Green M. The maximal sniff in the assessment of diaphragm function in man. *Clin Sci* 1985; **69:** 91–96.
17. Laroche CM, Cairns T, Moxham J, Green M. Respiratory muscle weakness in hypothyroidism. *Am Rev Respir Dis* 1988; **138:** 472.
18. Mier AK, Brophy C, Wass J, Moxham J, Green M. Respiratory muscle strength in myasthenia gravis. *Am Rev Respir Dis* 1988; **138:** 867.
19. Mier AK, Laroche CM, Green M. Respiratory muscle weakness in Addison's disease. *BMJ* 1988; **297:** 457–458.
20. Laroche CM, Carroll N, Moxham J, Stanley NN, Courtenay Evans RJ, Green M. Diaphragm weakness in Charcot–Marie–Tooth disease. *Thorax* 1988; **43:** 478.
21. Laroche CM, Mier AK, Spiro S, Newsom–Davis J, Moxham J, Green M. Respiratory muscle function in the Eaton Lambert myasthenic syndrome. *Thorax* 1989; **44:** 913–918.
22. Davison A, Mulvey D, Currie D, Green M. Idiopathic diaphragmatic weakness. *BMJ* 1992; **34:** 492–494.
23. Mier AK, Brophy C. Measurement of twitch transdiaphragmatic pressure: Surface versus needle electrode stimulation. *Thorax* 1991; **46:** 669–670.
24. Simolowski T, Fleury B, Launois S, Cathala HP, Bouche P, Derenne JP. Cervical magnetic stimulation: a painless method for bilateral phrenic nerve stimulation in conscious humans. *J Appl Physiol* 1989; **67:** 1311–1318.
25. Aquilina R, Wragg S, Moran J, Goldstone J, Green M, Moxham J. Magnetic stimulation as a simple and reliable method for stimulating the phrenic nerves in the neck. *Thorax* 1991; **46:** 754 (abstract).
26. Moxham J. Respiratory muscle weakness – its recognition and management. *Respir Dis Pract* 1991; **April–May**: 12–17.
27. Bellemare F, Grassino A. Effect of pressure and timing of contraction on human diaphragm fatigue. *J Appl Physiol* 1982; **53:** 1190–1195.
28. Goldstone JC, Allen K, Green M, Moxham J. Sequential measurement of the inspiratory effort quotient during weaning. *Eur Respir J* 1990; **3:** 334S (abstract).
29. Moxham J. Respiratory muscle fatigue – mechanisms, evaluation and therapy. *Br J Anaesth* 1990; **65:** 43–53.
30. NHLBI Workshop Respiratory Muscle Fatigue: Report of the respiratory muscle fatigue workshop group. *Am Rev Respir Dis* 1990; **142:** 474–480.
31. Edwards RHT. Physiological analysis of skeletal muscle weakness and fatigue. *Clin Sci Mol Med* 1978; **54:** 463–470.
32. Bigland-Ritchie B, Jones DA, Hosking GP, Edwards RHT. Central and peripheral fatigue in sustained maximum voluntary contractions of human quadriceps muscle. *Clin Sci Mol Med* 1978; **54:** 609–614.

33. Bellemare F, Bigland-Ritchie B. Central components of diaphragmatic fatigue assessed by phrenic nerve stimulation. *J Appl Physiol* 1987; **62:** 1307–1316.
34. Bigland-Ritchie B. EMG and fatigue of human voluntary and stimulated contractions. In: Porter R, Whelan J, eds. *Human Muscle Fatigue (Ciba Foundation Symposium 82)*. London: Pitman Medical, 1981; 130–148.
35. Merton PA. Voluntary strength and fatigue. *J Physiol (Lond.)* 1954; **128:** 553–564.
36. Aldrich TK. Transmission failure of the rabbit diaphragm. *Respir Physiol* 1987; **69:** 307–319.
37. Edwards RHT. Biochemical basis of fatigue in exercise performance: catastrophic theory of muscular fatigue. In: Knuttgan HG, Vogel JA, Poortmans JC, eds. *Proceedings of the Fifth International Symposium on the Biochemistry of Exercise*. Champaign, IL: Human Kinetics Publishers Inc., 1983; 3–28.
38. Gribben HR, Gardiner IT, Heinz CJ, Gibson GJ, Pride NB. The role of impaired inspiratory muscle function in limiting ventilatory response to CO_2 in chronic airflow obstruction. *Clin Sci* 1983; **64:** 487–495.
39. Goldstone, J, Allen K, Green M, Moxham J. Respiratory muscle fatigue during weaning from mechanical ventilation. *Eur Respir J* 1990 ; **3** (Suppl. 10): 664 (abstract).
40. Green M, Moxham J. Respiratory muscles. In: Flenley DC, Petty TL, eds. *Recent Advances in Respiratory Medicine*. Edinburgh: Churchill Livingstone, 1983; 1–20.
41. Edwards RHT, Hill DK, Jones DA, Merton PA. Fatigue of long duration in human skeletal muscle after exercise. *J Physiol (Lond.)* 1977; **272:** 769–778.
42. Moxham J, Wiles CM, Newham D, Edwards RHT. Contractile function and fatigue of the respiratory muscles in man. In: Porter R, Whelan J, eds. *Human Muscle Fatigue (Ciba Foundation Symposium 82)*. London: Pitman Medical, 1981; 120–129.
43. Newham D. The consequences of eccentric contractions and their relationship to delayed onset pain. *Eur J Appl Physiol* 1988; **57:** 353–359.
44. Wilson SH, Cooke NT, Moxham J, Spiro SG. Sternomastoid muscle function and fatigue in normal subjects and in patients with chronic obstructive pulmonary disease. *Am Rev Respir Dis* 1984; **129:** 460–646.
45. Rochester DF, Martin LL. Respiratory muscles rest. In: Roussos C, Macklam PT, eds. *The Thorax: Lung Biology in Health and Disease, Vol. 28*. New York: Marcel Dekker, 1985; 1303–1328.
46. Gutierrez M, Beroiza T, Contreras G, Diaz O, Cruz E, Moreno RC. Weekly cuirass ventilation improves blood gases and inspiratory muscle strength in patients with chronic airflow limitation and hypercarbia. *Am Rev Respir Dis* 1988; **138:** 617–623.
47. Elliott MW, Mulvey DA, Moxham J, Green M, Branthwaite MA. Domiciliary nocturnal nasal intermittent positive pressure ventilation in COPD: mechanisms underlying changes in arterial blood gas tensions. *Eur Respir J* 1991; **4:** 1044–1052.
48. Moxham J. Respiratory muscle fatigue: central, peripheral, or both? In: Jones NL, Killian KJ, eds. *Breathlessness: Campbell Symposium*. Hamilton, Ontario: Dekker 1992; 45–51.
49. Koulouris N, Vianna LG, Mulvey DA, Green M, Moxham J. Maximal relaxation rates of esophageal, nose and mouth pressures during a sniff reflect inspiratory muscle fatigue. *Am Rev Respir Dis* 1989; **139:** 1213–1217.
50. Mulvey D, Koulouris NG, Elliott MW, Laroche CM, Moxham J, Green M. Inspiratory muscle relocation rate after voluntary maximal isocapnic ventilation in humans. *J Appl Physiol* 1991; **70:** 2173–2180.
51. Tobin MJ, Pres W, Guenther SM *et al.* The pattern of breathing during successful and unsuccessful trials of weaning from mechanical ventilation. *Am Rev Respir Dis* 1986; **134:** 1111–1118.

Index